NERVE REPAIR AND REGENERATION

its clinical and experimental basis

Edited by

DON L. JEWETT, M.D., D.Phil.

Associate Professor of Orthopaedic Surgery and Lecturer in Physiology,
University of California School of Medicine,
San Francisco, California

H. RELTON McCARROLL, Jr., M.D.

Vice Chairman, Department of Hand Surgery,
Presbyterian Hospital, Pacific Medical Center,
San Francisco, California

with 324 illustrations

with 47 contributors

The C. V. Mosby Company

ST. LOUIS • TORONTO • LONDON   1980

Copyright © 1980 by The C. V. Mosby Company

All rights reserved. No part of this book may be reproduced in any manner without written permission of the publisher.

Printed in the United States of America

The C. V. Mosby Company
11830 Westline Industrial Drive, St. Louis, Missouri 63141

Library of Congress Cataloging in Publication Data

Main entry under title:

Nerve repair and regeneration.

    Bibliography: p.
    Includes index.
    1. Nervous system—Regeneration.   2. Nerves,
peripheral—Growth.   3. Nervous system—Surgery.
4. Nerves, Peripheral—Transplantation.
I. Jewett, Don L., 1931-   II. McCarroll,
H. Relton, 1936-   III. Title.
[DNLM: 1. Nerve regeneration.   2. Peripheral
nerves—Surgery.   WL500 N455]
QP365.5.N47   599'.01'88   79-19276
ISBN 0-8016-2507-6

C/CB/B 9 8 7 6 5 4 3 2 1   02/D/240

CONTRIBUTORS

Albert J. Aguayo, M.D.

Professor of Neurology, Department of Neurology and Neurosurgery, McGill University; Division of Neurology, Montreal General Hospital, Montreal, Quebec, Canada

Kenneth C. Archibald, M.D.

Associate Clinical Professor, Department of Orthopaedics (Physical Medicine), University of California, San Francisco, California

Bert Bratton, M.D.

Chief Resident, Department of Neurosurgery, Louisiana State University Medical Center, New Orleans, Louisiana

Garth M. Bray, M.D.

Associate Professor, Department of Neurology and Neurosurgery, McGill University; Division of Neurology, Montreal General Hospital, Montreal, Quebec, Canada

Harry J. Buncke, M.D.

Associate Clinical Professor of Surgery, University of California, San Francisco; Staff, Ralph K. Davies Medical Center, San Francisco, California

Richard P. Bunge, M.D.

Professor of Anatomy and Neurobiology, Department of Anatomy and Neurobiology, Washington University School of Medicine, St. Louis, Missouri

P. R. Burgess, Ph.D.

Professor, Department of Physiology, University of Utah, College of Medicine, Salt Lake City, Utah

H. Edward Cabaud, M.D., MAJ, MC, USA

Letterman Army Institute of Research, Presidio of San Francisco, San Francisco, California

D. Charles

Electronics Technologist, Department of Physiology, University of Alberta, Edmonton, Alberta, Canada

L. A. Davis, M.D.

Clinical Professor, Department of Surgery, University of Alberta, Edmonton, Alberta, Canada

Jack Diamond, M.D., Ph.D.

Professor, Department of Neurosciences, McMaster University Medical Center, Hamilton, Ontario, Canada

James R. Doyle, M.D.

Assistant Clinical Professor, Department of Orthopedic Surgery, University of Hawaii, Honolulu, Hawaii

Thomas B. Ducker, M.D., F.A.C.S.

Professor and Head, Division of Neurosurgery, University of Maryland School of Medicine, Baltimore, Maryland

Svante Edshage, M.D.

Associate Professor and Chief, Department of Hand Surgery, University of Gothenburg, Göteborg, Sweden

David S. Forman, Ph.D.

Research Physiologist, Division of Applied Physiology, Naval Medical Research Institute, National Naval Medical Center, Bethesda, Maryland

T. Gordon, Ph.D.

Research Associate, Department of Physiology, University of Alberta, Edmonton, Alberta, Canada

J. A. Hoffer, Ph.D.

Formerly Post-Doctoral Fellow of the Muscular Dystrophy Association of Canada, Department of Physiology, University of Alberta, Edmonton, Alberta, Canada; Currently Staff Fellow, Laboratory of Neural Control (NINCDS), National Institutes of Health, Bethesda, Maryland

K. W. Horch, Ph.D.

Assistant Professor, Department of Physiology, University of Utah, College of Medicine, Salt Lake City, Utah

Alan R. Hudson, M.B., Ch.B., F.R.C.S. (Ed), F.R.C.S. (C)

Chairman, Division of Neurosurgery, University of Toronto, Toronto, Ontario, Canada

Daniel Hunter

Electronmicroscopy Technician, Department of Neurosurgery, St. Michael's Hospital, Toronto, Ontario, Canada

Patrick C. Jackson

Research Assistant, Department of Neurosciences, McMaster University Medical Center, Hamilton, Ontario, Canada

Don L. Jewett, M.D., D.Phil.

Associate Professor of Orthopaedic Surgery and Lecturer in Physiology, University of California School of Medicine, San Francisco, California

E. N. Kaplan, M.D.

Associate Professor of Surgery, Department of Surgery, Division of Plastic and Reconstructive Surgery, Stanford University, Stanford, California

David Kline, M.D.

Professor and Chairman, Department of Neurosurgery, Louisiana State University Medical Center, New Orleans, Louisiana

G. Lundborg, M.D., Ph.D.

Laboratory of Experimental Biology, Department of Anatomy and Division of Hand Surgery, Department of Orthopaedic Surgery I, University of Göteborg, Göteborg, Sweden

H. Relton McCarroll, Jr., M.D.

Vice Chairman, Department of Hand Surgery, Presbyterian Hospital, Pacific Medical Center, San Francisco, California

Harold D. McDonald, M.D.

Microsurgery Fellow, Ralph K. Davies Medical Center, San Francisco, California

W. G. McLean, Ph.D.

Lecturer, School of Pharmacy, Liverpool Polytechnic, Liverpool, England

U. J. McMahan, Ph.D.

Professor of Neurobiology, Department of Neurobiology, Stanford University School of Medicine, Stanford, California

Lawrence M. Marshall

Research Fellow, Department of Neurobiology, Harvard Medical School, Boston, Massachusetts

Hanno Millesi, M.D.

Professor of Plastic Surgery, University of Vienna; Head of the Plastic Surgical Service, I. Chirurgische Universitatsklinik Wien; Head of Ludwig Boltzmann Institute of Experimental Plastic Surgery, Vienna

José Ochoa, M.D., Ph.D.

Associate Professor of Neurology Division of Neurology, Dartmouth Medical School, Hanover, New Hampshire

Sidney Ochs, Ph.D.

Professor of Physiology and Medical Biophysics, Department of Physiology, Indiana University School of Medicine, Indianapolis, Indiana

George E. Omer, Jr., M.D., M.S. (Orthopaedic Surgery)

Professor and Chairman, Department of Orthopaedics and Rehabilitation; Chief, Division of Hand Surgery, Department of Surgery, University of New Mexico Medical Center, Albuquerque, New Mexico

Michael G. Orgel, M.D.

Associate Professor of Surgery (Plastic), University of New Mexico School of Medicine, Albuquerque, New Mexico

Norman K. Poppen, M.D.

Chief, Hand Surgery Service, Department of Orthopaedic Surgery, David Grant USAF Medical Center, Travis AFB, California; formerly Sterling Bunnell Fellow in Hand Surgery, Department of Hand Surgery, Pacific Medical Center, San Francisco, California

Michael Rasminsky, M.D., Ph.D.

Division of Neurology, Montreal General Hospital; Associate Professor, Department of Neurology and Neurosurgery, McGill University, Montreal, Quebec, Canada

William G. Rodkey, D.V.M., CPT, VC, USA

Letterman Army Institute of Research, Presidio of San Francisco, San Francisco, California

Joseph M. Rosen, M.D.

Post-Doctoral Research Fellow in Surgery, Department of Surgery, Division of Plastic and Reconstructive Surgery, Stanford University, Stanford, California

Annelise Rosenfalck, Ph.D.

Professor, Institute of Electronic Systems, Aalborg University Centre, Aalborg, Denmark

B. Rydevik, M.D., Ph.D.

Laboratory of Experimental Biology, Department of Anatomy, University of Göteborg, Göteborg, Sweden

Joshua R. Sanes, Ph.D.

Assistant Professor of Physiology, Washington University Medical Center, St. Louis, Missouri

J. Sjöstrand, M.D., Ph.D.

Institute of Neurobiology and Department of Ophthalmology, University of Göteborg, Göteborg, Sweden

R. B. Stein, Ph.D.

Professor, Department of Physiology, University of Alberta, Edmonton, Alberta, Canada

Sir Sydney Sunderland

Professor Emeritus of Experimental Neurology, University of Melbourne Medical Centre, Melbourne, Australia

Jack W. Tupper, M.D.

Associate Clinical Professor of Orthopaedic Surgery, University of California, San Francisco, California; Director of Highland Alameda County Hand Clinic, Oakland, California

Stephen G. Waxman, M.D., Ph.D.

Professor of Neurology, Stanford University School of Medicine; Chief, Neurological Unit, Veterans Administration Medical Center, Palo Alto, California

PREFACE

Each year the Department of Orthopaedic Surgery of the University of California, San Francisco, commemorates the work of Dr. Sterling Bunnell by means of the Sterling Bunnell Memorial Lectureship. Lecturers are selected whose achievements are of particular significance to the field of upper extremity reconstructive surgery. Sir Sydney Sunderland of the University of Melbourne was chosen as the Thirteenth Sterling Bunnell Memorial Lecturer. His two presentations as guest lecturer served as the catalyst for a symposium on peripheral nerve injury that was held in November, 1977. The faculty included leaders from the basic sciences and clinical fields with a particular interest in the problems of peripheral nerve regeneration and repair.

This volume is based in part on that symposium. In many instances contributors were asked to include additional material in the published paper to cover their topic more completely than was possible in the brief time each was allotted at the symposium. In addition, several discussants kindly provided short papers. Some portions of the discussion that relied heavily on slides were not included and the discussion was edited to correlate with the appropriate chapters of this book.

The symposium was planned not only to review our current knowledge but also to stimulate new thought and discussion among clinicians and researchers. This same goal explains the publication of this volume. Any book of such a scope has lapses. One such untouched area has become obvious to us as we asked contributors to comment on what might be happening at the suture line of a repaired nerve. Since the work of Ramon y Cajal, very little additional knowledge has been gained concerning what happens to axons as they cross a repair site and by what means they persist and grow distally. By its virtual absence in the discussion, this topic declares itself ripe for further endeavors.

Don L. Jewett
H. Relton McCarroll, Jr.

CONTENTS

Contents

NERVE REPAIR AND REGENERATION

its clinical and experimental basis

1

A brief history of nerve repair and regeneration

Sidney Ochs

Advances in nerve repair today are closely linked with the understanding of nerve physiology as revealed by animal experimentation and clinical experience. So it was in the past. This chapter will trace the history of nerve regeneration as the concept developed, with observation leading to experimentation and in turn experimental conclusions conditioning the clinical expectation of nerve repair.

EARLY PRACTICE OF NERVE REPAIR

Ancient authority before Galen is silent on the possibility of nerve regeneration. Galen (130-200, AD) described medicaments to treat nerve wounds, warning that nerve lesions might lead to convulsions.[15] In cases where convulsions seemed imminent, he advised that the nerves be cut to forestall that event. Possibly the occurrence of tetanic infections may have been the basis for such a proscription. Galen's treatment of nerve wounds was based on his mastery of nerve anatomy, but it was confounded by the then unknown effects of infection and a humoral physiology hampered by lack of understanding of the circulation. It is not clear whether he used sutures or believed that nerves could regenerate. Galen remained the great authority for the Middle Ages, and at least some of his commentators and followers considered that he sanctioned treatment aimed at bringing about an "agglutination" or regeneration of the wounded nerve. Paul of Aegina in the 7th century[22] used medicaments to promote "agglutination," but it is evident that he also used sutures:

After the exposed nerve has been covered over, we must apply externally pledgets, with some of those things which are fitting for narrow wounds, such as that from euphorbium, or that from pigeon's dung, taking in also much of the sound parts. When the wound is transverse there is greater danger of convulsions, but everything relating to the cure is in this case the same, except that while the wound is recent some have used sutures and certain of the agglutinative applications; but the sutures must not be applied very superficially lest the part below remain ununited, but more deeply, taking care however that the nerve be not punctured by the needle. It is to be known once for all, that in wounds of the nerves the medicine which cures punctures being of a bitter nature, it is not possible to cure with it the division of the nerve, as the parts cannot endure pungency and inflammation. And neither does the medicine which cures incisions answer with punctures. For its strength does not reach the bottom of it, the incision of the skin being narrow.

Adams, who translated the books of Paul into English, considers in his commentary that Paul closely follows Galen as did also Avicenna, Rhazes, Lanfrancus and Paré.[22]

In the 13th century, Roger of Parma[29] advised the use of galenic medicaments, including egg albumin, to aid the process of agglutination. Possibly its use had a rationale that fit the humoral theory. Also its binding properties were known from cooking experience. In a compendium written between 1230 and 1264, Roger's student Gilbert of England[11] stated that he had seen treated nerves healed (conglutinari) and regenerated (consolidari). In the case of a puncture of a nerve, it is to be divided to relieve pain and

1

prevent tetanus. Roland[30] who edited a later edition of Roger's work rejected the use of egg albumin, favoring instead the use of the cautery to aid agglutination.

Guy de Chauliac, considered the most eminent authority on surgery in the 14th and 15th centuries, gave clear evidence that the suturing of nerves was practiced, and he observed that an excellent functional restoration can occur in the young.[9]

The incision of nerves apart from the three intentions above mentioned has need of three or four other particular intentions. The first is that if it is without any loss of substance it may be sutured with the flesh; the second that a drain should be put gently in the place which is lowest; the third, that some sedative and incarnative medicament proper to nerves should be placed over it; the fourth that it should be bandaged above with a compress of soft wool.

Now that such suture is useful is proved thus: because by the suture the parted ends are approximated and preserved together; beyond this by the covering of the skin of the flesh the nerve is protected from cold which injures it. And thus Avicenna, when he says in the Fourth: If the nerve is torn in its length then it is necessary to sew it, and without that it is not agglutinated. William of Salicet and Lanfranc testify the same. Notwithstanding that some say that Galen does not command to suture nerves, inasmuch that they would not be consolidated and that the pricking of the needle is provocative of convulsion. But (save their reverence) Galen has not forbidden it; but if he is silent, yet he has otherwise affirmed it. What is even more he seems to consent to it in the Sixth of the Therapeutics Chapter III, when he says: The nerve being quite cut there is no longer any danger of convulsion, but part of it will be mutilated, and the treatment will be similar to that of other wounds. Now it is certain that other wounds are sutured in order that one should keep their parts approximated. He has signified the same thing when in the Third of the Techni, he does not make any difference in treatment of wounds in nerves, from that of other wounds unless in the punctate wound alone. Nor in the Sixth of the Therapeutics unless of that same and of wounds of the exposed nerve, and of the accident of that alone which is either wholly incised or not, and of their attrition. It is by this means that according to the same author, by such suture, that nervous parts of the abdomen are agglutinated. What they

say, concerning puncture of the nerve by the needle is of no value because the nerve is already pierced, seeing that the puncture penetrates all the substance. Nor what they object that nerves do not consolidate, because if they do not consolidate according to the first intention at least they consolidate according to the second as has been said before. If one replies that such does not profit anything, because as well since the nerve is cut (seeing that it is only consolidated according to the second intention which is made by the intervention of some foreign substance) it loses its continuity so that vitality is not conveyed through it and thus the movement of the part is lost, then I say that it profits in two ways: first in children in which the nerves are consolidated almost truly and if one part loses its action all is not lost. In the young, also, when the parts of the nerves are more approximated, there is less intervention of foreign substance; and by this some vitality can travel by it and hence the limb is more useful. I have seen and heard it said that in several cases, cut nerves and tendons have been so well restored by suture and other remedies that afterward one could not believe that they had been cut.

Paré (1510-1590) relates that it was the doctrine of ancient physicians in treating wounds of nerves that an early agglutination was to be avoided. The parts above are to be cut and the wound kept open so that the "filth may freely pass forth and the medicine applied to it to enter well."[21] Paré's course was, to the contrary, to apply medicaments to the wound to aid agglutination, indicating that he could have believed in regeneration. Salves or emplastrums were applied on the humoral theory so as to "draw" out the humors. "Sharp" and more so "drying" medicaments were favored, particularly in nerves laid bare. Prescriptions were compound and might include various balsams, oil of terebinth, aqua vitae (brandy), various roots powdered, euphorbia (spurges, plants with a milky sap that are vesicant and rubefacient, one species of which Dunglison[5] notes that the natives of Brazil use as a remedy for the bites of serpents—an interesting parallel to Paré's use of this substance for drawing humors from the injured nerve). Paré also notes that others have used animal fats or greases, plant oils, rosin, aqua vitae, or vinegar. In his cure of Charles the IX, who suffered a punctured nerve (a lesion most highly feared), Paré used oil of turpentine warmed and mixed with aqua vitae dropped into the wound. This was employed to penetrate to the bottom and "exhaust and dry up the serous and virulent humor which sweats from the substance of the pricked nerves," thus mitigating the pain. An emplastrum was also applied to dissolve the humor that had "already fallen down into the arm." In addition, the limb was bound and later in the course of treatment dissolving and drying medicaments were applied.

In such wounds if the pain increased, scalding oil was to be used or the nerve burned with a hot cautery. Escharotics powder of alum, mercury, and so forth were also used for this purpose. Paré warns that if in spite of all such aids "a contumacie, an imminent danger of convulsion exists, it is better to cut the nerve, tendon or membrane in order to preserve the whole body," a course of action clearly traced back to Galen.

Apparently the use of sutures had fallen from favor toward the end of the Middle Ages, and by the late 18th century it was the established opinion that nerves did not regenerate. As an example, de la Roche[4] in his book on nerve function states that a nerve when cut, "loses forever its ability to transmit movement between the separated portions even though they can join and form a cicatrix." He refers also to Munro who had confirmed this in animal experiments.

In a footnote to that passage, de la Roche notes that "a medical scientist of London doubts this as a general principle and believes that regeneration may occur in large nerves at least but probably not in the smaller branches." The reference to the medical scientist of London was certainly to Cruikshank whose work was then unpublished. Cruikshank had acted as an assistant to William Hunter and carried out his pioneer work on nerve regeneration in Hunter's laboratory in 1776. The paper was not published until 1795 because there were doubts at the time that it was indeed a true regeneration of nerve.[19] Nevertheless, it was with the exper-

iments of Cruikshank that the modern era of experimental study of nerve regeneration opened.

NERVE REGENERATION STUDIES BASED ON VAGOTOMY

It had been known at least since the time of Willis that a bilateral section of both vagus nerves in the neck of a dog leads within a short time to its death.[41] Cutting one of the vagus nerves was not, however, lethal. When Cruikshank cut the vagus nerve in the neck of a dog on one side, the animal soon after experienced some difficulty in breathing and exhibited an inflammation of the eye on that side.[3] This passed, and by the eighth day the animal had recovered. When, thereafter, the vagus nerve on the opposite side was cut, the animal's breathing became labored, it vomited, and copious salivation from the mouth took place. Later the animal ate and drank, passed stools, and recovered somewhat, but 7 days after the second operation it died. Cruikshank examined the nerves and found a substance the same color as nerve appearing to unite the two ends, which he inferred was regenerated nerve. Considering that the time allowed for regeneration had been too short, he waited for 3 weeks before cutting the second vagus nerve in a similar experiment. The animal survived for a period of $2^1/_2$ weeks before it died. The nerves appeared to be firmly united with a "kind of callous" substance. The prolongation of the animal's life indicated to him that the reunited nerve had been restored in its function so that later, when the vagus nerve on the other side was cut, death did not occur so soon. He analogized this apparent nerve regeneration to the healing of a broken bone, a subject of intense interest to Hunter and his colleagues. Nevertheless, doubts were raised by Hunter and others that the substance uniting the ends was true regenerated nerve rather than scar tissue. The nerves were removed from the animal along with the trachea and the preparation placed on exhibit in Hunter's museum.

In 1778 the Abbe Fontana, in the course of a visit to the museum, viewed the nerve preparation and discussed Cruikshank's experiments with him. Fontana was inspired to make a further study of nerve regeneration in spite of some earlier studies he had made using the sciatic nerve that had proved fruitless. Fontana turned his attention to the vagus nerve and removed a portion of the vagus nerves from a dozen rabbits. After waiting some days he found that the ends indeed had united in accord with Cruikshank's observation. Most importantly, Fontana made a microscopical study of the material present between the previously cut ends and observed a "spiral" or "banded" appearance of the matter between the ends, a banding similar to the banding he found present in normal nerve.[6] Fontana was convinced on this basis that a true regeneration of nerve substance had taken place. However, the time allowed by Fontana and Cruikshank was too short for the restoration of nerve function by regenerating vagal nerve fibers reaching the heart, lung, or the gastrointestinal tract. Cruikshank and Fontana were overly impressed by the apparent prolongation of the life of the animal from a matter of a day or so to a time of several weeks. Their observations fell within the variable range of survival following a bilateral vagotomy. Animals are able to live from a few days to several weeks after a bilateral vagotomy.[19]

Haighton[10] found, as had Cruikshank, that cutting one vagus nerve in a dog gave rise to relatively minor symptoms, cutting the other vagus nerve caused death 4 days later. When in another experiment Haighton prolonged the time before cutting the second vagus nerve to 9 days, the animal died after a delay of 13 days. This indicated to him that a "partial regeneration" of the nerve had occurred. In Haighton's next experiment the second vagus nerve was cut 6 weeks after cutting the nerve on one side, and the animal then lived for over 19 months. Haighton's work led to the belated appearance of Cruikshank's paper that was printed in the *Philosophical Transactions of the Royal Society of London* just before Haighton's paper in 1795. Haighton's observation received additional support from Prévost's[24] studies carried out in kittens. He found that a delay in the cutting of the second vagus nerve for even up to 1 or 2 months afterward might be insufficient to allow for an adequate nerve regeneration to occur, but when 4 months were allowed, the animals lived for a long time.

LATER STUDIES OF DEGENERATION AND REGENERATION

The variability in the time of death of an animal following a two-stage vagotomy, with multiple causes of death, added uncertainty as to whether a true regeneration of nerve was produced. The concept was not universally accepted on either experimental or clinical grounds. Richerand[28] expressed his rejection of the idea of nerve regeneration in most forceful terms:

This paralysis, produced by a complete section of a nerve is incurable where it occurs with or without a loss of substance. In the first case, regeneration is impossible; in the second, reunion which operates in favor of cellular tissue can hardly reconnect the nerve canals of which each fiber consists. The prognosis of lesions in which a large nerve is cut, would be less favorable if one could give some credence to those physiologists who pretend to have seen a reproduction of nerves. How is it that the opinion that nerves could reproduce themselves came to be established and enjoys a certain favor? It is that neither the authors of this strange opinion or their sectarians have repeated the observations they support. The sciences, which we pardon in this comparison, have their simpletons as does politics; such people who lie in wait for novelties and recieve without examination all that comes from Germany, Italy or England. The thing is absurd. Duped myself by the pretended regeneration of nerves, I have repeated without success the experiments of d'Aighton [sic, Haighton]. On reflexion a little later, I know that I ought to have foreseen this result.

Investigators turned from the use of the vagus nerve to study the sciatic nerve, where they could better look for the return of sensation and motor function as indices of regeneration. Müller[17] divided the sciatic nerve of rabbits and found a loss of sensation in the lower portion and a lack of movement on stimulating the nerve above the transection with electrical current. Three months later these functions returned and regenerated fibers were found microscopically below the transection by his colleague Schwann.

After transecting cat sciatic nerves, Steinrück[34] also studied the course of nerve regeneration by the return of sensation and motion. He found that some functional recovery had occurred after 5 weeks, with a full restitution requiring as much as 1 to 2 years. Steinrück considered that regeneration involved an exudate of "lymph" from the neurilemma of cut ends that formed a favorable medium in which new primitive nerve fibers arose. His concept of regeneration was that nerve fiber growth occurred by a process of "reunion" of the transected fibers. As will be shown in a later section, the confusion produced by this concept took considerable time and much effort to eradicate.

"MONISTIC" AND "DUALISTIC" VIEWS OF NEURAL ELEMENTS

To understand the context in which the concept of reunion had found such ready acceptance, we must turn to the view of nerve structure current at the time. Most investigators accepted a "dualist" neural view championed by Valentin and Purkinje. The histological investigations of Valentin convinced him that two independent nerve "elements" existed, nerve cell bodies and fibers.[35] The nerve fibers were generally believed to develop from the union of individual cells as shown by Schwann.[32] The cell bodies were by their shape and their contained nucleus analogized by Valentin and Purkinje to an egg. In the dorsal root ganglia and the central nervous system where the cell bodies and fibers were intertwined, the two nerve "elements" appeared to be closely opposed but without a true connection between them.

In opposition to that view, Remak[27] took a "monistic" position. He saw nerve fibers arising from, and thus integrally connected with, the nerve cell bodies. He was in fact the first exponent of what might be called an "early neuron theory." However, the term "neuron" was only announced at the end of

the 19th century by Waldeyer-Hartz[36] when much evidence for the concept of the neuron as a cell with long processes had accumulated. Even then, it was still challenged by Bethe and other "reticularists," and opposition to the neuron doctrine was only laid to rest in the early part of the 20th century. In the middle of the 19th century, those investigators who took a "dualist" position were in the majority. They considered that a divided nerve fiber might revert to its embryonic state, allowing the separated ends to undergo the same union as occurs in development. A "monist" on the other hand would view regeneration as an outgrowth of nerve fibers from the cell body.

WALLER'S VIEW OF DEGENERATION AND REGENERATION

Waller, who may or may not have accepted a "monistic" view, was the first to give evidence for regeneration as an outgrowth of nerve fibers. It was Waller's clear understanding of degeneration that allowed him to describe the course of regenerated fibers. After nerve transection, Waller found that the normally cylindrical-shaped nerve fibers break up distally, the myelin sheath becoming beaded and then much later absorbed.[37] While Stannius[33] had earlier found that the degenerative changes were not confined to the immediate neighborhood of nerve transections, it was Waller, using the frog glossopharyngeal nerve, who showed that the nerve fibers degenerated all the way from the site of transection down to the fungiform papillae of the tongue. The part of the nerve fiber still connected to the center containing the cell bodies retained its normal form. Waller showed this in a clear fashion. In a group of kittens he cut the dorsal root of the second cervical ganglion in one animal; in another he cut the ventral root, in another he cut the dorsal root distal to the ganglia; and in yet another he cut the nerve distal to the ganglion.[39] In each case degeneration occurred only in the fibers separated from the cells. Waller announced as a law that those portions of the nerve fibers still connected to their cell bodies retained their normal appearance, while fibers separated from the cell bodies degenerated. And, most significantly, he stated that some "trophic" influence is continually passing from the cell bodies to supply the nerve fibers with materials required to maintain their viability. The trophic influence of cell on fiber was viewed by Waller as a "rivulet supplied by a river," the forerunner of our modern understanding of axoplasmic transport of material in nerve fibers.[18] Among the degenerated nerves Waller found small diameter pale fibers. Nasse had earlier reported similar fibers smaller in diameter than normal nerve fibers; Guenther and Schoen[8] also saw them, supposing that they arose from the distal and proximal ends of the transected fibers. Waller described these small fibers as, "being one quarter to one-eighth the normal diameter, pale without the double contour indicative of myelination and with fusiform nuclei positioned at intervals along their length."[38] The new regenerating fibers were found to lay among, but not within, the tubes of the degenerated fiber. Then, remarkably, Waller found the new fibers at increasingly distal positions at successively later times, as would be expected of their slow centrifugal growth in the degenerated nerve. It took 9 months for the new fibers to eventually reach the papillae of the frog's tongue.

CONFLICTS CAUSED BY THE "REUNION" CONCEPT

In spite of Waller's clear description of regenerating fibers growing into the distal stump, the reunion concept gained support. Some clinical observations had added apparent strength to that view. Paget[20] recounted the case of a boy in whom the median and radial nerves had been divided slightly above the wrist. The nerves were not sutured, but nevertheless a functional return was seen beginning 10 days later and it was nearly complete in a month. Another case he reported was that of a boy whose hand had been almost severed at the wrist with the median and radial nerves divided. After their surgical apposition, sensation returned in 10 to 12 days. These cases were referred to by Paget as

examples of healing by "immediate union" or "primary adhesion."

Additional experimental studies also gave support to the concept of reunion. Schiff[31] carried out a series of studies on cats and dogs and found an early recovery of function after nerve transections, much too soon to be due to an outgrowth of regenerating fibers and therefore he supported the concept of the reunion of transected nerves. Schiff considered that the fibers that Waller had reported as regenerating were, in fact, the axis cylinders of fibers that were better seen after they had been deprived of their myelin. Fascicles of normal appearing fibers found by Schiff in the distal nerve portions 3 to 4 weeks after transecting the lingual and intraorbital nerves, were interpreted as being caused by a reunion of the axons followed by a restoration of their myelin. Bruch[2] also found a quick recovery of nerve function after dividing the sciatic nerves of cats. In a number of cases he reported that little or no trace of scarring at the site of transection might be seen with a slight constriction of the sheath of Schwann revealed by stretching the nerve. Lent[16] also considered that myelin disappeared in the degenerated part of the fiber leaving behind the empty sheaths of Schwann. The axis cylinders then reverted to their embryonic form, reuniting and reforming their myelin sheaths.

Still more support came from the investigation of Philipeaux and Vulpian[23] who in microscopical examination of the nerve showed the presence of numerous new "in situ regenerated nerve fibers." Ranvier[26] pointed out that fine strands of nerve fibers growing into the isolated piece of nerve might very well have been missued by Philipeaux and Vulpian, but the evidence favoring reunion remained strong. Even Waller retreated from his earlier correct view of regeneration in the face of apparently overwhelming evidence.[40]

At the end of the 19th century support for the idea was still forthcoming. Kennedy[14] on reviewing the history of regeneration took a strong reunionist position. He cited his own clinical cases where sensation returned within 2 to 5 days following the repair of severed nerves in the forearm. Such a rapid recovery was, as he pointed out, incompatible with the regrowth of fibers. When delays and shortcomings in the course of recovery of motor function were found, they were ascribed to atrophic changes in the muscles.

From our point in time we have no clear explanation for the ready acceptance of an early return of function as described by Kennedy, Laugier, Paget, and others. One explanation is that there is often an overlap in the distribution of adjacent nerve territories. A lesion of one nerve allows the intact nerves to partially take over the function of the lost nerve. While cases of apparently early reunion continued to be reported,[13] with accumulating clinical experience they gradually became rarer.

NEURON DOCTRINE AND PRESENT VIEWS

Around the turn of the 19th century and early 20th century, additional experimental investigations finally turned the tide against the reunion concept. The neuron doctrine was made the basis of Barker's[1] monograph on the nervous system, and the neurobiological studies of Harrison[12] showing the outgrowth of fibers from cells in tissue culture had considerable influence. The importance of his findings was indicated by a letter from Gaskell written to Starling on August 8, 1910. Gaskell wrote how he welcomed Harrison's findings and stated, "The idea of a chain of cells forming a nerve fibre has always seemed to me absurd and I imagine is universally discredited although at the same time the sheath cells may assist in providing pabulum for the young nerve."[7] The incisive studies of Ramon y Cajal[25] finally established the neuron doctrine, and the view of regeneration as a growth of fibers from the part of the fiber connected with the cell body was accepted incontestably.

Axoplasmic transport (see Chapter 7) is required to carry needed materials into the regenerating fibers. We now ask what special materials might be required by the growing fibers and if some substances are present that

participate in directing the course of regenerating fibers toward their normal target sites. The identification and use of such tropic materials to guide motor and sensory fibers back to their original channels (a problem that, as noted previously, had already been recognized by Richerand in 1812) would open a new exciting chapter in the history of nerve repair with the promise of a fuller functional restitution.

ACKNOWLEDGMENT

I am most grateful for the kindness and help of the librarians of the University of Indiana Medical School of Medicine. The assistance of the History of Medicine Division of the National Library of Medicine, Washington, D.C., is most appreciated. The quotation from the letter of Dr. Gaskell[7] is by kind permission of the Royal College of Physicians of London.

REFERENCES

1. Barker, L. F.: The nervous system and its constituent neurones, New York, 1899, Appleton-Century-Crofts.
2. Bruch, C.: Über die Regeneration durchschnittenen Nerven, Zt. Wiss. Zool. **6:**135, 1855.
3. Cruikshank, W.: Experiments on the nerves, particularly on their reproduction; and on the spinal marrow of living animals, Philos. Trans. R. Soc. Lond. (abridged version) **85:**512, 1795.
4. de la Roche, F. G.: Analyse des fonctions du système nerveux (2 vols.), Geneva, 1778, Du Villard and Nouffer.
5. Dunglison, R.: A new dictionary of medical science and literature, Boston, 1833, Bowen.
6. Fontana, F.: Treatise on the venom of the viper; on the American poisons; and on the cherry laurel and some other vegetable poisons to which are annexed, observations on the primitive structure of the animal body; different experiments on the reproduction of the nerves; and a description of the nerves; and a description of a new canal of the eye (Translated from the French by J. Skinner) (2 vols.), London, 1778, Murray.
7. Gaskell, W.: Autograph letter signed. To: E. H. Starling. Cambridge, August 8, 1910. In possession of the Royal College of Physicians of London.
8. Guenther, A. F., and Schoen, J. M. A.: Versuche and Bemerkungen über Regeneration der Nerven und Abhangigkeit der peripherischen Nerven von den Central-organen, Müller's Arch. pp. 270-286, 1840.
9. Guy de Chauliac: On wounds and fractures (Translated by W. A. Brennan), Chicago, 1923, Published by translator.
10. Haighton, J.: An experimental inquiry concerning the reproduction of nerves, Philos. Trans. R. Soc. Lond. (abridged version) **85:**519, 1795.

11. Handerson, H. E.: Gilbertus Anglicus. Medicine of the thirteenth century, Cleveland, 1918, Medical Library Association.
12. Harrison, R. G.: The outgrowth of the nerve fiber as a mode of protoplasmic movement, J. Exp. Zool. **9**:787, 1910.
13. Holmes, W.: The repair of nerves by suture, J. Hist. Med. **6**:44, 1951.
14. Kennedy, R.: Degeneration and regeneration of nerves: an historical review, Proc. R. Philos. Soc. Glasg. **29**:193, 1898.
15. Kuhn, K. G.: Claudii Galeni Opera Omnia, vol. XIII. De compositione medicamentorum secundum locus, libri X, de compositione medicamentorum per genera libri XII, Hildesheim, 1965, Olms.
16. Lent, E.: Beitrage zur Lehre von der Regeneration durchschnittener Nerven, Zt. Wiss. Zool. **7**:145, 1856.
17. Müller, J.: Elements of physiology (Translated from the German by W. Baly) (2 vols.), London, 1838, 1842, Taylor and Walton.
18. Ochs, S.: Waller's concept of the trophic dependence of the nerve fiber on the cell body in the light of early neuron theory, Clio Med. **10**:253, 1975.
19. Ochs, S.: The early history of nerve regeneration beginning with Cruikshank's observations in 1776, Med. Hist. **21**:261, 1977.
20. Paget, J.: Lectures on surgical pathology delivered at the Royal College of Surgeons of England, vol. 1 (Revised and edited by W. Turner), London, 1863, Longman, p. 282.
21. Paré, A.: The workes of that famous chirurgeon Ambrose Parey translated out of Latine and compared with the French (Translated by T. Johnson, London, 1634), Republished, Kennebunkport, 1968, Milford House.
22. Paulus Aegeneta (Paul of Aegina): The seven books (Translated by F. Adams) (2 vols.), London, 1844-1847, Sydenham Society.
23. Philipeaux, J., and Vulpian, A.: Note sur des expériences démontrant que les nerfs separés des centres nerveux peuvent apres être altérés complètement se régénérer tout en demeurant isolés des ces centres, et recouvrir leurs propriétés physiologiques, C. R. Hebd. Acad. Sci. (Paris) **59**:507, 1859.
24. Prévost, J. L.: Über die Wiedererzeugung des Nervengewebes, Froriep's Notizen **17**:113, 1827.
25. Ramon y Cajal, S.: Degeneration and regeneration of the nervous system (Translated by R. M. May) (2 vols.), 1928, Reprinted New York, 1968, Hafner.
26. Ranvier, M. L.: Lecons sur l'histologie du Système Nerveux (2 vols.), Paris, 1878-1879, Savy, pp. 270-278.
27. Remak, R.: Observationes anatomicae et microscopicae de systematis nervosi structura, Reims, 1838, Berolini.
28. Richerand, A.-B.; Nosographie chiricale, ed. 3, vol. 2 (Translated from the quotation given by Holmes[13]), p. 197.
29. Roger of Parma: Quoted by Handerson, H. E.: Gilbertus Anglicus. Medicine of the thirteenth century, Cleveland, 1918. Medical Library Association.
30. Roland of Parma: Quoted by Handerson, H. E.: Gilbertus Anglicius. Medicine of the thirteenth century, Cleveland, 1918, Medical Library Association.
31. Schiff, M.: Sur la régéneration des nerfs et sur les altérations qui surviennent dans des nerfs paralysés, C. R. Hebd. Acad. Sci. (Paris) **38**:448, 1854.
32. Schwann, T.: Microscopical researches into the accordance in the structure and growth of animals and plants (Translated from the German by H. Smith), London, 1847, Sydenham Society. Reprinted New York, 1969, Kraus Reprint Co.
33. Stannius, H. F.: Untersuchungen über muskelreizbarkeit, Muller's Arch. pp. 443-462, 1847.
34. Steinrück, C. O.: De nervorum regeneratione, Berlin, 1838, Decker. Abstracted in Schmidt's Jahrbuch der in-und Ausland, Med. **26**:102, 1840.
35. Valentin, G.: Über den Verlauf der letzenden Enden der Nerven, Breslau, 1836, Barth.
36. Waldeyer-Hartz, H. W. G.: Ueber einige neure Forschungen im Gebiete der Anatomie des Centralnervensystems, Dtsch. med. Wochenschr. **17**: 1213; 1244; 1267; 1287; 1331; 1352; 1891.
37. Waller, A. V.: Experiments on the glossopharyngeal and hypoglossal nerves of the frog, and observations produced thereby in the structure of their primitive fibres, Philos. Trans. Roy. Soc. Lond. **140**:423, 1850.
38. Waller, A. V.: Nouvelles recherches sur la régéneration des fibres nerveuses, C. R. Hebd. Acad. Sci. (Paris) **34**:675, 1852.
39. Waller, A. V.: "Septième mémoire sur le système nerveux". C. R. Hebd. Acad. Sci. (Paris) **35**:301, 1852. Huitième mémoire sur le système nerveux, Ibid. **35**:561. Nouvelle méthode anatomique pour l'investigation du système nerveux, Bonn, 1852, Georgi.
40. Waller, A. V.: The nutrition and separation of nerves; being the substance of a lecture delivered at the Royal Institution of Great Britain, May 31, 1861.
41. Willis, T.: The description and uses of the nerves, 1681. Reprinted in Feindel W., ed.: The anatomy of the brain and nerves, Montreal, 1965, McGill University Press.

2

Various approaches to the field of nerve repair and regeneration

Don L. Jewett and Joseph M. Rosen

It is certainly remarkable that nerves regrow after injuries. Given such a marvelous capacity for repair, we can reasonably ask why the clinical results are, overall, so poor (Chapter 30). How are we to approach our bad results so that we can learn from them and improve our treatment? Should we look to experimental techniques for insight? How should we organize our search for answers? It is to this last question that this chapter is addressed.

The extensive clinical and basic science knowledge of nerve repair can be organized into a variety of classifications and compilations, each of which emphasizes different aspects of our knowledge and ignorance. For example, we can classify nerve repair according to normal anatomical structures, the histopathology of different injuries, or the phase of recovery. Alternatively, we can compile lists based on the presumed pathophysiology of malfunctioning nerves, the type of nerve repair, or the method of evaluating functional return after nerve injury.

We present here the contents of this book arranged according to these alternative classifications and compilations in a series of tables. The letter "D" following a chapter number indicates that a given topic is to be found in the discussion portion of that chapter.

ANATOMICAL CLASSIFICATION

A time-honored and useful starting point is classification according to the gross and microscopical anatomy of the structures involved in nerve regeneration. We have done this in

Table 2-1. Anatomical classification of the chapters of this book

Structure	Chapter
Peripheral nerve	
Gross anatomy	3,34
Microscopical anatomy	23
Peripheral neuron	1
Cell body	10
Axon/myelin	18,19
Synaptic connection	11,12,13
Schwann cell	5,6
Myelin portion	4,18
Connective tissue	3,7,8,25,34,35
Blood vessels	4D,8
End-organs	
Sensory	11,12
Motor	13
Central nervous system	—

Table 2-1, which lists the chapters of this book that deal directly with the changes in these anatomical structures during injury and repair.

HISTOPATHOLOGICAL CLASSIFICATION

A step beyond the anatomical classification is one based on different types of injury and the structures that show histological changes in response to these injuries. The injury classifications of Sunderland and Seddon serve as the basis for Table 2-2. Personally we have found the "compression/crush/cut" terminology shown in Table 2-2 to be a useful shorthand method of distinguishing between the

Table 2-2. Histopathological classification of the chapters of this book based on type of injury

Seddon—type:	Neurapraxia	Axonotmesis	Neurotmesis		
Sunderland—degree:	First	Second	Third	Fourth	Fifth
Structures showing histological changes					
Myelin	X	X	X	X	X
Axon		X	X	X	X
Endoneurium			X	X	X
Perineurium				X	X
Epineurium					X
Mechanism	Compression	Crush	Cut		
Consequence	Segmental demyelination	Wallerian degeneration	Wallerian degeneration		
Experimental chapters	4,19	4,19	4,19		
		9,11,12,13	9,11,12,13		
	8,18,20		1,6,10,14,15,16,17,23, 24,25		
Clinical chapters			26,27,28,29,30,31,32,34, 35,36,37		
	21,22	21,22	21,22		

Table 2-3. Pathophysiological compilation of possible altered function after nerve injury

Possible altered function	Chapter
Altered cellular metabolism	
Central	10
Axonal transport	7,8,9,12
Schwann cell nutrient support	5
Changed vascular support	4,8
Altered excitability after regeneration	
Central	—
Axonal	
Decreased dynamic range	20
Conduction block	
Caused by altered structure	19
Caused by ionic changes	4D,7
Ectopic foci	
Myelinated fibers	4,18
Unmyelinated fibers	—
Ephaptic transmission	4
Peripheral	11,12
Altered growth/regrowth patterns	
End-organ/nerve terminal	11,12,13
Schwann cell/nerve fiber	6

pathological conditions and their consequences.

PATHOPHYSIOLOGICAL COMPILATION

Since altered function can occur without detectable histological change, a compilation of possible pathophysiological conditions in nerve fibers after injury is shown in Table 2-3. At this stage in our knowledge it is not possible to directly correlate this listing with the classification scheme of Table 2-2, desirable as this may be.

NERVE REPAIR COMPILATION

Moving toward more clinical concerns, it is feasible to organize according to the various alternative treatment decisions that must be faced in nerve repair as indicated in Table 2-4. This approach has the advantage of focusing on the practical issues faced by the surgeon, but its deficiency is that the solutions to these decision dilemmas may have to be sought outside this compilation.

Table 2-4. Nerve repair compilation of the chapters of this book

Treatment decisions	Alternatives	Chapter
Overview		29,36,37
Timing	Primary or secondary	10,30,32,34,35
Level of repair	Epineurial or perineurial (funicular or fascicular)	3,23,24,30,32,33,34,35
Technique	Suture or sutureless	1,3,25,32,33
Tension/gaps	End-to-end, grafts, or cross-anastomosis	6,24,30,32,33,34,35
Materials and methods		32,33,34,35
Nonsurgical	Reeducation	11,26,34
	Chemical factors	5,9
	Therapeutic crush	12
	Microtelemetry	33
	Electromagnetic field	36

Table 2-5. Clinical evaluation classification of the chapters of this book

Phase of recovery*	Description	Testing method	Chapter
Phase 1	Axonal regeneration and reconnection with the periphery	Histological Physiological	4,14,15
		Axon	8,9,14,15,17,20
		Motor	21
		Sensory	22
Phase 2	Return of simple function	Sensory	26,28,30,31,34, 35
		Motor	30,34
		Autonomic	26,28D
Phase 3	Return of complex function	Pickup test	26,27
		Clinical impressions	30,36,37

*Based on Sunderland, Chapter 37.

CLINICAL EVALUATION CLASSIFICATION

Methods of evaluating clinical results must differ according to the phase of recovery, as described by Sunderland in Chapter 37. A classification based on different evaluation methods applicable to different recovery phases is presented in Table 2-5. Some of the techniques developed for experimental purposes can also be applied to clinical cases.

STRONG INFERENCE CLASSIFICATION AND COMPILATION

Faced with such an array of classifications, it seems redundant to add yet another approach to this chapter. However, all of the preceding tables have been formulated around broad issues, rather than by focusing on specific hypotheses devised to explain a single, pertinent observation. Platt[1] has argued that a "strong inference" approach can

Table 2-6. Strong inference approach to the chapters of this book

Anatomical site of functional difference	Hypotheses: "Recovery from cut injury is worse than recovery from crush injury because . . ."	Chapter
Axonal pathway and repair site	. . . fewer axons make useful connection across the repair site owing to one or more of the following:	3,36
	(a) failure to grow distally,	16,25
	(b) functionally inappropriate regeneration,	11,13
	(c) spatially disorganized regeneration.	11,13
	. . . branching at the repair site gives decreased sensory and motor specificity.	15
	. . . structural changes (for example, scarring, distal endoneurial tube shrinkage, proximal axonal shrinkage) along the axonal pathway and at the repair site result in complete or functional conduction block or decreased dynamic range.	3,14,16,19,20
	. . . biochemical changes secondary to altered axonal transport adversely affect conduction and/or peripheral synaptic function.	7,8,9
	. . . the increased period of denervation affects Schwann cell–axon interaction (for example, nerve growth factor) with subsequent decreased axonal function.	5,5D,6
Central connections and cell body	. . . cell body denervation hypersensitivity, chromatolysis, or central synaptic "disuse atrophy" is greater during prolonged regeneration.	3,10,29
	. . . of altered central sensory and reflex pathways owing to abnormal impulse patterns(hyperalgesia) and/or ectopic foci from more severe scarring in cut nerve.	4,26
	. . . reeducation is unable to compensate for the greater central, axonal, and peripheral effects in cut nerve.	11,26,29,37
Terminal connections and end-organs	. . . of increased atrophy of end-organs during longer regeneration time.	11,12D,13, 29,36,37
	. . . of invasion of nerve fibers from adjacent areas that "occupy" available end-organs with subsequent decreased somatotopic specificity.	11,12

speed evolution of a field of knowledge by delineating crucial issues and the experiments necessary to resolve major problems. Following his suggestions, we take one observation of special interest and then list as many hypotheses to explain the observation as seem appropriate for the present state of our knowledge.

We have chosen as the starting point the clinical observation that nerve crush injuries have greater functional recovery than do injuries involving transections of nerves. We find this point interesting for a number of reasons: (1) the observation rules out the possibility that poor results after nerve injury are caused solely by wallerian degeneration distal to the injury; (2) the histological consequences of the two types of injury are well established; (3) these injuries are both clinically and histologically distinct and form a major distinction in classifications of nerve injuries (Table 2-2); (4) the comparison of the two types of injuries is readily accomplished in animal experimentation; and (5) experiments that can explain the difference between the two injuries will provide an explanation for at least some of the poor results seen after nerve repair. Table 2-6 is a partial compilation of hypotheses, classified according to anatomical site, to explain the differences in recovery between cut and crush injuries. The hypotheses vary from the purely speculative to the more likely; some have been disproved with varying degrees of certainty. The range of hypotheses indicates the extent of experimentation needed to "explain" a single observation. The reader is encouraged to add additional hypotheses to the list.

REFERENCE

1. Platt, J. R.: Strong inference, Science **146**:347, 1964.

3

The anatomical basis of nerve repair

Sir Sydney Sunderland

While it is true that the limits of nerve repair will ultimately prove to be biochemical and physiological, there is always the danger that the broad morphological basis of the subject will become obscured by the more rapidly growing biochemical and physiological literature. For this reason I take this opportunity to review the clinically relevant parts of nerve morphology.

However, before proceeding to the development of this central theme there are some general points that call for comment. The first point concerns a question of terminology and relates to the often misleading use of the terms "endoneurium," "perineurium," and "epineurium" (Figs. 3-1 and 3-2). These tissues collectively represent the supporting connective tissue of the nerve trunk, although each has different structural and functional features. These terms need to be defined in order to remove any possible lingering confusion over their use.

Endoneurium

The endoneurium is the connective tissue framework of the interior of the funiculus. Here the fine collagen fibrils separate and encircle each nerve fiber to form an external definitive sheath. It has tensile strength and resists axonal pressure. When the axon and myelin degenerate, the endoneurium contracts about the surviving Schwann cells to outline an atrophied endoneurial tube. This atrophy is maximal by the third to the fourth month and leaves few denervated nerve fibers greater than 2 to 3 μ in diameter (Fig. 3-3).

Perineurium

The perineurium is the thin but dense lamellated layer composed of specialized perineurial cells, interspersed with fine collagen fibrils, that encircle each funiculus. The perineurium has the following properties.
1. It imparts tensile strength to the nerve trunk.
2. It constitutes a diffusion barrier.
3. It resists the spread of infection across it.
4. It resists and maintains an intrafunicular pressure.

With wallerian degeneration and the removal of the axon and myelin, the perineurium contracts around the atrophied endoneurial tubes and the funiculus is reduced in diameter.

Epineurium

The epineurium is the areolar connective tissue that encloses and forms a protective packing for the funiculi. The collagen fibrils of this tissue are thicker than those of the endoneurium and perineurium and there is some evidence that the fibroblasts elaborating them are the main offenders in causing fibrosis following nerve injury.

• • •

The second point I should like to make is that while we are interested in devising methods to accelerate axonal growth, an outstanding problem in nerve regeneration is to prevent axonal regrowth where it is undesirable. Regenerating axons have a remarkable

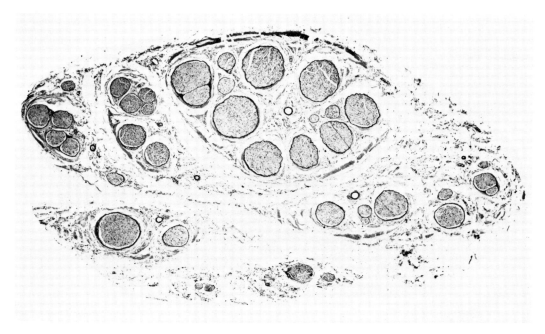

Fig. 3-1. Gross histological features of peripheral nerve trunk revealed in transverse section of nerve. Traces of funicular groupings are outlined by arrangement of epineurial connective tissue. (From Sunderland, S.: Nerves and nerve injuries, ed. 2, Edinburgh, 1978, Churchill-Livingstone.)

capacity for crossing, unaided, considerable gaps to reach and reinnervate the distal segment of a severed nerve or to otherwise grow in search of tissue to innervate as will be confirmed by those clinicians who are involved in the treatment of painful amputation stump neuromas and those experimentalists who are concerned with maintaining muscles in a denervated state.

Finally, I wish to call attention to the core of the problem of nerve repair, which is not only axon regeneration but also the restoration of what, to the patient, is *useful function.*

Now let us turn to morphology as it relates to nerve repair. The internal structure of the nerve shown in Fig. 3-1 is not constant along its length because its constituent funiculi are repeatedly dividing and uniting to form complicated funicular plexuses (Fig. 3-4). Variations in the internal structure of the nerve introduced in this way affect:

1. The size and number of the bundles
2. The funicular pattern as seen in a transverse section of the nerve trunk
3. The relative cross-sectional area of a nerve devoted to epineurial and funicular tissue
4. The funicular rearrangement and redistribution of nerve fibers representing individual branches

With very few exceptions human nerves are multifuniculated structures in which the size and the number of the bundles are inversely related. However, in some nerves the nerve fibers are sometimes collected into a single funiculus for a short distance in certain regions, such as in the radial nerve in the spiral groove, the lateral popliteal nerve in the distal part of the thigh, and the ulnar nerve behind the medial humeral epicondyle. These morphological features just outlined have considerable relevance to nerve repair as shall be demonstrated in the following.

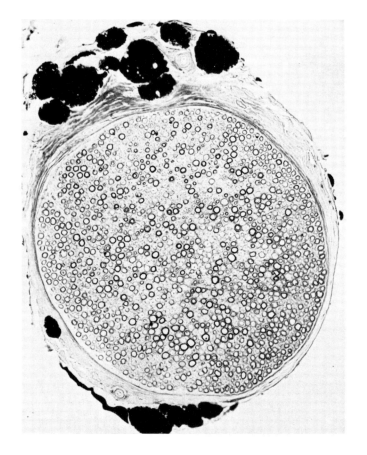

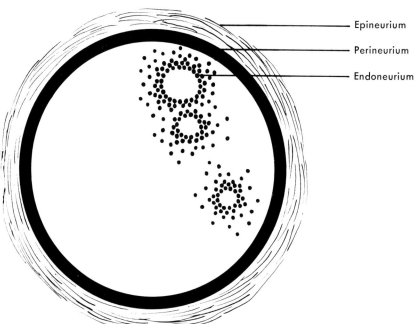

Fig. 3-2. Transverse section of monofunicular nerve trunk with matching diagram, accentuating arrangement of endoneurium, perineurium, and epineurium. Dark areas in epineurium are collections of adipose tissue. (From Sunderland, S.: Nerves and nerve injuries, ed. 2, Edinburgh, 1978, Churchill-Livingstone.)

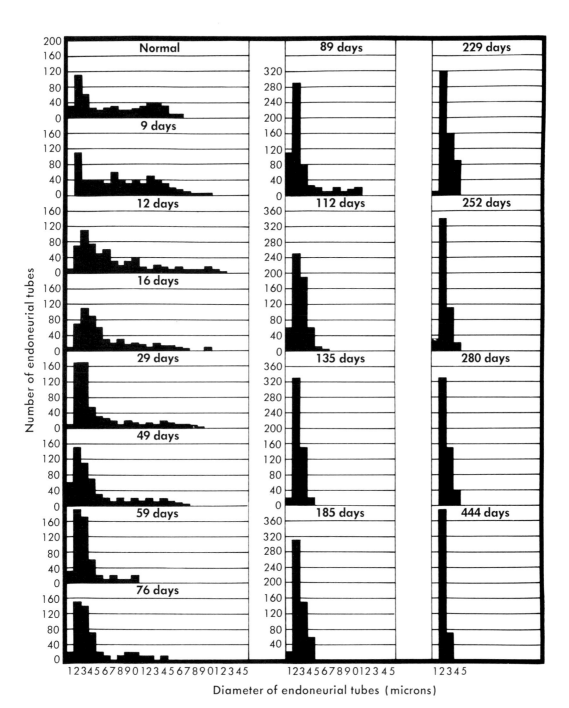

Fig. 3-3. Histograms illustrating progressive atrophy of endoneurial tubes that have been denervated for periods ranging from 9 to 444 days (Australian opossum *Trichosurus vulpecula*). (From Sunderland, S.: Nerves and nerve injuries, ed. 2, Edinburgh, 1978, Churchill-Livingstone.)

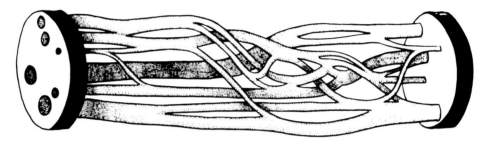

Fig. 3-4. Reconstruction of funicular arrangement in 3 cm length of specimen of musculocutaneous nerve of arm illustrating complexity of funicular unions and divisions. (From Sunderland, S.: Nerves and nerve injuries, ed. 2, Edinburgh, 1978, Churchill-Livingstone.)

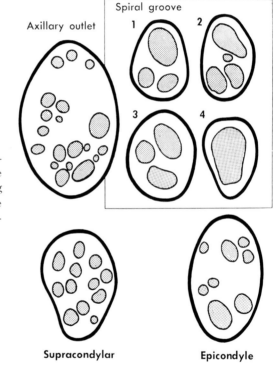

Fig. 3-5. Transverse sections from specimen of radial nerve taken at levels indicated to illustrate variations in size and number of funiculi along nerve. (From Sunderland, S.: Nerves and nerve injuries, ed. 2, Edinburgh, 1978, Churchill-Livingstone.)

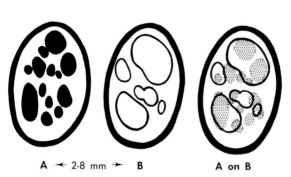

Fig. 3-6. Two transverse sections of specimen of radial nerve 2.8 mm apart to illustrate rapid change in size of component funiculi over short length of nerve. (From Sunderland, S.: Nerves and nerve injuries, ed. 2, Edinburgh, 1978, Churchill-Livingstone.)

FUNICULAR SIZE

At any given level, while the funiculi may be uniform in size, they more often vary considerably in size (Fig. 3-5). Funicular diameters range from about 0.04 to 2 mm with an occasional funiculus reaching 4 mm in diameter.

There is a linear relationship between funicular diameter and perineurial sheath thickness, the latter varying from 1.3 μ to 100 μ. Finally, funicular plexus formations often result in quite rapid changes in funicular size over short distances (Fig. 3-6).

Significance

While the larger funiculi are easily detected at the nerve end, the finest are particularly difficult to detect and, in any event, are too thin to take even the finest sutures without causing irreparable damage to the contained nerve fibers. Differences in the size of funiculi at the nerve ends constitute one of the factors that make funicular nerve repair on a funiculus-to-funiculus basis an impracticable proposition.

The size of a funiculus is also relevant to its survival when the nerve is being used as an autogenous graft. The revascularization of a graft across the suture lines and from its bed is in itself a fascinating problem. Suffice it to say that the thicker the bundle, the greater the risk of central necrosis. In this respect there must be a critical funicular diameter. We do not know what it is or the factors that influence the limit.

It is of interest that Seddon and his associates cautioned against the use of the lateral popliteal nerve as an autograft because of central funicular necrosis, which they attributed to full-thickness grafting.[6] However, there is another explanation to account for the failure of such grafts. It has already been noted that the site where this nerve is selected as a donor graft is often composed of either a solitary or major funiculus that is too thick to be adequately revascularized in time to ensure its survival. Such grafts may have failed not because they were full-thickness grafts but because of the size of the funiculus. The chances of a full-thickness graft surviving

are increased if it is composed of many small funiculi, an arrangement that resembles a cable graft.

In general the largest funiculi in the cutaneous nerves usually used for autografting have dimensions that do not put them at risk, but this must be regarded only as a generalization for there could be occasions when the critical size would be exceeded.

FUNICULAR NUMBERS

The divisions and unions of the funiculi that occur repeatedly along the nerve are responsible for affecting frequent changes in their number. Such is the nature of the changes produced in this way that the numbers of funiculi at levels even a short distance apart may differ considerably. Some idea of the numbers of funiculi comprising the major peripheral nerves is shown in the following data from human nerves.

Nerve	Number of funiculi
Median	3 to 37
Radial, ulnar, and lateral popliteal	1 to 36
Sciatic nerve in the gluteal region	43 to 137
Medial popliteal	11 to 93

The number of funiculi is always greater where the nerve crosses a joint than in the intervening regions. For any given specimen, the following examples will indicate the range of variation in funicular numbers along the nerve:

Nerve	Number of funiculi
Median	3 to 22, 5 to 16, 4 to 13, 15 to 36
Ulnar	1 to 8, 1 to 18, 3 to 8, 12 to 36
Radial	1 to 20, 2 to 13, 2 to 36, 8 to 29
Medial popliteal	11 to 27, 16 to 33, 28 to 93, 32 to 83
Lateral popliteal	1 to 15, 1 to 21, 5 to 20, 8 to 24

Significance

The fact that funicular numbers can change quite rapidly over short distances means that the numbers at the ends of a severed nerve are unlikely to correspond except with clean transections or the destruction of segments of less than about 1 cm (Fig. 3-6). In such situations, therefore, attempts at the funicular repair of a nerve by uniting funiculus to funiculus will inevitably leave some funiculi unmatched.

VARIATIONS IN FUNICULAR PATTERN

Funicular plexus formations produce such rapid changes in the size, number, and arrangement of the funiculi that sections taken more than a few millimeters apart will fail to show precisely the same patterns (Fig. 3-7). Dissimilarities arising in this way mean that when the two sections are opposed in epineurial nerve suture, much of the funicular tissue in one end of the cut nerve is opposed to interfunicular tissue in the other. In a large series the longest section of any nerve with an identical pattern has been 15 mm, although individual bundles and bundle groups may remain unchanged for greater distances.

Significance

This morphological feature of peripheral nerves means that, except after clean transections, the chances of obtaining precise and total funicular apposition at the nerve ends during repair are very remote indeed.

VARIATIONS IN RELATIVE CROSS-SECTIONAL AREA OF A NERVE DEVOTED TO FUNICULAR AND EPINEURIAL TISSUE

The cross-sectional area of a nerve devoted to funiculi on the one hand and epineurial tissue on the other is subject to considerable variation not only from nerve to nerve but also at different levels along the same nerve. Generalizing, the following may be stated.

1. The amount of epineurial tissue ranges from 22% to 88% of the cross-sectional area of the nerve.
2. The epineurium is relatively more abundant where the nerve is composed of numerous small bundles as distinct from few and large bundles.
3. Multiple funiculi are, regardless of their

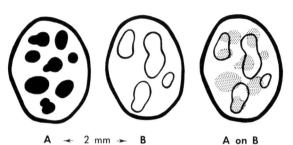

A ← 2 mm → B   A on B

Fig. 3-7. Two transverse sections of specimen of radial nerve 2 mm apart to illustrate rapid changes that occur in size, number, and arrangement of funiculi over short length of nerve. (From Sunderland, S.: Nerves and nerve injuries, ed. 2, Edinburgh, 1978, Churchill-Livingstone.)

number, more compactly arranged in some regions and in some nerves than in others.

Significance

These findings have a bearing on nerve repair in three ways. The first way concerns the behavior of the distal stump after nerve section. The cross-sectional area of the proximal stump of a severed nerve undergoes little change. On the other hand, the distal stump undergoes a series of significant changes as follows: Following the disintegration and removal of the axons and myelin, the endoneurial tubes shrink as the endoneurium contracts around the surviving Schwann cells. This shrinkage occurs rapidly at first and then more slowly until a stable state is reached about the third to the fourth month when few endoneurial tubes larger than 2 to 3 μ are seen (Fig. 3-3). As the endoneurial tubes shrink, the perineurium, in turn, contracts about the remaining contents of the funiculus, the overall effect being a progressive and corresponding reduction in the cross-sectional area of the funiculi. In contrast, the supporting epineurial connective tissue, other than that in the traumatized zone, remains essentially unchanged.

Since the funicular and epineurial tissues react quite differently to denervation, it follows that nerve trunk atrophy will be influenced not only by the duration of dener-

Table 3-1. Nerve trunk and funicular atrophy with increasing periods of denervation (Australian opossum)*

Nerve	Duration of denervation (days)	Percentage funicular atrophy	Percentage nerve trunk atrophy
Ulnar	16	37	6
Median	44	64	49
Ulnar	59	67	28
Median	59	50	31
Median	76	50	13
Median	76	54	58
Median	135	62	34
Ulnar	224	63	54
Median	229	59	33
Ulnar	485	66	56
Ulnar	335	72	22
Ulnar	335	74	42

*Because of differences in the cross-sectional areas of the distal stump devoted to funicular and epineurial tissue, nerve trunk atrophy does not bear a constant relationship to funicular atrophy.

vation but also by the relative amounts of the funicular and epineurial tissues comprising the nerve. Thus nerve trunk atrophy will be greater where the funiculi represent the major component of the nerve trunk. On the other hand, where the funiculi are well separated by large amounts of epineurial tissue and so occupy a smaller proportion of the cross-sectional area of the nerve, the overall effect will be one in which the nerve trunk does not atrophy to the same degree. This explains why the reduction in the cross-sectional area of the entire nerve does not correspond with the funicular atrophy but fluctuates irregularly in a manner determined by the factors previously mentioned (Table 3-1). All this means that a stump showing little atrophy can be masking marked funicular atrophy.

A second way in which variations in amount of epineurial tissue affect nerve repairs relates to the value of encasing the suture site with a cuff to protect it from harmful fibrosis and adhesions; this subject remains a controversial issue. Such cuffs do not exclude the interfunicular epineurial tissue that may occupy the bulk of the nerve at the site of the repair. It is from this epineurial tissue that intense and damaging intraneural fibrosis oc-

curs. Although the cuff may prevent the development of adhesions that would fix the suture line to the nerve bed, it will not prevent intraneural fibrosis. With variations in the ratio of epineurial tissue to funiculi, variations in intraneural fibrosis could be expected even though cuffs are utilized in an attempt to reduce fibrosis.

Finally, as to the importance of epineurial tissue, regardless of any dissimilarities in funicular patterns at the nerve ends, the chances of obtaining funicular apposition at the nerve ends during repair are enhanced when the funiculi are closely packed, while the chances are reduced when the bundles are widely separated by large amounts of interfunicular epineurial tissue.

CHANGES IN BRANCH FIBER COMPOSITION OF FUNICULI AND DISTRIBUTION OF DIFFERENT BRANCH FIBER SYSTEMS WITHIN THE NERVE TRUNK

Another morphological feature attributable to funicular plexuses is the funicular redistribution and regrouping of the nerve fibers representing different branches as they pass along the nerve (Fig. 3-8). For some distance above its origin, each branch is represented

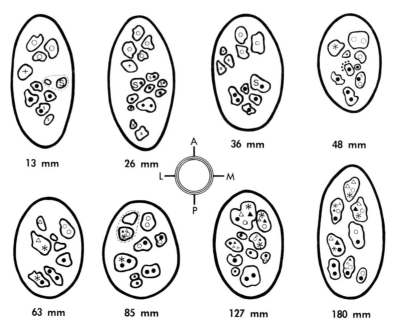

13 mm   26 mm   36 mm   48 mm

63 mm   85 mm   127 mm   180 mm

Fig 3-8. Selected transverse sections from serially sectioned specimen of radial nerve to illustrate funicular redistribution of nerve fibers representing individual branches as these are followed centrally within nerve. Symbols representing fibers of individual branches are: ○, superficial radial; ●, posterior interosseous; S, supinator; +, extensor carpi radialis brevis; ×, extensor carpi radialis longus; *, combined radial extensors of the wrist; △, brachioradialis; and ▲, brachialis. Measurements represent level of section in millimeters above lateral humeral epicondyle. Compass symbols A, P, L, and M represent anterior, posterior, lateral, and medial aspects of the nerve, respectively. (From Sunderland, S.: Nerves and nerve injuries, ed. 2, Edinburgh, 1978, Churchill-Livingstone.)

in the nerve by a funiculus, or group of funiculi, which is sharply localized and superficially situated.

When multiple branches from a muscle enter different aspects of a nerve at different levels, the bundles often migrate considerable distances through the nerve or along the surface of the nerve before uniting. It is also usual for funiculi from different muscles having similar actions to fuse before participating in further intercommunications. There is often considerable intraneural movement of one or both bundle systems, before fusion is effected, as one moves proximally along the nerve.

Funiculi representing individual branches subsequently intercommunicate with adjacent bundles composed of fibers from different branches. This results in an intermingling of the fibers of systems originally separate in the periphery. Further scattering and mixing of the fibers gradually continue as the intercommunications are repeated at successive levels until proximally in the nerve the various branch systems come to be widely represented over the funiculi in varying combinations and proportions, although each bundle does not necessarily contain fibers from every branch.

Thus the arrangement is one in which the fibers of any particular branch system are at first discretely localized in the nerve; then, moving proximally, they are in turn discretely localized but now mixed with other fibers and then only predominantly localized until, finally, fiber scattering reaches a degree where there is no recognizable localization.

Finally, with regard to their fiber composition, the funiculi are of two main types: (1) simple funiculi composed solely of fibers serving a particular muscle or cutaneous area

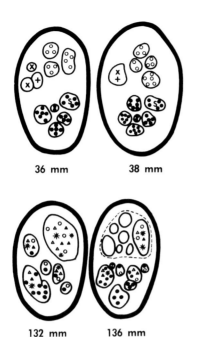

36 mm   38 mm

132 mm   136 mm

Fig. 3-9. Adjacent sections, a few millimeters apart, taken at two widely separated levels of specimen of radial nerve to illustrate effect of branch fiber composition of funiculi on chances of regenerating axons entering functionally related endoneurial tubes in distal stump of sutured nerve. Symbol code is same as that given in legend for Fig. 3-8. (From Sunderland, S.: Nerves and nerve injuries, ed. 2, Edinburgh, 1978, Churchill-Livingstone.)

and (2) compound funiculi composed of fibers from several sources in varying combinations and proportions.

Significance

The fiber content of the funiculi at the level where a nerve is repaired has a significant influence on the reconstitution during regeneration of functionally useful pathways (Fig. 3-9). When surgically opposed funiculi contain fibers from only one source or from functionally related structures (for example, the extensor muscles of the wrist), the consequences of the erroneous cross-shunting of regenerating axons into foreign endoneurial tubes at the suture line are minimized because the arrangement is one that ensures that an axon entering an endoneurial tube will at least reach a function-

ally related, if not the original, end-organ innervated by the fiber. On the other hand, when surgically opposed funiculi are composed of fibers from several different and functionally unrelated sources (for example, muscle and skin), the pattern of reinnervation may be so distorted because of the wasteful fiber mixing occurring during regeneration that recovery is seriously impaired.

CROSS-SECTIONAL AREA OF THE FUNICULI OCCUPIED BY NERVE FIBERS OF INDIVIDUAL BRANCHES

Another morphological feature of relevance to nerve repair concerns the proportion of nerve fibers in the individual branches in relation to the total number of fibers in the funiculi of the nerve trunk.

The task of counting the total number of fibers representing each branch in a peripheral nerve would be formidable. The cross-sectional area of a funiculus in an individual branch may, however, be accepted as a rough measure of the number of fibers the branch will contribute to the nerve trunk, although other factors, such as the caliber of the nerve fibers and the amount of endoneurial connective tissue, affect the accuracy of the calculation.

The percentage of funicular cross-sectional area occupied by the fibers representing any given individual branch naturally depends on the level at which the analysis is made. This point is illustrated by reference to the percentage funicular areas of a median and an ulnar nerve trunk occupied by the cutaneous and the muscular fibers *from the hand*, measured at the wrist and above the elbow as follows:

Nerve	At wrist		Above elbow	
	Muscular	*Cutaneous*	*Muscular*	*Cutaneous*
Median	6	94	4	66
Ulnar	44	56	28	35

The fibers of the median and ulnar branches in the hand occupy a greater proportion of their respective nerves in the lower forearm than in the upper arm, where fibers innervating the forearm muscles lie within the trunk.

Significance

This morphological feature has a bearing on the restoration of useful connections with the periphery during regeneration. Thus, where there is no branch fiber localization at the level of the repair, the chances of regenerating axons entering functionally related endoneurial tubes will, other things being equal, favor those axonal types that are numerically greater. This explains why, for example, following repair of the median nerve in the forearm, the recovery of sensation in the hand, no matter how imperfect, is far superior to the recovery of the affected thenar muscles.

BEHAVIOR OF NERVE TRUNKS UNDER TENSION

The nerve trunk runs an undulating course in its bed; the funiculi run an undulating course in the epineurium; and the nerve fibers run an undulating course inside the funiculi (Fig. 3-10). This means that the length of nerve fibers between any two fixed points on the limb is considerably greater than the distance between those points.

The initial effect of stretching the nerve is to take out the undulations in the nerve trunk. With continued stretching this is followed by the elimination of the undulations in the funiculi and finally the undulations in the nerve fibers. It is only at this last point that the nerve fibers are subjected to tension. With further stretching, conduction in the nerve fibers is next impaired, then fails, until finally the nerve fibers fracture inside the funiculi. The perineurium is the last component to fail structurally.

These structural features of nerve trunks mean that during limb movements the deli-

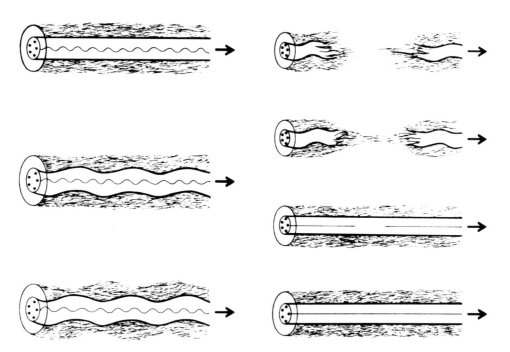

Fig. 3-10. Diagrammatic representation of behavior of different components of nerve trunk as it is stretched to and beyond limit of elasticity. For simplification only one funiculus and one nerve fiber are shown (lower left). Traction first eliminates undulations in nerve trunk (middle left). As deforming force increases, undulations in funiculi are lost (upper left), followed by those in nerve fibers (lower right) until finally all protective undulations in system have been removed and all components of nerve trunk are under tension. Beyond this point increasing stretch damages and then ruptures nerve fibers inside funiculi (right, second from bottom). In final stage funiculi rupture and nerve ends are drawn apart. (From Sunderland, S.: Nerves and nerve injuries, ed. 2, Edinburgh, 1978, Churchill-Livingstone.)

cate conducting elements of the nerve are adequately protected against traction deformation.

When a nerve is subjected to a gradually increasing tensile load, once the undulations in the funiculi have been removed and the funiculi begin to take the load, there is a linear relationship between the load and elongation until a certain point is reached beyond which the nerve ceases to behave as an elastic structure. The principal component imparting elasticity to the nerve trunk and giving it tensile strength is the perineurium. The percentage elongation has been recorded for a number of nerves at the elastic limit and at the point of mechanical failure. Data from tensile tests on nerves followed through to their destruction are shown in Table 3-2.

The rate of deformation is an important factor determining the point of mechanical failure. Nerves will tolerate considerable deformation providing they are stretched sufficiently slowly. In the experiments referred to, the rate of elongation was 7.5 cm/min.

Significance

The pattern of structural change that occurs when a peripheral nerve is stretched should be kept in mind when considering the consequences of applying tension at the suture line and of the postoperative stretching of nerves sutured under tension. The anatomical arrangement is one that protects the nerve fibers over a limited range when applying gentle traction on the nerve ends to bring them together. However, if traction is excessive, there is a serious risk of rupturing nerve fibers inside the funiculi. Again, should the nerve have been ill-advisedly sutured under considerable tension with the limb flexed, then during postoperative extension of the limb there is a serious risk of either (1) rupturing the suture line or (2) rupturing nerve fibers inside the funiculi if the suture line holds. The risk is even greater if the extension is effected too early or too rapidly.

RETROGRADE EFFECTS OF NERVE INJURY

This is an appropriate point at which to stray from the morphological path in order to mention that neurons are particularly sensitive to injury to their peripheral processes. It is not generally recognized that many parent cells may suffer irreparable damage as the result of the loss of their axon. Such a loss means the elimination of a quota of axons from the system, while persisting residual defects could affect the capacity of the cell to regenerate a new process. The severity of these retrograde effects is influenced by several factors, important among which are the severity of the peripheral injury and its proximity to the parent cell body.

NERVE REPAIR

When the morphological information outlined in the first part of this lecture is assembled, it provides essential background material for any rational examination and discus-

Table 3-2. Percentage elongation of human nerve trunks under tensile loading (rate of elongation 7.5 cm/min)

Nerve	At elastic limit		At mechanical failure	
	Range	Mean	Range	Mean
Ulnar	8 to 21	15	9 to 26	18
Median	6 to 22	14	7 to 30	19
Medial popliteal	7 to 21	17	8 to 32	23
Lateral popliteal	9 to 22	15	10 to 32	20
Anterior spinal roots	9 to 15	11	9 to 21	15
Posterior spinal roots	8 to 16	12	8 to 28	19

sion of many of the controversial issues that continue to harass the clinician.

Three main types of nerve repair are available to the surgeon:

1. The restoration of nerve trunk continuity by end-to-end union
2. The restoration of nerve trunk continuity by some form of grafting
3. Nerve cross-anastomosis in which axons are provided from another source

However, regardless of the method employed, the repair involves a suture line, and it is at this interface that many of the problems of nerve repair are to be found.

It is worth noting at this point that nerve grafting still further complicates the issue by introducing an additional suture line as well as a further set of hazards associated with the survival of the graft and its effectiveness in conveying regenerating axons to the distal stump.

For nerve repair to be effective regenerating axons must enter not only the distal stump but also the funiculi of the distal stump and, more importantly, appropriate endoneurial tubes in the funiculi.

Where there is complete correspondence between the funicular patterns of the opposed nerve ends, such as occurs with clean or almost clean nerve transection, all that is needed is accurate, matching coaptation of the nerve ends by superficial epineurial sutures. In making this statement I am deferring any consideration of the relative merits of epineurial and funicular repair until later.

Usually, however, a segment of nerve trunk is lost and this, together with the preparation of the nerve ends for repair, creates a situation in which:

1. The nerve ends may or may not correspond in size.
2. The funiculi will probably not correspond in size and number.
3. The funicular patterns will be dissimilar.
4. There will be no localization of branch fiber systems except in certain regions.

As a result of such discrepancies, some axons will fail to enter the distal stump; others will fail to enter funiculi, and still a

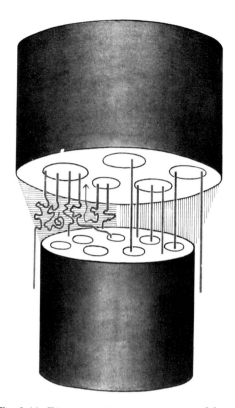

Fig. 3-11. Diagrammatic representation of factors operating at suture line that adversely affect passage of axons into endoneurial tubes in distal stump and restoration of functionally useful pathways. (From Sunderland, S.: Nerves and nerve injuries, ed. 2, Edinburgh, 1978, Churchill-Livingstone.)

third group will fail to enter functionally related endoneurial tubes (Fig. 3-11).

A further obstacle to regeneration is scarring at the suture line. While axon sprouting offsets, to some extent, the wasteful regeneration occurring in this way, it is clear that many axons fail to reestablish useful connections with the periphery so that recovery is inevitably imperfect and incomplete.

Under these circumstances the best the surgeon could do in the past was to maintain correct axial alignment of the nerve ends during repair in order to take advantage of any fiber localization existing at that level. Even here, however, he could be defeated by the movement of some funiculi from one sector of the nerve to another so that when the nerve ends were opposed these particular bundles would not be in corresponding sectors.

The question of improving on this unfavorable state of affairs introduces for consideration the feasibility of undertaking a funicular repair with the object of: (1) confining regenerating axons to funiculi and (2) taking advantage of any localization of branch fiber systems where this is present. These two objectives will, for convenience and simplification, be considered separately.

Funicular repair designed to confine regenerating axons within funiculi

The anastomosis of individual funiculi is technically possible for all but the very finest funiculi. However, the complete restoration of funicular continuity in this way is, with very few exceptions, an impossibility because of disparities in the size and number of the funiculi at the nerve ends, which are aggravated by any funicular atrophy present in the distal stump. However, it has already been noted that some funiculi may run long courses in the nerve before participating in plexus formations with neighboring funiculi. This feature means that, depending on the length of nerve destroyed, it is possible for the same funiculus to be present at both nerve ends where it can be accurately identified and continuity restored by direct anastomosis.

Attempts at individual funicular anastomosis are contraindicated where the nerve is composed of many small funiculi. This would leave the junctional zone bristling with sutures, each of which, no matter how fine, would excite a fibroblastic reaction thereby aggravating harmful scarring at the suture line that obstructs and constricts regenerating axons.

The question now arises as to whether there is any merit in the technique of gently freeing the funiculi for a short distance from the epineurium at the nerve ends and then grouping them during repair in a manner designed to achieve the best possible funicular apposition, the object being to reduce the number of axons lost by wasteful regeneration into interfunicular epineurial tissue. The

techniques involved in group funicular repair will be discussed further in this volume.

At this point it should be noted, however, that if reducing the loss of axons by wasteful regeneration into epineurial tissue were the sole reason for performing group funicular repair, then the method would be a sound alternative to epineurial repair only when the funiculi are widely separated by large amounts of epineurial tissue. The method would confer no advantage on the repair when the bundles are closely packed, an arrangement that in itself would offset dissimilarities in the funicular patterns.

Funicular repair designed to assist regenerating axons to enter functionally related endoneurial tubes

Group funicular repair has particular merit when it comes to the question of assisting regenerating axons to enter functionally related endoneurial tubes. In this respect two criteria must be satisfied before the method can be considered worthwhile.

1. There should be a degree of fiber localization at the nerve ends that is worth exploiting by this technique.
2. It should be possible to identify, positively and accurately, specific individual funicular groups at the nerve ends.

The potential of the method for assisting regeneration can best be explained by examining the feasibility of applying it at three levels in the limbs: distally, proximally, and at intermediate levels. These will each be discussed in the following.

Distal funicular repair

In the peripheral part of the limb the terminal branch systems are localized to specific funiculi in a manner that offers excellent prospects for group funicular repair. The following examples will illustrate the advantages of this method in the distal portion of the limb.

Ulnar nerve

At the wrist the fibers destined for the deep division of the ulnar nerve are confined to a group of funiculi occupying the medial and posteromedial portion of the nerve (fibers labeled "M" in Fig. 3-12, 36 mm level). This group can be easily identified and separated from the remaining bundles, which are devoted to the fibers continuing as the superficial division of the nerve (Fig. 3-12). The individual digital branch fibers are confined to their own funiculi in the latter group, but the bundles are usually too small and the line of demarcation between the subgroups not sufficiently distinct to permit their identification. The superficial (predominantly cutaneous) and deep (predominantly muscular) divisions can, however, be readily identified at the nerve ends.

Although the funicular localization obtaining at this level naturally favors the entry of axons into functionally related tubes following conventional end-to-end repair, it would be wise to suture or graft the two bundle systems separately in order to eliminate all possibility of motor regenerating axons entering sensory endoneurial tubes and sensory processes entering motor tubes.

In the mid forearm the bundle group representing the dorsal cutaneous nerve of the hand occupies the medial and posteromedial portion of the nerve (fibers labeled "O" in Fig. 3-12). The group can be identified and isolated from the point where the branch joins the trunk for a distance of 15 to 20 cm,

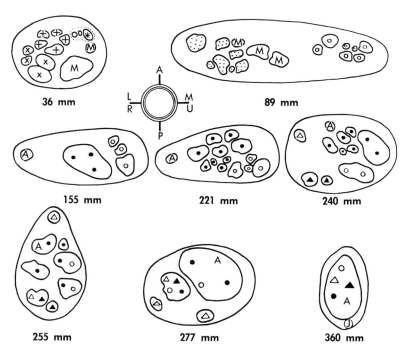

Fig. 3-12. Selected transverse sections from serially sectioned specimen of ulnar nerve to illustrate funicular redistribution of nerve fibers representing individual branches as these were followed centrally within nerve. Symbols representing fibers of individual branches are: +, cutaneous fibers from ulnar side of little finger; ×, cutaneous fibers from fourth digital interspace; *, cutaneous fibers from hypothenar eminence; M, deep (muscular) division fibers; ⦂·⦂, combined terminal cutaneous fibers; ○, dorsal cutaneous fibers of hand; ●, combined terminal and muscular cutaneous fibers; A, fibers to ulnar artery; △, flexor carpi ulnaris fibers; and ▲, flexor digitorum profundus fibers. Nerve divided into its terminal, superficial, and deep divisions 20 mm below radial styloid level; measurements give level of section above site of this branching. Compass symbols A, P, L-R, and M-U represent anterior, posterior, lateral-radial, and medial-ulnar aspects of nerve, respectively. (From Sunderland, S.: Nerves and nerve injuries, ed. 2, Edinburgh, 1978, Churchill-Livingstone.)

the number of bundles over this length varying from one to eight. Importantly, this sensory bundle group is situated immediately medial to that containing motor fibers.

The isolation and separate repair of the dorsal cutaneous bundle group are indicated in order to prevent regenerating sensory processes of this group straying into motor endoneurial tubes and to prevent motor regenerating axons from entering sensory funiculi.

Fig. 3-13 shows two sections taken 25 mm apart from a serially sectioned specimen of an ulnar nerve. If the blackened segment of the nerve were destroyed, the proximal and distal stumps would present the funicular patterns illustrated. The funiculi for the dorsal cutaneous fibers (labeled "*D*" in Fig. 3-13) would be present in the proximal stump but not in the distal stump. If the nerve were repaired by simple end-to-end union or continuity restored by the insertion of a graft, these cutaneous bundles would be brought into close relationship with those in the distal stump that are destined for the deep terminal (muscular) branch (labeled "*M*"). In such a situation the dorsal cutaneous bundle group should be isolated, mobilized, and transferred to supplement the reinnervation of sensory funiculi in the distal stump.

Median nerve

At the wrist the median nerve usually consists of a large number of small bundles (Fig. 3-14) in which the terminal branches are precisely localized in terms of specific bundle groups representing the individual digital branches from medial to lateral with the motor group located anteriorly. It is sometimes possible to identify these separate bundle groups because they are sufficiently spaced to permit this while slight encircling condensations of epineurial tissue may also assist in identifying separate bundle groups. When, however, there is uncertainty about the identification of bundles, the entire

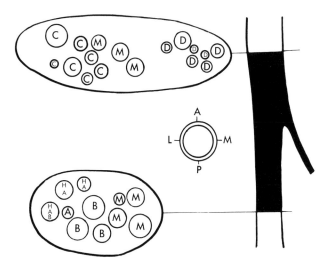

Fig. 3-13. Diagram of specimen of ulnar nerve with 25 mm segment in lower forearm missing. Branch fiber composition of funiculi at proximal and distal nerve ends is indicated by following symbols: *H, A,* and *B,* cutaneous fibers from hypothenar eminence, ulnar side of little finger, and fourth digital interspace, respectively; *C,* combined superficial division (cutaneous) fibers; *M,* deep terminal division (muscular) fibers; *D,* dorsal cutaneous hand fibers. Compass symbols *A, P, L,* and *M* represent anterior, posterior, lateral, and medial aspects of nerve, respectively. (From Sunderland, S.: Nerves and nerve injuries, ed. 2, Edinburgh, 1978, Churchill-Livingstone.)

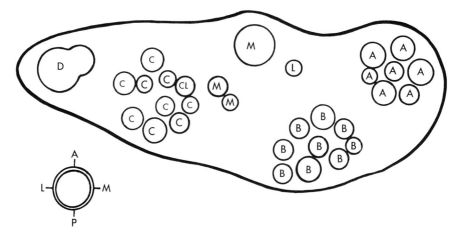

Fig. 3-14. Transverse section of specimen of median nerve at wrist to illustrate terminal branch fiber composition of funiculi comprising nerve at that level. *A*, *B*, and *C*, cutaneous fibers from third, second, and first interdigital spaces, respectively; *D*, cutaneous fibers from radial side of thumb; *M*, thenar muscular fibers; *L*, lumbrical fibers. Compass symbols *A*, *P*, *L*, and *M* represent anterior, posterior, lateral, and medial aspects of nerve, respectively. (From Sunderland, S.: Nerves and nerve injuries, ed. 2, Edinburgh, 1978, Churchill-Livingstone.)

posterior bundle system may be divided arbitrarily into four groups—one for each digital branch.

Radial nerve

At and just above the lateral humeral epicondyle the superficial radial fibers are always contained in a bundle group (one to four in number) that is sharply localized on the anterior surface of the nerve where it can be readily identified and isolated in a transverse section of the nerve (fibers labeled "*O*" in Fig. 3-8). Approximately 50 mm above the epicondyle, however, this bundle group commences to engage in plexus formations with neighboring motor funiculi. When repairing the radial nerve at and just above the epicondyle, advantage should be taken of this funicular arrangement to repair the cutaneous bundle group separately.

Proximal funicular repair

In the proximal part of the limb the fiber composition of the funiculi is such that, excluding the fibers of high branches, each funiculus in the nerve contains, in varying proportions, fibers representing most, if not all, of the peripheral branches.

Thus the fibers of any particular branch are widely distributed over the funiculi of the nerve.

Under these circumstances, there is clearly no point in attempting group funicular suture with the object of assisting regenerating axons to enter functionally related endoneurial tubes. Aiding regenerating axons to enter funiculi then becomes the essential object of the exercise. If the degree of separation of the funiculi at the nerve ends did justify group funicular suture, then the bundles would be arranged into groups on an arbitrary basis to achieve the best possible correspondence of funicular tissue to funicular tissue while still, however, maintaining quadrantal relationships between the funicular groupings so that advantage is taken of any trace of branch fiber localization that might conceivably be present at that level. The procedure may mean grouping two, three, or four small funiculi to match a large one, three to match two, and so on. However, where the funiculi are closely packed, the situation would be covered just as well by a simple, less demanding epineurial end-to-end repair with correct axial alignment of the nerve ends.

Funicular repair at intermediate levels

Between the two extremes represented at distal levels, where the funicular localization of branch fibers is discrete, and proximally, where there is no fiber localization, there is partial localization in which the fibers of a particular branch are scattered over several funiculi in combination with other fiber systems. These compound funiculi are, however, confined to a particular sector of the nerve although the area occupied by them exceeds that occupied by the branch in question at distal levels. This means that the localization of the fibers in the nerve is no longer total and sharp but involves a greater area of the nerve and an admixture with other fibers. Nevertheless the overall arrangement could be one that is worth exploiting by group funicular suture.

In summary, expectations that group funicular suture will assist regenerating axons to reestablish functionally useful connections with the periphery will only be realized where there is total, or at least a reasonable degree of, funicular fiber localization at the level of the repair. Prospects for the application of this technique are excellent at distal levels, particularly for the median and ulnar nerves, fair at intermediate levels, but negligible at proximal levels. The success of the method is, however, critically dependent on the accurate identification of specific funicular groups at the nerve ends. This remains a problem.

IDENTIFICATION OF SPECIFIC FUNICULAR GROUPS AT NERVE ENDS

Anatomical, electrophysiological, and histochemical methods are available for this purpose but each has its limitations.

Anatomical methods

Information is available on the funicular distribution and localization of branch fiber systems at different levels along peripheral nerves. However, there are bound to be individual variations in this regard, and, in any event, only in certain regions is the localization sufficiently precise, obvious, and characteristic to be of value.

Electrophysiological methods

The electrophysiological technique, which has been investigated experimentally by Vandeput and associates[7] and Grabb and associates[2] and used clinically by Hakstian[5], involves stimulating the funiculi at the nerve ends with the object of identifying and differentiating between those that are sensory and those that are motor. The procedure follows: The funiculi in the distal stump are stimulated individually. In the absence of a motor response the funiculus is tagged as sensory. A motor response does not, however, exclude the presence of sensory fibers in the funiculus. Depending on the nature of the response, Grabb and co-workers[2] have attempted to classify funiculi as predominantly motor or sensory. They have also stimulated digital nerves at the fingertips with the object of detecting the evoked sensory responses at the ends of sensory funiculi in the distal stump. Because severed nerve fibers degenerate and cease to conduct within 72 hours of the transection, the method is limited to this time interval. Funicular screening of the proximal stump requires a conscious and cooperative patient because it is based on his response to funicular stimulation. The absence of a response indicates a motor funiculus. However, a sensory response does not exclude the coexistence of motor fibers in the funiculus.

Electrophysiological testing is of no clinical value at levels where mixed funiculi predominate. It works best following clean transection of the median and ulnar nerves at the wrist where fiber localization in terms of separate motor and sensory funiculi is good. However, this is a region where the bundle group systems can be readily identified from a knowledge of funicular anatomy. Grabb and co-workers[2] investigated, in the monkey, the relative merits of funicular suture based on the alignment of funiculi according to their size and position and on their electrical properties. Because the results were similar, they decided in favor of the more simple anatomical method.

Histochemical methods

It has been shown[3,4] that sensory nerve fibers differ from motor nerve fibers with regard to content of acetylcholinesterase. This feature prompted Freilinger and co-workers[1] to devise a histochemical method for distinguishing between sensory and motor funiculi at the ends of a severed nerve. Biopsy transverse sections must be taken from the nerve ends within 72 hours of the injury. The sections are treated for acetylcholinesterase, which requires 25 to 30 hours incubation by which time the motor axons are stained while the sensory fibers are not. This information is then used to match corresponding motor and sensory funiculi at a later operation. In addition to requiring a second operation the method is also limited to regions where the funiculi are exclusively motor or sensory. Finally, the nerves selected for the investigation of this method were the median and the ulnar nerves at the wrist, and the results have only served to confirm the validity of anatomical data that provide a more practical guide during group funicular suture. At present the histochemical method is only of theoretical interest.

GENERAL COMMENT ON FUNICULAR REPAIR

When funiculi are widely separated by much epineurial tissue, group funicular repair should be effective in reducing the loss of regenerating axons into the interfunicular epineurial tissue. However, when the bundles are closely packed, the method has no advantage over conventional epineurial repair. Expectations that group funicular suture will assist regenerating axons to reestablish functionally useful connections with the periphery will only be realized when there is a total or reasonable degree of funicular fiber localization at the level of the repair. Group funicular repair has most to offer in the surgical treatment of severed median and ulnar nerves in the lower forearm and at the wrist. Elsewhere this method is subject to a number of limitations and these should be recognized and understood. It is important not to make demands on the method that it cannot possibly meet, and it is pointless to embark on a long, complicated and demanding group funicular suture at a level where a simple epineurial repair would be just as effective.

GROUP FUNICULAR SUTURE IN NERVE GRAFTING

In comparison with the use of group funicular suture for end-to-end repair, the use of this technique in nerve grafting is a distinct improvement on previous methods. This is because the planned union of selected funicular groups at the nerve ends to funicular groups in the cable strand ensures the best possible funicular apposition at the nerve graft junctions. The loss of regenerating axons into epineurial tissue, which would otherwise occur at two suture lines, is thereby reduced. Whether or not this method also aids the entry of axons into functionally related endoneurial tubes in the distal stump is, as in the case of end-to-end repair, determined by the degree of fiber localization present at the nerve ends.

Regarding terminology, "group funicular cable grafting" seems more appropriate than "fascicular" or "interfascicular grafting" because the graft is still of the cable variety and is not composed solely of funicular tissue, while the term "fascicular" relates more to the method of attaching the graft at the nerve ends.

In the past, the ends of the graft strands in a simple cable graft were applied to the ends of the recipient nerve without reference to funicular structure. The same applied to full-thickness grafting where the graft was attached by conventional epineurial sutures. In each case the importance of funicular matching at the nerve-graft junctions was not appreciated. Both should now be discontinued in favor of group funicular cable grafting or group funicular full-thickness grafting. In this respect the cable variety has a distinct advantage over the full-thickness variety. Apart from considerations of graft revascularization and survival, the combined strands of a cable graft confer other advantages that will now be considered.

The alignment of the strands of a cable graft means that axons growing down one strand of a cable cannot be widely scattered

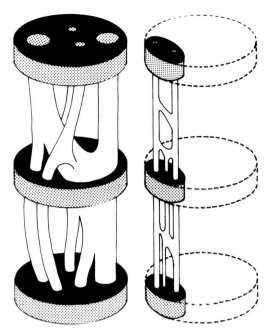

Fig. 3-15. Diagrammatic representation of full-thickness and cable nerve grafts to illustrate how regenerating axons from particular sector of proximal nerve end would be directed by strand of cable graft to corresponding sector of distal nerve end, whereas regenerating axons descending down endoneurial tubes in full-thickness graft may be directed across graft and so into very different sector in distal stump. (From Sunderland, S.: Nerves and nerve injuries, ed. 2, Edinburgh, 1978, Churchill-Livingstone.)

as they advance, while those entering a bundle in a full-thickness graft may, because of interfunicular communications, undergo a considerable shift from one part of the graft to another (Fig. 3-15). This bestows on the cable variety an advantage that increases with the number of separate strands. A stage is reached, however, when such an advantage is offset by the greatly added amount of epineurial tissue.

At the proximal and distal nerve ends the funicular patterns will differ, although some bundles may correspond, since all funiculi are not simultaneously involved in plexus formations; in addition the branch fiber arrangement may or may not correspond depending on the level and on the length of nerve destroyed. However, the need to graft usually implies the loss of a substantial length

of the nerve in which case the branch fiber arrangement at the nerve ends will probably not be identical, owing to the redistribution of fibers that has occurred in the lost nerve segment.

As regards the funicular nerve fiber arrangement at the nerve ends there are four possibilities (Fig. 3-16).

1. The sector of the host nerve, above and below in Fig. 3-16, can contain one or more funiculi, presenting either the same or dissimilar patterns but composed of fibers from the same source (Fig. 3-16, *1a* and *1b*). Funicular plexuses in the cable strand will produce some rearrangement of axons as they grow through the funiculi, but this is not of major functional significance in this case, since it involves only fibers of the same branch system.

2. The funiculi in the sector of the distal stump contain fibers from different sources, but the fibers in any single funiculus are from one source (Fig. 3-16, *2a* and *2b*). In the corresponding sector of the proximal end some funiculi are composed of fibers from one source, while others contain fibers from several of the funiculi in the sector of the distal stump; despite this a predominant localization still obtains. Here there is some chance of restoring useful functional connections.

3. Each of the funiculi in the opposing sectors contains fibers from several branches, and there is no fiber localization (Fig. 3-16, *3*). Under these conditions the graft, other than conveying axons to funiculi in the distal stump, probably makes no contribution to the restoration of useful connections; "probably" is used advisedly because there is always the chance that the fibers of a particular branch system may outnumber others with which they are mixed, and this would give them an advantage in any competition for endoneurial tubes.

4. The sector in the central stump contains fibers not represented in the distal sector. Here there is no way of redirecting regenerating axons into their old paths down a lost branch (Fig. 3-16, *4*).

The funicular arrangements described in 1, 2, and 3 above are common at distal levels

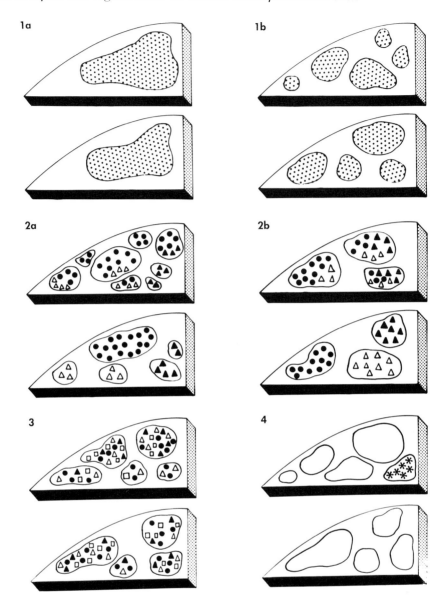

Fig. 3-16. Corresponding sectors (above and below in each pair, respectively) of proximal and distal ends of nerve that are to be linked by strand of cable graft. Branch fiber composition of funiculi at nerve ends ranges from one in which there is discrete localization of branch fiber systems to one in which there is no localization. This variable anatomical feature is one factor that affects restoration of functionally useful pathways and connections with periphery. (From Sunderland, S.: Nerves and nerve injuries, ed. 2, Edinburgh, 1978, Churchill-Livingstone.)

and are progressively replaced at proximal levels by 2, 3, and 4, respectively.

The ideal graft would be one in which the funicular arrangement was identical with that of the destroyed segment so that, after traversing the graft, the axons would be automat-ically directed to the appropriate endoneurial tubes in the distal segment. This would go a long way toward restoring the original fiber pattern. Although this ideal can never be realized, it is clear that the next best thing is a cable graft, which minimizes the dispersion of regenerating axons as they grow through the graft, and group funicular anastomosis at the nerve graft junctions, which minimizes the wasteful regeneration of axons into epineurial tissue and may, under favorable conditions, go some way to help restore useful connections with the periphery. The greatly improved recoveries that are now coming from group funicular cable autografting in the hands of Millesi and others are the result of meticulous attention to funicular anatomy and to improvements in effecting the junctional union.[6] This represents the greatest advance in nerve repair in recent years.

CROSS-ANASTOMOSIS TO RESTORE NERVE FUNCTION AFTER DESTRUCTIVE NERVE LESIONS THAT PRECLUDE END-TO-END REPAIR

The final method of nerve repair to be considered in the context of the present discussion relating to group funicular repair is cross-anastomosis for the restoration of nerve function.

Here again a knowledge of funicular anatomy can be helpful in designing the procedure. A good illustration in point is provided by those injuries in which there has been extensive destruction of the median nerve in the arm or forearm. Reparative procedures include cable grafting, free vascularized nerve grafting, and nerve cross-anastomosis using, as the donor nerve, the dorsal cutaneous nerve of the hand branch of the ulnar nerve. Based on the knowledge of the funicular anatomy of the median and ulnar nerves at the wrist, it is possible to devise a procedure in which the ulnar dorsal cutaneous branch and its bundle group in the ulnar nerve trunk are mobilized, and the funiculi of the branch are united to those

bundles in the median nerve representing the digital branches innervating importantly the thumb and index finger (Figs. 3-12 and 3-14). The advantages of this method of nerve repair will be discussed in Chapter 36.

Although the foregoing account by no means exhausts the list of factors contributing to the quality of the recovery after nerve repair, sufficient has been said to emphasize the importance of funicular anatomy and to highlight the difficulty of isolating each of the many involved variables for separate study and evaluation.

ACKNOWLEDGMENT

The illustrations in the text are from my book *Nerves and nerve injuries*[6] and are published with the permission of Churchill Livingstone, Edinburgh.

REFERENCES

1. Freilinger, G., et al.: Differential funicular suture of peripheral nerves. Transactions of the Sixth International Congress of Plastic and Reconstructive Surgery, Paris, 1975, Masson et Cie, Editeurs, p. 123.
2. Grabb, W. C., et al.: Comparison of methods of peripheral nerve suturing in monkeys, Plast. Reconstr. Surg. **46**:31, 1970.
3. Gruber, H., Zenker, W., and Hohenberg, E.: Untersuchungen über die Spezfität der Cholinesterasen im peripheren Nervensystem der Ratte, Histochemistry **27**:78, 1971.
4. Gruber, H., and Zenker, W.: Acetylcholinesterase: histochemical differentiation between motor and sensory nerve fibres, Brain Res. **51**:207, 1973.
5. Hakstian, R. W.: Funicular orientation by direct stimulation: an aid to peripheral nerve repair, J. Bone Joint Surg. **50A**:1178, 1968.
6. Sunderland, S.: Nerves and nerve injuries, ed. 2, Edinburgh, 1978, Churchill Livingstone. (This reference contains the details on which statements made in the text are based.)
7. Vandeput, J., Tanner, J. C., and Huypens, L.: Electrophysiological orientation of the cut ends in primary peripheral nerve repair, Plast. Reconstr. Surg. **44**:378, 1969.

4

Histopathology of common mononeuropathies

José Ochoa

The results of collaborative work on local nerve lesions done at Queen Square in London and at Dartmouth in the United States with Drs. Gilliatt, Fowler, Rudge, Neary, and Marotte will be reviewed here. It is not my intention to engage in an exhaustive review of the microscopical pathology of local nerve lesions of all sorts, but rather simply to focus on those that have been the subject of our research interests over the past decade and that happen to be the most common. Thus emphasis will be on local nerve lesions underlying acute compression, chronic entrapment, and painful traumatic neuromas. The neuropathies of leprosy and those caused by primary disease of the vasa nervorum such as acute diabetic mononeuropathy and the mononeuropathies of collagen-vascular disease are beyond the scope of this review (see Asbury[3] and Sabin and Swift[49]).

It should be obvious that the common denominator behind the family of pathological conditions about to be discussed is physical injury, more explicitly, mechanical injury. Traumatic neuromas, characterized by axonal division, are the direct consequence of mechanical violence on the structural components of peripheral nerves. However, when it comes to the *demyelinating* lesions underlying acute compression (neurapraxia) and chronic nerve entrapment, the situation is less straightforward. Indeed, in addition to the simple possibility that mechanical phenomena might be directly responsible for the nerve lesion, it is conceivable that compression operates indirectly by interfering

with the blood supply of the nerve: both hypotheses have their supporters, and it could well be that here we have an example where scientific debate between opposing schools is perpetuated—because everyone is right. Having conceded that proviso, one can now present, for all intents and purposes, incontrovertible evidence that the primary lesion of myelinated fibers underlying neurapraxia is primarily mechanical in origin and that the distinct lesion of myelinated fibers underlying chronic entrapment also recognizes a mechanical cause. This is not the same as stating that the vasa nervorum escape damage in those conditions, nor that nerve ischemia is noncontributory to some transient clinical manifestations in entrapment syndromes. Nevertheless, the lesions described in the following are in themselves sufficient to account for their corresponding electrophysiological defects and for most of their corresponding clinical phenomena. Moreover, recent studies directed to assess the separate contribution of ischemia in the development of neurapraxia have come with a negative answer.[65]

TRANSIENT ISCHEMIC NERVE INJURY

Of course, ischemia does affect peripheral nerve function and may affect peripheral nerve structure. The histopathology of acute experimental nerve ischemia following ligation of the main arterial supply to a limb has been dramatically illustrated by light and electron microscopy.[26] Under those circumstances, nerve fibers undergo the typical

36

changes of axonal (wallerian) degeneration. In the human, overt pathology has been described in nerve specimens obtained from lower limbs of patients suffering chronic obstructive arterial disease.[10,18] Such changes involved both demyelination and axonal degeneration, leading to progressive dropout of nerve fibers.

The utterly predictable fact that ischemia may affect nerve function was most elegantly documented in the 1930's by Sir Thomas Lewis and his collaborators. In their classical studies, where they offered themselves for human experimentation, Lewis, Pickering, and Rothschild[28] made observations of permanent value concerning negative und positive sensory phenomena and of ascending paralysis following compression of the upper arm, at suprasystolic pressure, with a pneumatic cuff. With ingenuity, they managed to sort out the effects of ischemia from those of direct compression of the nerve: having placed the cuff and waited the traditional 20 to 30 minutes until sensorimotor paralysis, they proceeded to place a second cuff at similar pressure proximal to the first one. On release of the first cuff, symptoms did not recover immediately, unlike the usual, indicating that sustained ischemia and not local nerve compression was responsible for the functional nerve defect.

The phenomenon described above is well known to the layman when he speaks of an arm or a leg having "gone to sleep." Lewis, Pickering, and Rothschild[28] spoke of "centripetal paralysis." Perhaps one should speak of "transient ischemic nerve block," that is, a transient ischemic attack of the peripheral nerve. An essential feature of this condition is its immediate reversibility on reestablishing circulation. Under such circumstances no structural change is to be expected: this held true for an isolated microscopical and ultramicroscopical observation in an animal experiment. (Ochoa, 1975, unpublished)

NEURAPRAXIA

Sustained local compression of a nerve or a whole limb may result in irreversible paralysis and sensory loss. If the physical injury has been very severe, the axons will be crushed and the sequence of wallerian degeneration with loss of nerve excitability distal to the lesion will follow inevitably. In Seddon's[51] classification this is "axonotmesis"; in Sunderland's[55,56] classification it is "second degree nerve injury." Functional recovery will be slow and rarely complete as it will require regrowth of new axons at a rate of 1 mm/day (under the best conditions) and correct guidance to their appropriate periphery.

Sometimes the clinical and electrophysiological features of sensorimotor paralysis that persist following compression are such that a local demyelinating block can be diagnosed as opposed to axonal division. The nerve will remain excitable throughout the symptomatic period when stimulated distal to the lesion, and there will be no evidence of denervation of the flaccid muscles.[11] This intermediate condition was defined electrophysiologically by Erb in 1876 and has been the subject of another important recent experimental study in primates by Fowler, Danta, and Gilliatt.[15] Seddon[51] called it "neurapraxia," and Sunderland[55,56] called it "first degree nerve injury." Recovery is nearly complete and often resolves in a matter of weeks. Common examples are acute radial palsy ("Saturday night paralysis") and tourniquet paralysis.

The demyelinating nature of the lesion underlying the intermediate type of nerve block under discussion was first demonstrated by Denny-Brown and Brenner[8,9] in their classical studies of "paralysis induced by direct pressure, by tourniquet and by spring clip." Although not entirely a new concept, at that time the idea of selective damage to myelin with sparing of axons was refreshing.

In the minds of Denny-Brown and Brenner[8,9] the demyelinating block underlying neurapraxia was a complication of the transient ischemic paralysis defined by Lewis, Pickering, and Rothschild[28]: prolonged ischemia would eventually cause structural damage to the myelin sheaths. Arguing in support of ischemia, Denny-Brown and Brenner[8,9] brought up the experiment of Grund-fest.[21] For unrelated purposes, Grundfest had compressed portions of nerves within pressure chambers and had observed that in an atmosphere of oxygen nerves continue to conduct the nervous impulse even under enormous pressures. Such observation was construed by Denny-Brown and Brenner[8,9] as sufficient evidence against a direct mechanical effect. However, this apparently impeccable analogy is not valid. As will be demonstrated, the demyelinating nerve lesion underlying acute nerve compression occurs selectively at the borderlines between compressed and uncompressed nerves and therefore cannot develop in stretches of nerves enclosed within a chamber and subjected to equal pressure throughout.

Demyelination was undoubtedly confirmed when Gilliatt, Fowler, Rudge, and Ochoa reexamined, at Queen Square, the neurophysiology and neuropathology of nerve lesions following local compression of various severities in lower limbs of baboons. Most studies were done with the tourniquet paralysis model but a model equivalent to "Saturday night paralysis" was also examined in detail.[13,42-44,48] With the advantage of modern morphological techniques, important differences became apparent compared with the original descriptions of Denny-Brown and Brenner.[8,9] First, the nerve fiber defects did not extend all along the area of compression as described originally. Instead, they were concentrated under the edges of the cuff, with sparing under the center almost without exception. A similar pattern was found in the much narrower lesion (equivalent to "Saturday night paralysis"): here again the center was spared. Second, there was a difference with the original description concerning the types of nerve fibers affected. Denny-Brown and Brenner[8,9] described uniform involvement of all fiber types, whereas our studies, which included electron microscopy, showed consistent sparing of small diameter fibers. This type of fiber dissociation affords a simple explanation for the clinical observation that pain and temperature sensation and autonomic

function tend to be preserved in tourniquet paralysis[33] and in "Saturday night paralysis."

The most significant discrepancy between the two studies concerned the features of the nodes of Ranvier of medium and large diameter fibers when examined early after compression. Denny-Brown and Brenner[8,9] interpreted them as normal, probably because at the original site of the nodes there will remain, in abnormal fibers, an indentation mimicking the light microscopical profile of the normal nodes. Modern techniques disclose a dramatic distortion of nodes and paranodal regions that precedes and leads into subsequent demyelination of the affected paranodes. In abnormal myelinated fibers microdissected from nerves fixed and osmicated in preparation for electron microscopy, it is possible to recognize, by light microscopy, that the normal gaps signaling nodes of Ranvier are indented but obliterated. A dark region is present toward one side at variable distance from the indentation. Only by single fiber electron microscopy is it possible to elucidate the lesion.[36] One myelin segment has partially invaginated the next with passage of myelin through the nodal gap (Fig. 4-1). The direction of invagination is reversed on opposite sides of the compressed region (Fig. 4-2).

The origin of such striking pathology must be mechanical since we are dealing with displacement of structures along the direction of mechanical forces and to a degree that is proportional to those forces. Obviously, compression has generated longitudinal forces that tend to drive the structures in opposite directions toward uncompressed tissue. In terms of the nerve fibers, the axonal contents would be squeezed away like toothpaste. However, the squeezed axoplasm seems to find an obstacle at the level of the nodes of Ranvier, where the axon is normally narrowed in the larger fibers. Under pressure, the axoplasm within a segment would project the nodal region forward, thus stretching its axonal membrane and invaginating the axonal membrane of the next segment to an equivalent degree. Myelin follows the axon passively, which seems to

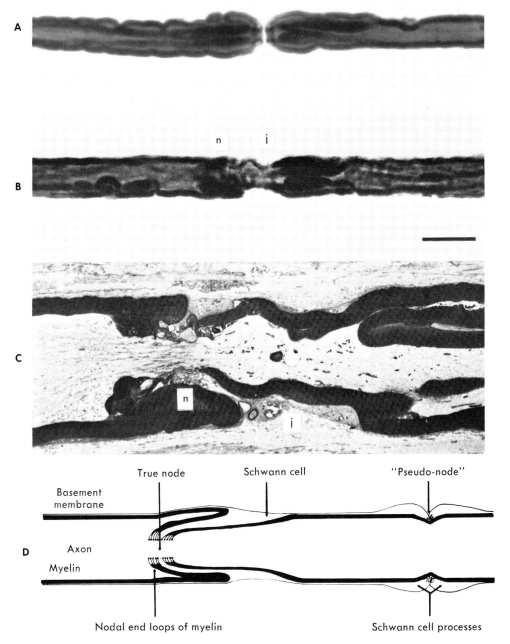

Fig. 4-1. A, Normal myelinated fiber microdissected from baboon tibial nerve after fixation in buffered glutaraldehyde and postfixation in osmium tetroxide. Note myelin gap at node of Ranvier. **B,** Occlusion of nodal gap with invagination (intussusception) of adjacent myelin segments. Myelin has stretched beyond original site of node marked by indentation *j* to reach *n*. Microdissected from baboon tibial nerve, early after acute compression with pneumatic cuff, leading to neurapraxia. Bar = 20 μm. **C,** Low-power electron micrograph of abnormal myelinated fiber from baboon ulnar nerve early after compression leading to neurapraxia. Original site of node is marked by indentation at site of Schwann cell junction *j*. Note new position of node covered by infolded myelin, *n*. **D,** Diagram describing primary lesion of myelinated fibers underlying neurapraxia. Myelin segment on right has partially invaginated segment on left. (**B** and **C** from Rudge, P., Ochoa, J., and Gilliatt, R. W.: J. Neurol. Sci. **23:**403, 1974; **D** from Ochoa, J., Fowler, T. J., and Gilliatt, R. W. In Desmedt, J. E., ed.: New developments in electromyography and clinical neurophysiology, vol. 2, Basel, 1973, Karger.)

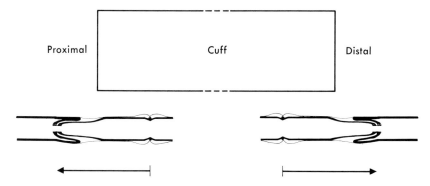

Fig. 4-2. Diagram illustrating reversal of direction of movement of paranodal regions in adjacent myelin segments under either edge of area compressed by pneumatic cuff. (From Ochoa, J., Fowler, T. J., and Gilliatt, R. W.: J. Anat. **113:**433, 1972.)

reflect a relatively firm attachment between those two structures. Like the axon, the myelin in the adjacent segment infolds to accommodate the dislocated structures. Fair comparison can be made with an intussusception of the intestine. The Schwann cell junction remains in place affording a useful point of reference for the microscopist wanting to measure the extent of dislocation of the node, which may reach up to a few hundred microns, depending on the amount and duration of action of the driving forces. The behavior of Schwann cells, which dissociate themselves from myelin rather than from their basal lamina and endoneurial environment, probably reflects a stronger attachment to the latter structures.

Reasons for sparing small myelinated fibers are less obvious, but two tenable interpretations emerge: Perhaps the fact that there is no axonal narrowing at their nodes makes all the difference. Alternatively, small myelinated fibers may escape damage simply because greater and greater force is required to displace axoplasm in smaller and smaller capillary tubes, and before the necessary force has been generated the nerve has already been crushed and the preparation destroyed. Actually, beyond a certain amount of duration of compression, progressive evidence of wallerian degeneration was found from interruption of myelinated and unmyelinated axons at the site of the lesion.[14,42]

The regions of invaginated myelin progressively disintegrate, probably because they have become extracellular with regard to their Schwann cells and perhaps also from configurational changes owing to stretch. Thus, by the second week following injury, one finds demyelinated stretches of axon arranged in orderly series substituting for the original paranodes. Demyelination of complete segments is decidedly unusual. Remyelination takes place by intercalation of proliferated Schwann cells that wind short new myelin sheaths (Fig. 4-3, *E*). Demyelination of the extent found in these lesions is sufficient to account for a block of conduction of the nervous impulse.[29,46] The idea that the conduction block occurring before demyelination is due to a blockade of ionic currents in the obliterated nodes is appealing but awaits confirmation by single fiber electrophysiology.

Clinical recovery evolves in good temporal harmony with recovery of nerve conduction and with remyelination, and under the usual experimental conditions of tourniquet paralysis in baboons, the fastest rates of recovery take place between the third and sixth weeks.[15] Human examples of very prolonged, and presumably demyelinating conduction blocks following local nerve compression have been the subject of recent interesting clinicoelectrophysiological reports.[24,47,59] The anatomicopathological substrate of the equivalent syndrome in severe

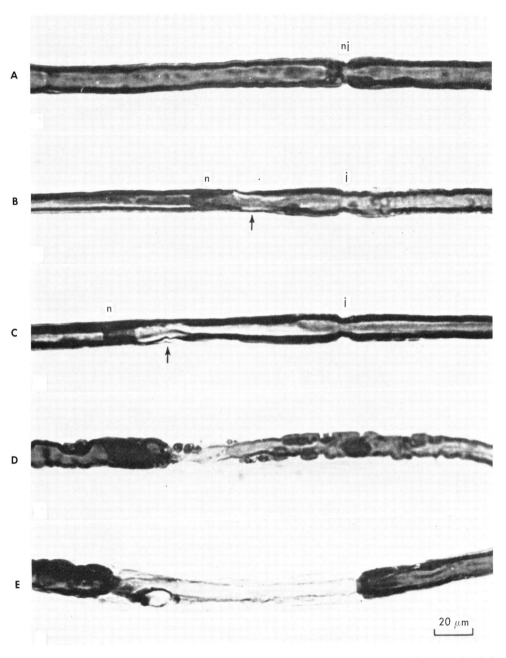

Fig. 4-3. A to **C,** Abnormal fibers, 4 days after compression, showing different degrees of nodal displacement (reaching 120 μm in **C**). *j,* Schwann cell junction; *n,* new position of node. Note thinning of myelin at arrows. **D,** Fiber, 15 days after compression, undergoing demyelination of paranodal region. There is tapering of myelin of paranode on right. **E,** Thinly myelinated intercalated segment, 61 days after compression. (From Ochoa, J., Fowler, T. J., and Gilliatt, R. W.: J. Anat. **113:**433, 1972.)

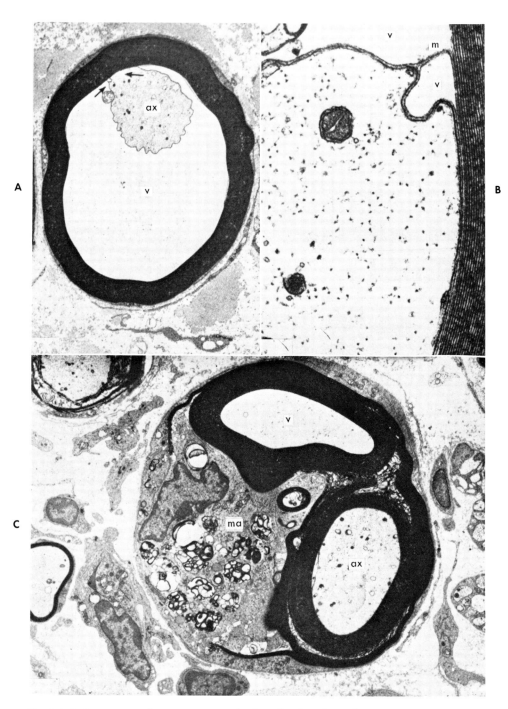

Fig. 4-4. A, Low-power electron micrograph of myelin sheath swelling 6 weeks after compression. Swollen inner tongue of Schwann cell cytoplasm, *v*, separates most of surface of axon, *ax*, from myelin sheath. Sector remains attached to sheath. (×3000.) **B,** Enlargement of area arrowed in **A.** Mesaxon, *m*, is seen with swollen Schwann cell cytoplasm, *v*, on either side of it. (×44,000.) **C,** Myelinated fiber from same nerve as above, showing axon, *ax*, and pocket of edema, *v*. Macrophage, *ma*, has penetrated basement membrane and broken into myelin sheath. (×4600.) (From Ochoa, J., Fowler, T. J., and Gilliatt, R. W.: J. Anat. 113:433, 1972.)

tourniquet paralysis in baboons was striking: edema within the myelin sheath and around the axon developed, mostly toward the extremities of the myelin segments adjacent to the demyelinated regions. Even though remyelination of the paranodal regions had taken place, conduction block would persist. Recovery following removal and remyelination of the swollen regions of myelin suggested an additional block at those levels[42] (Fig. 4-4).

CHRONIC NERVE ENTRAPMENT

Refined studies of the nerve fiber pathology of entrapped nerves have only become available very recently in the mid 1970's. Nevertheless, the concept that the nerve damage is due to ischemia has been built into the context of nerve entrapment for decades. A basis for this assumption can probably be found in gratuitous extrapolation from the widely known experiments of Lewis, Pickering, and Rothschild,[28] demonstrating that ischemia and not direct mechanical pressure is responsible for transient paralysis during tourniquet application; from those of Denny-Brown and Brenner,[8,9] claiming a similar origin for the demyelinating block persisting after tourniquet application; and also, from the apparently suggestive fact that ischemia precipitates symptoms relatively quickly in patients with carpal tunnel syndrome.[16,19]

When it was discovered that guinea pigs, 2 years of age and older, develop a carpal tunnel syndrome,[2,17] the comfortable opportunity arose to study the pathology of entrapped median nerves. Although the authors elected not to speculate with regard to etiology, the demonstration of prominent demyelination under the site of entrapment in these animals brought no challenge to the ischemic theory, since such pathology was in keeping with Denny-Brown and Brenner's findings.[8,9] When Fullerton, Gilliatt, and their associates explored the guinea pig model of median entrapment, they did stop to illustrate and comment on a striking distortion of the myelin segments proximal to the wrist: the segments were bulbous at one end and tapered toward the other end. The abnormal

segments were consistently polarized, the bulb pointing away from the wrist. Ochoa and Marotte,[40] working in Gilliatt's department at Queen Square, reexamined the guinea pig model of chronic entrapment of the median nerve. It appeared reasonable to search for evidence of "intussusception" of myelin segments, since chronic entrapment might have well represented the additive result of repeated minor acute compressions. But signs of acute dislocation of myelin segments were not found after a dedicated search in many nerves from animals of different ages. During the study there was plenty of opportunity to confirm the descriptions of Fullerton, Gilliatt, and Anderson concerning polarized distortion of myelin segments: they looked like regiments of sperms touring away from the wrist toward the elbow. An original observation from Ochoa and Marotte[40] prompted reassessment of the pathology of local nerve entrapment without the traditional bias: distal to the wrist there was clear-cut reversal of polarity of the distorted myelin segments (Fig. 4-5). Looking at nerves from younger animals it became apparent that such deformity, which in older animals was adjacent to the region of demyelination, was not an awkward consequence of local demyelination, since it preceded demyelination. Indeed, in young animals there was pure deformity without demyelination and the turning point could be shown under the carpal tunnel. With increasing age the distortion grew more and more exaggerated, and demyelination and remyelination emerged strikingly. Loss of axons from wallerian degeneration starting at the site of entrapment and attempts at repair by thin axonal outgrowths became increasingly prominent with age (Fig. 4-5). As with the unexpected lesion of myelinated fibers underlying neurapraxia, the fine structure of distorted myelin segments from entrapped nerves is revealing of its pathogenesis (Fig. 4-6). At the tapered ends of the myelin internodes, myelin lamellae end short of their normal attachment sites, as though they had slipped away. Often, myelin thickness changes more or less abruptly in a stepwise

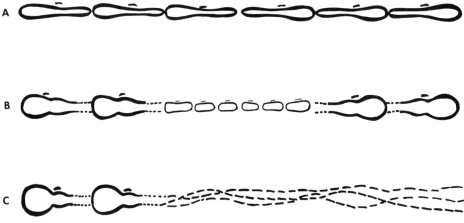

Fig. 4-5. Diagrammatic representation of primary lesion of myelinated fibers underlying chronic entrapment and its progression. **A,** Distorted myelin segments from median nerve of young guinea pig. Polarity is reversed at wrist, represented at center of figure. **B,** Increased deformity of myelin segments with partial exposure of axon toward tapered ends of internodes. Thinly remyelinated segments repair extensive local demyelination at wrist. **C,** Grotesque bulbous ends of distorted internodes and signs of wallerian degeneration and regeneration at wrist. (Modified from Ochoa, J. In Omer, G., and Spinner, M., eds.: Management of peripheral nerve problems, Philadelphia, 1978, W. B. Saunders Co.)

fashion. A series of myelin lamellae can be found orderly arranged under each step. Displacement progresses in consistent order, in that the innermost myelin lamellae are those found further from the node. At the bulbous ends there is excess myelin. In small-sized bulbs, some innermost myelin lamellae are seen inturning, suggesting their reaccommodation following slippage. Ingrowth seems to be their only alternative since the outermost lamellae remain attached to the axon, thus preventing prolapse of inner lamellae between axon and myelin sheath at the nodal region. Bulbs grow bigger as more and more redundant myelin lamellae contort between axon and myelin. Grotesque bulbs stuffed with displaced myelin are formed eventually. Axons may become locally narrowed and progressively drop out.

It is perhaps inaccurate to talk of "demyelination" unqualifiedly in this lesion. It seems clear that initially we are seeing simple slippage of myelin lamellae with partial exposure of the axon rather than myelin disintegration. In advanced stages, however, myelin may disintegrate, particularly at the bulbs

where invading phagocytes may be seen occasionally. The fact that "demyelination" is, at least initially, confined to the tapered ends supports the interpretation mentioned above (Fig. 4-7). Further, this fact questions the alternative proposition that demyelination here is due to ischemia: why should ischemia affect selectively one and the same end of the internodes on one side of the compressed nerve and the opposite end on the other? Our current and still tentative interpretation of the changes described above is as follows: Repeated minor mechanical trauma, or perhaps repeated minor stretching or friction against tough neighboring tendons or joints, determines propagation of pressure waves in opposite directions along the axons. Inner myelin lamellae would be shattered, detached, and would relentlessly slip away. Sunderland,[57] on the other hand, contends that the initial problem is obstruction of the venous return leading to local nerve edema, persistently raised intraneural pressure, and secondary interference with blood supply; consequently, anoxia would cause the nerve fiber lesion.

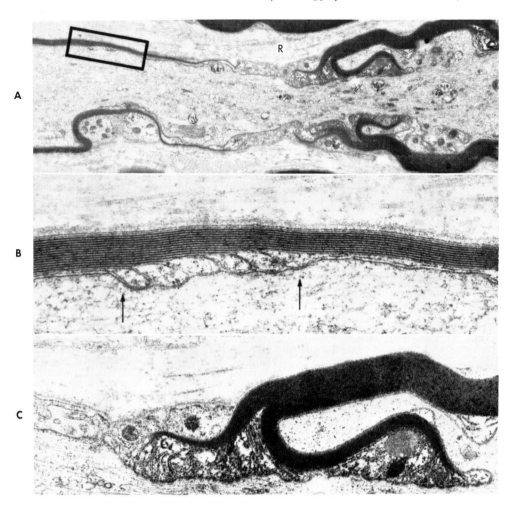

Fig. 4-6. A, Low-power electron micrograph of moderately abnormal fiber taken from guinea pig median nerve above wrist. Paranode on left is tapered. Bulbous paranode on right shows inturning of group of inner lamellae. *R*, Node of Ranvier. (×7000.) **B,** Enlargement of area enclosed in rectangle in **A.** Six myelin lamellae end in cytoplasmic loops between arrows. (×48,000.) **C,** Detail of bulbous paranode. (×20,000.) (From Ochoa, J., and Marotte, L. R.: J. Neurol. Sci. **19:**491, 1973.)

Vasa nervorum certainly do not escape anatomical damage, and as anticipated earlier, probably contribute to the pathogenesis in a way that is still obscure. Impressive changes in epineurial blood vessels of compressed nerves have been demonstrated in plantar "neuromas" by Lassmann, Lassmann, and Stockinger.[27] In my opinion, endoneurial vessels are abnormal in entrapped nerves, and Renaut bodies[4] are strongly suspicious of being degenerated vessels.

The pathology of entrapped nerves *in man* has only been the subject of occasional reports. In 1913, Marie and Foix[30] first became aware of the fact that a sufficient cause for some forms of wasting of thenar muscles was a lesion of the median nerve at the level of the wrist. With the primitive histological means available at the time they showed that myelin disappeared under the carpal tunnel. Whether this meant local demyelination or axonal degeneration cannot be established in

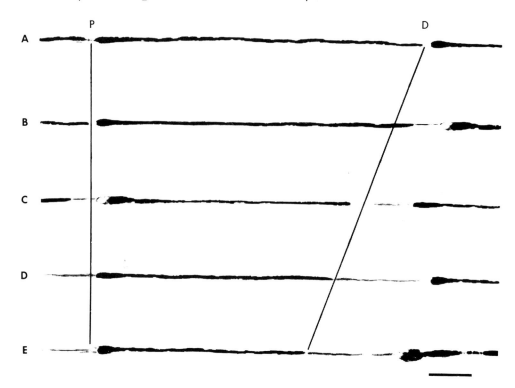

Fig. 4-7. Five consecutive internodes, *a* to *e*, taken from above wrist, displayed to emphasize asymmetry of internodes and progressive "demyelination" of tapered ends. *P*, Proximal; *D*, distal. Bar = 100 μm. (From Ochoa, J., and Marotte, L. R.: J. Neurol. Sci. **19:**491, 1973.)

retrospect, especially since the authors did not examine the median nerve distal to the wrist. Half a century later, Thomas and Fullerton[58] examined at autopsy the median nerve of a patient with a carpal tunnel syndrome suggested clinically and confirmed electrophysiologically. Local myelin loss under the carpal ligament was again a feature, but some myelin reappeared distally. The element of demyelination was obvious although not clearly spelled out at that time: the concept of demyelination was still incipient. A few years ago, Neary, Ochoa, and Gilliatt[34] examined a number of fresh adult autopsy specimens of median nerves at the wrist and ulnar nerves at elbow, confirming local demyelination and all the changes described earlier in the guinea pig.[40] Changes of identical character have been observed recently in specimens of lateral cutaneous nerve of the thigh from under the inguinal ligament in cases of meralgia paresthetica.[39]

In advanced cases of chronic entrapment the component of wallerian degeneration is prominent and all fiber types are affected. In milder cases, however, unmyelinated fibers are selectively spared, at least structurally[31]: the significance of such a dissociated anatomical pattern in terms of the accompanying sensory disorder is intriguing.[39]

From the consistency of the anatomical changes found underlying chronic nerve entrapment in median, ulnar, and thigh nerves, it seems legitimate to regard the lesions described by Ochoa and Marotte[40] in the guinea pig as the *primary* nerve fiber pathology underlying chronic entrapment in general. It is likely that similar lesions occur at other common sites of entrapment, as for example, the peroneal nerve at the head of the fibula and the posterior interosseus nerve in the vicinity of the supinator muscle.[54]

Entrapped nerves may be enlarged locally and so profoundly distorted microscopically that they may be confused with a neoplasm.[41]

TRAUMATIC NERVE LESIONS CAUSING PAIN IN MAN

Although there are several conflicting theories to explain neuralgia from local nerve lesions and although such theories imply quite different pathological substrates, we know little about the mechanisms behind neuralgia and very little about its pathology.

The idea that at the site of a painful nerve injury an "artificial synapse" may be created, where normal ongoing ascending or descending impulses may cross-excite the afferent pain pathway, has been entertained for decades. An early proposal along these lines came from Granit, Leksell, and Skoglund[22] and Granit and Skoglund[21] who demonstrated ephaptic excitation between motor and sensory nerve fibers at the level of an acute violent nerve injury in animals. Wall, Waxman, and Basbaum,[62] however, failed to observe perpetuation of the cross-excitation beyond short periods following the acute experiment. On the other hand, abnormal electrical events, best explained as a consequence of ephaptic cross-excitation, have been observed to occur naturally in abnormally myelinated nerve fibers in the spinal roots of dystrophic mice,[45] and so credibility has been restored to the concept that activity across artificial synapses might be responsible for abnormal motor and sensory phenomena, inclusive of pain.

Another well-established theory to explain neuralgia from nerve disease was put forward by Noordenbos,[35] the "fiber dissociation theory." Selective loss of large-diameter fast conducting afferents, concerned with various sensory modalities other than pain, would release small fibers carrying impulses from noxious stimuli. The theory was inspired in Henry Head's concept of two conflicting peripheral nervous systems and was reciprocally supportive with the gate control theory of pain.[32] Noordenbos' concept was based on clinical and histological observations in postherpetic neuralgia: the histology, performed by Weddell in Oxford, seemed to indicate selective or predominant loss of large myelinated fibers in the intercostal nerves supplying the abnormal dermatomes.

A third, more novel theory to explain neuralgia from nerve injury blames spontaneous electrical discharges generated in abnormal nerve fibers. Wall and Gutnick[60, 61] have produced convincing evidence toward spontaneous impulse generation at the level of experimental neuromas in animals, having identified sprouts from small-diameter parent fibers as the sources of the electrical discharges. Another interesting observation from Wall and Gutnick[60] has been the arrest of spontaneous impulse generation for up to an hour or so following electrical nerve stimulation, suggesting that antidromic invasion of the sprouts may have induced a voltage-dependent change in their ability to generate action potentials and affording a new interpretation for the effect of nerve stimulation in some peripheral pain states. Axonal sprouts need not be the only example of abnormal impulse generators: nerve fibers with defective myelin have been incriminated also by Rasminsky[45] and Calvin, Loeser, and Howe.[7]

The "fiber dissociation" and the "pacemaking sprout" theories represent a straightforward challenge to quantitative nerve morphology. The ephapse, on the other hand, would appear to be more of a qualitative issue, difficult to assess if not beyond morphological confirmation. Indeed, no serious attempt appears to have been made to identify the structural correlates of "artificial synapses." On the anecdotal side, Seddon writes, "and J. Z. Young once showed me some striking photomicrographs of axons that had fused laterally over a short distance."[52]

Among the range of local nerve lesions, only some are the source of neuralgia. Rarely are entrapped nerves accompanied by spontaneous chronic pain; the same applies to neurapraxia. Amputation neuromas and traumatic neuromas-in-continuity are common but not consistent sources of pain, as is the invasion of nerves and nerve roots by cancer. Thus it is not possible to predict pain from the etiology of the nerve lesion. This, added to the uncertainties involved in the communication of subjective experience, makes it preferable to explore the anatomical substrate of painful nerve lesions in the human rather than experimental animals.

Classical histology describes painful amputation neuromas in man as composed of abundant tangled nerve fibers amidst increased fibrous tissue, but no quantitative studies have been performed and possible differences between painful and nonpainful amputation neuromas have not been analyzed. Features of amputation neuromas in animals are the formation of small fascicles outside the original perineurial confines as well as nerve fiber branching and the abundance of small-diameter nerve fibers.[53] Distended growth cones and the recurrent nerve fibers described by Cajal[6] were also noted in the comprehensive animal study by Spencer.[53] Quantitative light- and electron-microscopical studies on painful local nerve lesions in man have already yielded some interesting results. In a series of plantar neuromas removed for *recurrent* pain, the pathology was usually so severe that opportunities to define a pattern were jeopardized. In the fortuitous mild case, there were indications of damage similar to that described for entrapped nerves.[37] One must assume that recurrent mechanical injury caused progressive destruction of the nerve trunks while continuing to be able to induce pain through irritation of (hyperexcitable?) amputated axons terminating further proximally. In a case of meralgia paresthetica, atypical in the sense that the injury of the lateral cutaneous nerve of the thigh had led to *constant* pain for several months, there were changes that might equally satisfy the fiber dissociation theory, abnormal impulse generation from demyelinated axons, and

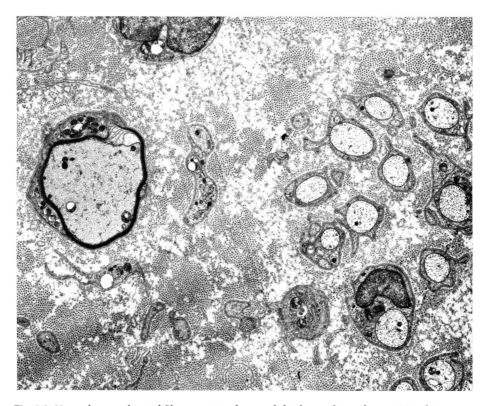

Fig. 4-8. Normal unmyelinated fibers next to abnormal thinly myelinated axon. Meralgia paresthetica. (×4800.)

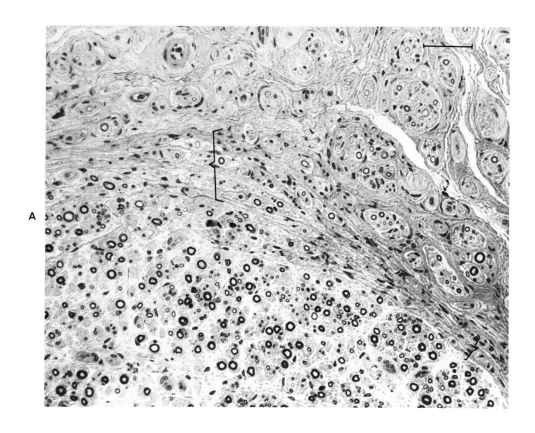

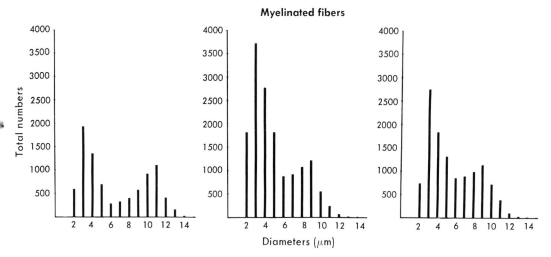

Fig. 4-9. A, Part of abnormal nerve fascicle, sectioned transversely, at neuroma underlying site of Tinel's sign. Multicellular perineurial sheath (bracketed) is disorganized and permeated by nerve fibers. Outside original fascicle (top half of figure) there occur many abnormal miniature fascicles containing mostly fibers of small diameter. Bar = 50 μm. **B,** Total numbers of myelinated fibers in injured nerve with neuroma-in-continuity, featuring Tinel's sign, chronic pain, and hyperalgesia. Left, Proximal to neuroma; center, at neuroma; right, distal to neuroma. Note excess numbers of small-diameter fibers at level of neuroma, including immature sprouts. Note robust population of large-diameter fibers at all levels.

even perhaps the "artificial synapse": selective (anatomical) sparing of small-diameter fibers and profuse demyelination was prominent[39] (Fig. 4-8). In a patient who had a Tinel's sign and complained of spontaneous pain and hyperalgesia at the site of a 33-year-old bullet injury of the superficial radial nerve, relieved by neurectomy, there were a number of revealing findings.[38] At the site of the neuroma-in-continuity, which exactly underlay the site of the Tinel's sign, there was massive outgrowth of immature nerve sprouts, satisfying the "pacemaking sprout" theory of neuralgic pain and affording a straight explanation for the Tinel's sign, in view of the low threshold to mechanical stimuli of immature regenerated sprouts[5, 25] (Fig. 4-9). Total counts of myelinated fibers proximal and distal to the lesion failed to support "fiber dissociation" (Fig. 4-9). A basis for hyperalgesia was not suggested by the morphological study. In more recent studies of the same nature in collaboration with Noordenbos, we have found consistently a marked local increase in the total numbers of small nerve fibers at the level of the neuroma-in-continuity. This excess suggests sprouts and their immaturity. Since breaches in the continuity of the perineurium at the site of the injury and outpouring of nerve fibers were found consistently, we believe that excess production of sprouts that fail to mature is a consequence of frustrated peripheral reconnection of regenerated fibers that have gone astray beyond the confines of the perineurial continent. Impaired maturation and overproduction of regenerated sprouts is a well-recognized event in disconnected nerves.[1, 12, 50, 63, 64]

REFERENCES

1. Aitken, J. T., Sharman, M., and Young, J. Z.: Maturation of regenerating nerve fibres with various peripheral connections, J. Anat. **81:**1, 1947.
2. Anderson, M. H., et al.: Changes in the forearm associated with median nerve compression at the wrist in the guinea-pig, J. Neurol. **33:**70, 1970.
3. Asbury, A. K.: Ischemic disorders of peripheral nerve. In Vinken, P. J., and Bruyn, G. W., eds.: Handbook of clinical neurology, vol. 8, Amsterdam, 1970, North-Holland Publishing Co., p. 154.
4. Asbury, A. K.: Renaut bodies: a forgotten endoneurial structure, J. Neuropathol. Exp. Neurol. **32:**334, 1973.
5. Brown, A. G., and Iggo, A.: The structure and function of cutaneous "touch corpuscles" after nerve crush, J. Physiol. **165:**28P, 1963.
6. Cajal, S. R.: Degeneration and regeneration of the nervous system, New York, 1928, Oxford University Press, Inc.
7. Calvin, W. H., Loeser, J. D., and Howe, J. F.: A neurophysiological theory for the pain mechanism of tic douloureux, Pain **3:**147, 1977.
8. Denny-Brown, D., and Brenner, C.: Paralysis of nerve induced by direct pressure and by tourniquet, Arch. Neurol. Psychiatry **51:**1, 1944.
9. Denny-Brown, D., and Brenner, C.: Lesion in peripheral nerve resulting from compression by spring clip, Arch. Neurol. Psychiatry **52:**1, 1944.
10. Eames, R. A., and Lange, L. S.: Clinical and pathological study of ischaemic neuropathy, J. Neurol. Neurosurg. Psychiatry **30:**215, 1967.
11. Erb, W.: Diseases of the peripheral cerebrospinal nerves. In Ziemssen, H. von.: Cyclopedia of the practice of medicine, vol. XI, London, 1876, Samson Low, Marston, Searle and Rivington.
12. Evans, D. H. L., and Murray, J. G.: A study of regeneration in a motor nerve with unimodal fibre diameter distribution, Anat. Rec. **126:**311, 1956.
13. Fowler, T. J.: Tourniquet paralysis in the baboon, D. M. Thesis, 1975, University of Oxford.
14. Fowler, T. J., and Ochoa, J.: Unmyelinated fibres in normal and compressed peripheral nerves of the baboon; a quantitative electron-microscopic study, Neuropathol. Appli. Neurobiol. **1:**247, 1975.
15. Fowler, T. J., Danta, G., and Gilliatt, R. W.: Recovery of nerve conduction after a pneumatic tourniquet: observations on the hind-limb of the baboon, J. Neurol. Neurosurg. Psychiatry **35:**638, 1972.
16. Fullerton, P. M.: The effect of ischaemia on nerve conduction in the carpal tunnel syndrome, J. Neurol. Neurosurg. Psychiatry **26:**385, 1963.
17. Fullerton, P. M., and Gilliatt, R. W.: Median and ulnar neuropathy in the guinea-pig, J. Neurol. Neurosurg. Psychiatry **30:**393, 1967.
18. Gairns, F. W., Garven, H. S. D., and Smith, G.: The digital nerves and the nerve endings in progressive obliterative vascular disease of the leg, Scot. Med. J. **5:**382, 1960.
19. Gilliatt, R. W., and Wilson, T. G.: Ischaemic sensory loss in patients with peripheral nerve lesions, J. Neurol. Neurosurg. Psychiatry **17:**104, 1954.
20. Gutmann, E., and Sanders, F. K.: Recovery of fibre numbers and diameters in the regeneration of peripheral nerves, J. Physiol. **101:**489, 1943.
21. Granit, R., and Skoglund, C. R.: Facilitation, inhibition and depression at the artificial synapse formed by the cut end of a mammalian nerve, J. Physiol. **103:**435, 1945.
22. Granit, R., Leksell, L. and Skoglund, C. R.: Fibre

interaction in injured or compressed region of nerve, Brain **67**:125, 1944.

23. Grundfest, H.: Effects of hydrostatic pressures upon the excitability, the recovery, and the potential sequence of frog nerve, Cold Spring Harbor Symp. Quant. Biol. **4**:179, 1936.

24. Harrison, M. J. G.: Pressure palsy of the ulnar nerve with prolonged conduction block, J. Neurol. Neurosurg. Psychiatry **39**:96, 1976.

25. Konorski, J., Lubinska, L.: Mechanical excitability of regenerating nerve fibres, Lancet **250**:609, 1946.

26. Korthals, J. K., and Wisniewski, H. M.: Peripheral nerve ischemia: Part 1. Experimental model, J. Neurol. Sci. **24**:65, 1975.

27. Lassmann, G., Lassmann, H. and Stockinger, L.: Morton's metatarsalgia: light and electron microscopic observations and their relation to entrapment neuropathies, Virchows Arch. Pathol. Anat. Histol. **370**:307, 1976.

28. Lewis, T., Pickering, G. W., and Rothschild, P.: Centripetal paralysis arising out of arrested bloodflow to the limb, including notes on a form of tingling, Heart **16**:2, 1931.

29. McDonald, W. I.: The effects of experimental demyelination on conduction in peripheral nerve: a histological and electrophysiological study. I. Clinical and histological observations, Brain **86**:481, 1963. II. Electrophysiological observations, Brain **86**:501, 1963.

30. Marie, P., and Foix, C.: Atrophie isolée de l' éminence thénar d'origine nevritique. Rôle du ligament annulaire antérieur du carpe dans la pathogénie de la lésion, Rev. Neurol. **26**:647, 1913.

31. Marotte, L. R.: An electron microscope study of chronic median nerve compression in the guinea-pig, Acta Neuropathol. **27**:69, 1974.

32. Melzack, R., and Wall, P. D.: Pain mechanisms: a new theory, Science **150**:971, 1965.

33. Moldaver, J.: Tourniquet paralysis syndrome, Arch. Surg. **68**:136, 1954.

34. Neary, D., Ochoa, J., and Gilliatt, R. W.: Subclinical entrapment neuropathy in man, J. Neurol. Sci. **24**:283, 1975.

35. Noordenbos, W.: Pain, Amsterdam, 1959, Elsevier.

36. Ochoa, J.: Ultrathin longitudinal sections of single myelinated fibres for electron microscopy, J. Neurol. Sci. **17**:103, 1972.

37. Ochoa, J.: The primary nerve fibre pathology of plantar neuromas, J. Neuropathol. Exp. Neurol. **35**:370, 1976.

38. Ochoa, J.: Neuralgia and hyperalgesia from local nerve lesions: pathophysiology, Electroencephalogr. Clin. Neurophysiol. **43**:597, 1977.

39. Ochoa, J., Meralgia paresthetica: quantitative electron-microscopy, Abstract 497, Fourth International Congress on Neuromuscular Disease, Montreal, 1978.

40. Ochoa, J., and Marotte, L.: Nature of the nerve lesion underlying chronic entrapment, J. Neurol. Sci. **19**:491, 1973.

41. Ochoa, J., and Neary, D.: Localised hypertrophic neuropathy, intraneural tumour, or chronic nerve netrapment? Lancet **1**:632, 1975.

42. Ochoa, J., Fowler, T. J., and Gilliatt, R. W.: Anatomical changes in peripheral nerves compressed by a pneumatic tourniquet, J. Anat. **113**:433, 1972.

43. Ochoa, J., Fowler, T. J., and Gilliatt, R. W.: Changes produced by a pneumatic tourniquet. In Desmedt, J. E., ed.: New developments in electromyography and clinical neurophysiology, vol. 2, Basel, 1973, Karger.

44. Ochoa, J., et al.: Nature of the nerve lesion caused by a pneumatic tourniquet, Nature **233**:265, 1971.

45. Rasminsky, M.: Abstract 595, Neurosci. Abstr. vol. 2, Part 1, 1976 (see also Chapter 18).

46. Rasminsky, M., and Sears, T. A.: Internodal conduction in undissected demyelinated nerve fibres, J. Physiol. **227**:323, 1972.

47. Rudge, P.: Tourniquet paralysis with prolonged conduction block: an electrophysiological study, J. Bone Joint Surg. **56**:716, 1974.

48. Rudge, P., Ochoa, J., and Gilliatt, R. W.: Acute peripheral nerve compression in the baboon. Anatomical and physiological findings, J. Neurol. Sci. **23**:403, 1974.

49. Sabin, T. D., and Swift, T. R.: Leprosy. In Dyck, P. J., Thomas, P. K., and Lambert, E. H., eds.: Peripheral neuropathy, Philadelphia, 1975, W. B. Saunders Co.

50. Sanders, F. K., and Young, J. Z.: Effect of peripheral connection on diameter of nerve fibres, Nature **155**:237, 1945.

51. Seddon, H. J.: Three types of nerve injury, Brain **66**:237, 1943.

52. Seddon, H. J.: Surgical disorders of the peripheral nerves, ed. 2, Edinburgh, 1975, Churchill Livingstone, p. 142.

53. Spencer, P. S.: Light and electron microscopic observations on localised peripheral nerve injuries, Thesis, University of London, 1971.

54. Spinner, M.: The orcade of Frohse and its relationship to posterior interosseus nerve paralysis, J. Bone Joint Surg. **50B**:809, 1968.

55. Sunderland, S.: A classification of peripheral nerve injuries producing loss of function, Brain **74**:491, 1951.

56. Sunderland, S.: Nerves and nerve injuries, Baltimore, 1968, The Williams & Wilkins Co.

57. Sunderland, S.: Nerve lesion in the carpal tunnel syndrome, J. Neurol. Neurosurg. Psychiatry **39**:615, 1976.

58. Thomas, P. K., and Fullerton, P. M.: Nerve fibre size in the carpal tunnel syndrome, J. Neurol. Neurosurg. Psychiatry **26**:520, 1963.

59. Trojaborg, W.: Prolonged conduction block with axonal degeneration, J. Neurol. Neurosurg. Psychiatry **40**:50, 1977.

60. Wall, P. D., and Gutnick, M.: Ongoing activity in peripheral nerves: the physiology and pharmacology

of impulses originating from a neuroma, Exp. Neurol. **43**:580, 1974a.

61. Wall, P. D., and Gutnick, M.: Properties of afferent nerve impulses originating from a neuroma, Nature **248**:740, 1974b.

62. Wall, P. D., Waxman, S., and Basbaum, A. I.: Ongoing activity in peripheral nerve: injury discharge, Exp. Neurol. **45**:576, 1974.

63. Weiss, P., and Taylor, A. C.: Further experimental evidence against "neurotropism" in nerve regeneration, J. Exp. Zool. **95**:233, 1944.

64. Weiss, P., Edds, M. V., and Cavanaugh, M.: The effect of terminal connections on the caliber of nerve fibres, Anat. Rec. **92**:215, 1945.

65. Williams, I. R., Gilliatt, R. W., and Jefferson, D.: Limb ischemia and acute nerve compression, Electroencephalogr. Clin. Neurophysiol. **43**:592, 1977.

DISCUSSION

Sunderland: Dr. Ochoa showed the results of his splendid work on compression syndromes, where the lesion is due to mechanical deformation. There is no doubt whatsoever about those dramatic changes that he has so convincingly demonstrated. But there are probably a host of other factors also operating in at least some compression injuries that can produce a block without in turn producing this marked degree of physical deformation at the node. For example, there can be vascular factors operating at the site of compression. The facial nerve in the facial canal is an unusual nerve in many respects. In particular, over a certain segment of its length it is composed of a single funiculus, with a clearly defined perineurial sheath. Occupying the facial canal with it are vessels that are going to vascularize this nerve. Remember that the largest vessels you will see inside a funiculus are capillaries and that the perineurium maintains the intrafunicular pressure. To maintain an adequate circulation to the nerve fibers in that part of the nerve, the intracapillary pressure, of course, must be greater than the intrafunicular pressure; otherwise, the capillaries would be collapsed. The veins in the facial canal must be at a still lower pressure. With an increase in pressure in the facial canal (or the carpal tunnel), the first structures to be affected as the pressure increases are the veins located in the tissue outside the funiculus. As the increased pressure in the veins is reflected back on the capillary circulation, there is decreased capillary blood flow. This ultimately leads to a lesion that is predominantly hypoxic in the initial stages and then anoxic. It was shown by physiologists some time ago that the larger caliber fibers are more susceptible to hypoxia and anoxia than are the finer caliber fibers. Hence the large fibers tend to suffer in the initial stages of this pathological process. If the pressure is not relieved, the capillary slowing ultimately reaches a level where the capillary endothelium begins to suffer. The subsequent changes have been spectacularly demonstrated by Dr. Lundborg and his colleagues in Göteborg: the endothelium now begins to leak protein. As a result of this, edema develops inside the funiculus itself with further increased intrafunicular pressure so that the nerve fibers are now suffering in a number of ways. As the entire process continues, the pressure continues to rise inside the funiculus and in this way a vicious circle is created. The edematous tissue that develops inside the funiculus is an excellent medium for the proliferation of fibroblasts, and this ushers in the terminal phase in which the contents of the funiculus are converted into fibrous tissue. The end result is one in which nerve fiber structure is completely destroyed in the affected region, and a proximal neuroma or swelling develops where nerve fibers are attempting to regenerate. There is also a slight swelling distally in the case of the carpal tunnel syndrome because, as the pressure in the carpal tunnel rises and this sequence of events follows, endoneurial fluid is forced both proximally and distally, and when that fluid reaches the level where the funiculi are not subjected to compression under the carpal ligament, they do swell slightly. But in addition, of course, not only is the endoneurial tissue becoming edematous but the epineurial tissue is likewise (since the median nerve is multifuniculated), so there will also be fibrosis in the epineurium.

This alternative explanation must remain somewhat speculative because we rarely get these nerves to study. However, where such specimens have become available, the histological findings support such a vascular hypothesis. Dr. Ochoa has a great advantage in that he can, in animal experiments, obtain these nerves. The controversial point is whether in chronic compressive lesions the primary pathology is based on vascular factors or is the result of physical deformation. Quite clearly, when the compressing force reaches a certain magnitude or is very acute in its onset, you do have the type of deformation that has been described, which leads to nodal intussusception and a slipping of myelin lamellae. But this is certainly not the entire story because patients with a carpal tunnel syndrome tend to be disturbed in the early hours of the morning with a distressing pain in the distribution of the median nerve. And what do they do? Almost without exception, they get up and wring the arm—they exercise the limb. Presumably the explanation of this reaction is that during sleep there is a stasis in the circulation in an immobile extremity that sets in train those changes that lead to hypoxia and anoxia of the nerve fibers and pain. By exercising the limb, you immediately restore the circulation and the symptoms subside. Furthermore, if you obstruct the venous circulation with a compression cuff, then you precipitate an attack of pain immediately. Finally, in the postoperative phase when you have decompressed the carpal tunnel, the patient will invariably tell you that the relief is dramatic and immediate. It would seem from such evidence that vascular factors must be crucial in causing the symptoms.

Ochoa: The elaboration by Dr. Sunderland makes sense, but I don't believe there is evidence available to support the view that the initial pathological lesion underlying local entrapment is venous stasis nor that the presumed venous stasis and subsequent endoneurial capillary wreckage and edema are responsible for the nerve fiber lesion. The earliest known pathological change in nerve fibers consists of displacement of inner myelin lamellae in opposite directions on either side of the site

of entrapment, almost certainly of mechanical origin. So we have important evidence to support the idea that the nerve fiber lesion is primarily mechanical and little to support an ischemic cause. However, it would be quite naive to confuse nerve pathology with clinical manifestations and ascribe every possible symptom and sign to the gross anatomical changes found in nerve fibers. It must be stressed that in addition to the stable negative symptoms and signs obviously derived from nerve conduction block and from actual dropout of nerve fibers, there are striking intermittent numbness, paresthesias, and weakness in these patients, which are almost certainly caused by intermittent ischemic and postischemic nerve fiber dysfunction. Such manifestations are identical to those experienced during the experiments so well described by Lewis, Pickering, and Rothschild in the 1930's. So, there should be no question that even nerves need oxygen, but it is conceivable that in addition to the intermittent transient manifestations, ischemia may be contributing to the structural change; however, I don't think we have a measure of that contribution at the moment.

Sunderland: There are other conduction block lesions that are due to pathology at the site of an original trauma that has led to fibrosis. The fibrosis almost certainly obstructs or constricts funiculi and their fibers. In these cases the onset of recovery is delayed for some considerable time, even months, and yet immediately on release of the pressure on the nerve, recovery follows within 48 hours. Originally there was controversy in peripheral nerve surgery as to whether either external neurolysis or internal neurolysis in these cases was in fact a beneficial surgical procedure. It was claimed by some that the delayed onset of recovery in a nerve lesion in continuity was due to fibrous constriction of the nerve. It was believed that the fibrotic tissue was responsible for the block and that the dramatic recovery following neurolysis was due to the removal of this constrictive scar tissue. Others maintained that the coincidence of the surgical procedure and the onset of recovery were quite fortuitous, and that if the surgeon had delayed a little longer, signs of spontaneous recovery would have appeared. There is no doubt that in about 70% of cases the latter is the correct explanation, namely, that neurolysis was performed prematurely and that the nerve would have recovered in the absence of any surgical decompression. On the other hand, there are unquestionably some cases where the surgical procedure is responsible for the immediate return of function over the entire field distal to the site of the lesion. We can only speculate on the nature of the lesion in these cases. I doubt very much if it is mechanical deformation of nerve fibers, because the onset of recovery following neurolysis is too dramatic. Neurosurgeons will know that with a spinal cord block giving rise to paraplegia immediately following a laminectomy and the removal of a tumor that has been pressing on the cord, within 48 hours the patient will tell you that he can move his toes. Quite clearly this recovery is not dependent on axon regeneration, which would take months. I would like to hear what the axon transport advocates have to say about this phenomenon, because it may be playing a role. Perhaps in some way the compression inhibits the distal transport of essential materials.

Ochs: I believe that the effects of anoxia can be directly explained by the lack of ATP, the energy that drives the materials in the transport system. We can explain much of what follows after that.

Aguayo: With regard to neurolysis, some nerves probably improve from the surgery, but there is also a good possibility that some may worsen after surgery. At least from experimental work done, well-documented by Dr. Spencer, if one does cut the epineurium, there can be extensive fibrotic demyelination at the site of the cut.

Sunderland: I think this illustrates the importance of terminology. Dr. Aguayo is quite correct when he mentioned that what is

done to the nerve may harm it. However, Dr. Spencer does not divide the epineurium; he divides the perineurium, and it is the division of the perineurium that creates the problem. Neurolysis is now falling into two categories: external neurolysis, where you meticulously remove the outer epineurium to relieve it of constrictive scar tissue, and internal neurolysis, which is only technically feasible with an operating microscope together with a recognition and appreciation of the complexity of the internal structure of nerves. The surgeon, in performing internal neurolysis, must never damage the perineurium. The perineurium is the critical element in a peripheral nerve trunk. It is the tissue that maintains the integrity of the contained nerve fibers.

Ochs: The perineurium is a functioning metabolic entity that maintains the proper ionic constitution around the fiber. If the perineurium is damaged, then we can speculate that changes in ionic composition can then show themselves in terms of failures in conduction, pain, and possibly, if the calcium level is interferred with, block in axoplasmic transport.

Editor: One might expect such damage to cause permanent impairment of function on a physiological basis, even with a good histological picture.

Edshage: The perineurium is a very important structure. To my knowledge, with the exception of what I will now mention, there is little evidence as to the healing of the perineurium after nerve suture. Does it become absolutely intact? Doctor Almgren has studied the distribution of fluorescent albumin injected intravenously or applied topically in traumatized rabbit nerves.

Albumin can be made fluorescent by tagging it with Evans Blue.* When placed about an intact nerve, the albumin does not penetrate the perineurium. If a defect is created in the perineurium, the albumin

---

*Lundborg, G., and Rydevik, B.: J. Bone Joint Surg. **55B**:390, 1973.

diffuses into the fascicle where it can be seen under ultraviolet light. If the tagged albumin is injected intravenously, it remains within the endoneurial capillaries of an uninjured nerve. After major nerve traumas it leaks out of the capillaries into the endoneural space.

In studying experimental transplantation in peripheral nerves, both techniques have been used. Both techniques show that there is a leakage at the suture line after epineurial suture up to the maximum time studied, 150 days, in rabbits. I think this means something: the perineurium may not heal completely, that is, so it will not leak albumin in and out.

Jewett: Would Dr. Ochoa indicate how the sprouting process at the level of a nerve repair may be similar or different from what he has described for neuromas-in-continuity?

Ochoa: I have no personal experience in nerve grafts, but from the classical work of J. Z. Young, Paul Weiss, and others during World War II, what seems clear is that there will be successful regeneration and maturation of the nerve provided there is good reestablishment of functional connection with the periphery, a point also stressed by Dr. Sunderland. If a nerve is allowed to grow across the graft and make contact with the periphery, then progressively the diameter histogram of the proximal stump is going to be practically reconstituted distally. However, if there are problems along the pathway of the regenerating fibers, such as fibrosis, then fibers will fail to reach the periphery, to muscle or sensory endings. Two consequences follow: (1) a marked excess in the number of axons regenerated and (2) an absence of maturation in diameter with failure of restoration of an appropriate thickness of myelin around the axon.

Niebauer: I was wondering if age differences might account for my impression that although children may have neuromas, they are very seldom painful.

Ochoa: We don't really know how neuromas that are not painful look in man histologi-

cally, hence we are at a loss to determine what factors determine whether a neuroma will be painful.

Sunderland: With regard to gross morphology it was our impression that the rather smaller, firmer neuromas were not tender, not as painful in any event, as the larger softer neuromas that can be exquisitely sensitive. That's the experience of others as well.

We attempted to equate the size of the neuroma with the internal morphology of the nerve, and it's our belief that where there is a considerable degree of overlap, funicular tissue to epineurial tissue, large numbers of regenerating axons grow into the epineurial tissue where they end blindly. This adds to the mass at the site of suture or injury, and the large numbers of very immature or fine unmyelinated axons in that abnormal situation give rise to the marked swelling and tenderness. If there is a reasonable degree of funicular apposition, then the neuroma is not as large. Perhaps a certain critical mass of fine endings is necessary to give a painful response to a mechanical stimulus.

Jewett: Is light microscopy adequate for us to classify and distinguish nerve lesions now, or must we move to electron microscopy?

Sunderland: I'm a very simple man and as that great Frenchman Maurice Chevalier reminded us, at our age we must be reasonable. I think that light microscopy in providing a simple sort of working classification is all that we need at the present time. But that doesn't mean that the search should stop short of the electron microscopical level. However, at the moment I think there is so much bothering us at the level at which we're operating, that the electron microscopy experts, although unquestionably adding valuable data, can't help us very much. I think we must define our clinical problems more clearly and specifically before they can really contribute to this issue: in terms of the classification of nerve injuries, in terms of what is happening at the site of trauma, in terms of axon sprouting, and so forth, then there is still a great deal to be done before we get down to electron microscopy. However, I must admit that I did see some of Dr. Kreutzberg's electron microscopy photographs from Munich that were just fantastic. At the end of a severed nerve there were literally not hundreds of axons but thousands of them. It was a very interesting demonstration of the way in which axoplasm can proliferate and sprout at that site.

Worther (Santa Clara): A question on terminology—a sensory fiber, strictly speaking, is a dendrite, and a motor fiber is, strictly speaking, an axon. Is the biology and regeneration process the same for both motor and sensory fibers? What does the term "axon" include in this context?

Sunderland: I think that for all purposes the long sensory processes of the dorsal root ganglia behave as axons. It is true that they are conducting in one direction and the motor axons are conducting in the other, but from the point of view of the behavior to trauma and from the point of view of regeneration rates they are the same. Histologically, they are indistinguishable and therefore I think that we only confuse the issue if we attempt to separately describe "dendrites" and "axons" in the periphery. If we all understand that we're dealing with a population of nerve fibers in a peripheral nerve trunk that are in terms of their physiological properties dendrites and axons but in terms of their morphological properties are essentially the same, then "axon" becomes a generic term so to speak and covers all fibers.

5

Some observations on the role of the Schwann cell in peripheral nerve regeneration

Richard P. Bunge

Many of the chapters of this volume will discuss specific factors that are known to influence the regeneration of peripheral nerves. My purpose in this chapter is to briefly review and emphasize some of the things we now know regarding the contribution of the Schwann cell to this process. In doing this I shall juxtapose observations from the older literature and some very new observations in order to develop the argument that certain of the "trophic" influences of the Schwann cell that so impressed the older workers may be related to a rather new and now well-known factor of known importance in nerve development, nerve growth factor (NGF). In general, the hypothesis I shall develop may be stated as follows.

Both in development and in regeneration, nerve fibers may grow for a period of several days or weeks rather autonomously, but for continued useful growth and maturation provision of trophic factors from the environment is necessary. During development these trophic factors may be provided by the target of the nerve fiber. Nerve regeneration in the adult, however, requires axon growth over great distances and for extended time periods; thus trophic materials from the target are not available for many weeks or months. During the period of regeneration the Schwann cells of the bands of Büngner within the peripheral stump may serve as a surrogate source of trophic factor, providing both guidance and trophic materials to foster axon growth.

SOME HISTORICAL ASPECTS

In 1928, in his extensive treatise on degeneration and regeneration in nervous tissue, Cajal[2] discussed the elements necessary for successful repair of peripheral nerves as follows:

The nervous reunion of the peripheral stump and restoration . . . of the terminal nerve structures, are the combined effect of three conditions: the neurotropic action of the sheaths of Schwann and terminal structures; the mechanical guidance of the sprouts along the old sheaths; and, finally, the superproduction of fibers, in order to insure the arrival of some of them at the peripheral . . . regions. Of all these conditions the most essential . . . is the trophism of the peripheral stump, motor plates and sensory structures.

To provide for the mechanical guidance offered by the connective tissue framework of the distal stump the surgeon must juxtapose the severed nerve ends or interpose a nerve graft to provide for bridging of extensive gaps. The severed nerve fibers of the proximal stump must express their capacity for extensive and multiple sprouting and growth. But, surprisingly, Cajal's emphasis is not on these conditions but on the trophic influences provided by the tissues within the distal stump, particularly by the orphaned Schwann cells that retain their residence and, in fact, expand their numbers within the endoneurial tubes.

The role of the Schwann cell in promoting axonal regrowth within peripheral nerves is repeatedly emphasized in Cajal's writings. He considered the Schwann cells aligned within the endoneurial tubes of the distal nerve stump as a "tutorial . . . cordon" guiding the regrowing nerve fibers toward their targets. He describes the apparent support for growth that regenerating axons receive with the distal stump as coming directly from the "nutritive placenta" of the cell of Schwann. To Cajal the distal stump not only contained the guiding bands of Büngner but vital cordons of Schwann cells providing nutritive assistance essential for the success of peripheral axon regeneration. This concept was a central theme also in the extensive review of peripheral nerve regeneration written by the eminent British anatomist J. Z. Young in 1945.[10]

THE CONCEPT OF TROPHISM

The concept that nerve fiber growth and neuronal welfare are dependent on substances in the periphery delivered to the neuron to provide trophic support derives its most compelling evidence from observations made during embryonic development. During a circumscribed period of embryonic life a large proportion of the neurons generated to provide innervation to a particular region die.[3] As reviewed elsewhere[8] this phenomenon has been observed in the development of many regions of both the central and peripheral nervous systems, including the ventral spinal cord, the dorsal root ganglion, the cervical visceromotor column, the ciliary ganglion, and the trigeminal nucleus, among others. The timing of this naturally occurring neuronal cell death during embryonic development generally coincides with the arrival of the axons of the developing neurons within their target territory. In several instances the amount of neuronal cell death has been observed to be increased by experimental removal of part of the target territory and decreased by implantation of tissue, such as additional limbs, to serve as additional peripheral territory for innervation.[5] The effects of peripheral deprivation are less dramatic when this deprivation is imposed after neural connections are well established.[6] These observations have been interpreted as indicating that generally during embryonic development an excess number of neurons is generated to provide innervation to a specific area. Those neurons that, on reaching the target area, fail to find target tissues with which to make permanent connections are lost. This embryonic event is considered a form of remodeling to allow the neuronal number to fit the functional needs of the embryo. During this embryonic period the neurons appear to be competing for peripheral sites of innervation and thus also for the trophic materials these sites provide. This competition is critical, for the failure to find access to the requisite trophic factor is a life-and-death matter for the embryonic neuron.

Reference to these embronic events within the concept of trophism is generally met with some resistance. The inability to define what the trophic factor provides in order to prevent the death of the neuron is awkward, yet the presence of the phenomenon is no longer questioned. This situation has, at least in part, been clarified by the discovery and recognition of one well-characterized trophic factor, nerve growth factor (NGF). This factor has retained its original name, implying its importance in nerve growth, but it is clear that its importance for the embryonic neuron is more comprehensive. This is most directly illustrated by the fact that NGF-sensitive neurons taken from embryos and grown without benefit of their normally associated supporting cells will survive in the presence of this factor and perish in its absence.[8]

In part, because of this manifestly critical role in the survival and well-being of certain neurons and its availability in large amounts (as purified from salivary glands), we now know a great deal about NGF and its role in the body. Some of this very considerable literature may be summarized as follows.[1,4,8]

1. NGF is a protein with a molecular weight of 13,250 daltons found in various regions

of the body as a dimer. Its amino acid sequence has certain analogies with the proinsulin/insulin peptides. It is generally purified from the male mouse submandibular gland.

2. The action of NGF is largely restricted to adrenergic autonomic and sensory neurons but may also affect selected neurons within the central nervous system. This conclusion derives in part from the following observations:
   a. Antibodies of NGF given during the perinatal period cause failure of adrenergic neuron development.
   b. NGF given during development may prevent normally occurring cell death in adrenergic autonomic neurons.
   c. Addition of NGF to media permits tissue culture of sensory or autonomic neurons in complete absence of supporting cells.
   d. There is no known effect of NGF on parasympathetic or somatic motoneurons.

3. There are many sources of NGF in the body other than the salivary glands, for when the salivary glands are removed blood levels of NGF return to preoperative levels within several weeks.

4. NGF is taken up by certain nerve terminals and transported by retrograde axonal transport to the nerve cell bodies.

5. Retrograde transport of NGF has only been demonstrated in neurons responsive to NGF.

6. Retrograde transport of NGF from axon terminals is quantitatively more substantial than uptake at the nerve cell body.

7. There is now considerable evidence that NGF has important functions in the adult, as well as in development, including:
   a. Removal of the submandibular gland in adult mice results in decreased activity of all enzymes involved in noradrenalin synthesis in related adrenergic neurons.
   b. The detachment of synapses from adrenergic neurons subjected to axotomy is prevented by either systemic or topical application of NGF.
   c. Chromatolytic changes induced by axotomy in adrenergic neurons can be, in part, prevented by application of NGF to the axotomy site.

From these considerations it is clear that NGF can be considered a trophic agent for both sympathetic and dorsal root ganglion neurons. A key point is that NGF is required for the survival of these neurons during a critical stage in their development and that it is involved in the maintenance of the well-being of at least sympathetic neurons throughout their lifetime. An illustration of this latter point is provided by the experiments of Hendry[4] in which he observed a reduction in tyrosine hydroxylase within the superior cervical ganglion after removal of one of the target tissues of this ganglion, the submandibular gland. This could be prevented by replacing the ablated gland with an artificial depot of NGF. This experiment shows that the rat submandibular gland provides a meaningful supply of NGF to the adult sympathetic neuron and establishes this gland as one example of a peripheral target organ as a source of a trophic factor.

Of particular interest to the present discussion is the direct evidence that NGF injected into the target tissues of autonomic neurons will be carried from the innervation field to the soma of the neuron.[7] It should be noted that these experiments may be carried out in adult rats and applied, in addition, to dorsal root ganglia, which are considered not to be sensitive to NGF in adult animals. Thus NGF-sensitive neurons have been shown to acquire this factor from their periphery both during development and in the adult. There is, in addition, evidence that NGF is taken up from iris tissue and transported retrogradely along sympathetic axons innervating the iris into the corresponding superior cervical ganglion.[8] Taken together with the evidence that NGF is produced within the iris, this system provides another example indicating that NGF provided from peripheral tissues is transported to the innervating neuronal soma in adult animals.

It should be emphasized at this point that NGF is clearly not a universal trophic factor for all of the neuronal types that have axons coursing through the peripheral tissues of the body. As we have discussed above, the somatic motoneurons of the ventral spinal cord show a similar dependence on trophic factors from their periphery during development. It seems clear, however, that this trophic material is not NGF for these neurons have no selective uptake mechanism for NGF and show no response to NGF when studied in tissue culture. It should be noted that parasympathetic neurons are manifestly dependent on trophic materials from peripheral fields during their development but that this trophic material is also known not to be NGF.[8] It seems reasonable to assume, however, that whatever these alternative trophic materials are, their principles of action may be similar to those of NGF.

Peripheral supporting cells as sources of trophic factors

There now exists a substantial body of literature indicating that NGF-sensitive neurons may survive in tissue culture in the absence of NGF provided that they are allowed to relate to supporting cells. In a series of studies Varon and his colleagues[8] have demonstrated that both dorsal root ganglia and sympathetic neurons taken from embryos at a time when they are very sensitive to NGF withdrawal will survive in culture when provided with non-neuronal cells derived from the same ganglionic source as were the neurons. This ability to support cultured neurons was not observed with a variety of nonganglionic cell populations. They also observed that purified antibody against beta NGF blocked the NGF-like activity of ganglionic non-neuronal cells even when the antibody treatment was applied before presentation of the supporting cells of the cultured neurons. These observations would seem to be best explained in terms of the production of and delivery by ganglionic non-neuronal cells of a trophic agent that is similar, if not identical, to NGF.

There is also now available direct proof that a variety of non-neuronal cell types in tissue culture may produce NGF-like proteins; these include rat glioma cells, human glioma cells, rat astrocytoma cells and normal human glial cells, and fibroblasts.[8] Unfortunately, this list of known cellular sources of NGF-like material does not yet directly include the cell of Schwann. Whereas the work from Varon and his collaborators discussed above implicates the Schwann cell, it is possible that other cell types derived from the trypsin dissociation of peripheral ganglia such as fibroblasts may be involved. Thus efforts to study the ability of pure populations of Schwann cells to provide trophic support for neurons are indicated.

We have recently undertaken experiments of this type. Utilizing purified cell populations[9] we have observed that the cell of Schwann is able to provide trophic support for a variety of cell types whose axons course within the peripheral nerve system. These observations have been made on dissociated neurons from dorsal root ganglia, autonomic ganglia, and ventral spinal cord neurons from embryonic rats.

For experiments involving dorsal root ganglia or adrenergic neurons these are first prepared under culture conditions using antimitotic agents and NGF to remove all supporting cells, leaving pure populations of neurons. These may then be dissociated and transferred to new culture dishes without NGF. If these recipient culture dishes contain pre-prepared populations of Schwann cells,[9] many of the neurons survive as they establish themselves among these cells; dissociated neurons placed in culture dishes without Schwann cells perish within several days.

In experiments involving ventral horn neurons, these may be prepared directly from 14-day rat embryos by enzymatic dissociation. If these are placed at low density into culture dishes, the larger neurons that represent the somatic motor population do not survive. If placed in culture dishes containing pure populations of Schwann cells, many neurons of this type survive, and in time their axonal processes may be myelinated by Schwann cells.

An example of this latter experiment is

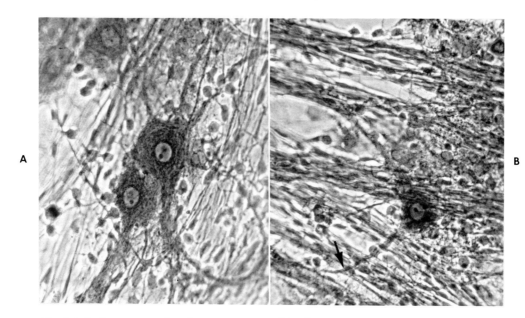

Fig. 5-1. Light micrographs of neurons prepared by dissociation of 14-day rat embryo spinal cord and seeded at sparse densities into culture dishes containing pure populations of Schwann cells. Embryonic neurons placed in dishes containing no Schwann cells do not survive. **A,** Contains portions of three neurons; many of the background cells derive from underlying Schwann cell population. **B,** Shows one neuron maturing on background Schwann cell population and containing a portion of axon that is beginning to be myelinated by Schwann cells provided. Background of Schwann cells still retains a fascicular arrangement reflecting lack of migratory activity in pure Schwann cell populations. Both photographs of Sudan black-stained fixed preparations 3 weeks after neuron addition. (×350.) (Preparation courtesy of Dr. Patrick Wood.)

given in Fig. 5-1. In this experiment regions of the ventral spinal cord from 14-day-old rats were dissociated by trypsin treatment and seeded into culture dishes either with or without a preestablished population of Schwann cells. Under the culture conditions used, only those dishes that contained Schwann cells supported the long-term survival after sparse seeding of these dissociated ventral horn cells.

Preparations of purified populations of Schwann cells have only recently become available,[9] and these have not yet been subjected to the types of analysis that allow direct demonstration of NGF production. It has been possible, however, to utilize Schwann cell populations as a type of "cellular substrate" for neuronal cell populations placed into culture after being separated from their native supporting cell components.

Trophism and regeneration

At the present state of our knowledge we must extrapolate from the observations cited previously, generally made on cultured embryonic tissues, to factors influencing the regeneration of nerve fibers in adult animals. This seems reasonable considering the evidence cited above that the known trophic factor, NGF, has important actions on adult tissues. The nerve fiber severed many centimeters from its target must undertake the process of regeneration over a period of weeks or months prior to the time when it will arrive in the region of the target to obtain sources of trophic materials available there. The evidence cited above suggests that the Schwann cell is able to provide continuing sources of trophic factor en route, throughout the extended period during which the axon is growing toward the target. By serving as a surrogate for the target as a source of trophic

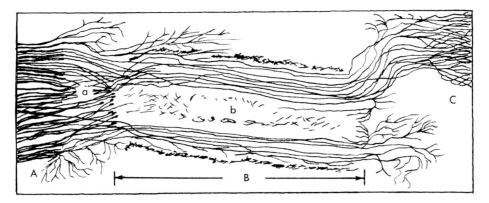

Fig. 5-2. Redrawing of figure presented by Cajal[2] to illustrate importance of vitality of cells of Schwann within nerve graft. Experiment was conducted on young cat killed 12 days after graft, *B*, had been inserted between proximal nerve stump, *A*, and somewhat misaligned distal stump, *C*. Central region of graft, *b*, had become necrotic, for Cajal had deliberately kept graft at room temperature for 4 hours prior to insertion. Regrowing nerve fibers, *a*, appear to avoid degenerate central portions of graft and course instead through viable cortical regions (see Fig. 139 in Cajal[2]).

material during the period of regeneration the cell of Schwann promotes regeneration at the same time that it aids in guiding the axon toward the target region.

The more recent observations discussed above would appear to support Cajal's concepts of the central role of the cell of Schwann in peripheral nerve regeneration. Cajal noted particularly the importance of the vitality of the Schwann cell in providing ongoing trophic support (Fig. 5-2). He felt that whatever substance was provided for the axon would need to be continuously provided by the metabolic activity of the Schwann cell. His description of the nature of the trophic substance could well serve today as a description of NGF. He concludes his extensive writing on the mechanisms of nerve tissue degeneration and regeneration with a description that reads as follows:

There is only a step between the recognition of the cells [of Schwann] as a nutritive placenta and the admission in them of secretions capable of stimulating and orienting the [nerve] sprouts. It is difficult . . . to imagine what is the nature of the stimulating substance . . . we have supposed that the substance contained in the sheaths of Schwann of the peripheral stump should be conceived, not as a fixed, quiescent principle, capable of being neutralized . . . within the cone of growth, but as a ferment or catalytic agent which stimulates the assimilation of the axonic protoplasm, and which does not become used up while acting on the nervous protoplasm.[2]

These words translated in English 50 years ago are still appropriate today, for the definition of the mode of action of trophic substances remains obscure. Our understanding of ways to promote peripheral regeneration would appear, at least in part, to depend on a better definition of the mode of action of trophic substances. We have the advantage of now having available at least one such substance, but as Cajal writes we need: ". . . a more precise knowledge of the elements or sources of neurotropic action; to isolate the attracting substances . . . to determine their nature and mode of action . . . ; to discover the laws which regulate their production and extinction; to explain, finally, the mechanism of chemical reactions and equilibria provoked in the receptor substances present in the young axon and terminal club . . ."

ACKNOWLEDGMENT

Work in my laboratory is supported by NIH Grant NS09923 and Grant 1118 from the National Multiple Sclerosis Society.

REFERENCES

1. Bradshaw, R. A., and Young, M.: Nerve growth factor—recent developments and perspectives, Biochem. Pharmacol. **25**:1445, 1976.
2. Cajal, R.: Degeneration and regeneration of the nervous system (Translated and edited by Raoul M. May), New York, 1959, Hafner Press/Macmillan.
3. Cowan, W. M.: Neuronal death as a regulative mechanism in the control of cell number in the nervous system. In Development and aging in the nervous system, New York, 1973, Academic Press, Inc., p. 19.
4. Hendry, I. A.: Control in the development of the vertebrate sympathetic nervous system, Rev. Neurosci. **2**:149, 1976.
5. Hollyday, M., and Hamburger, V.: Reduction of the naturally occurring motor neuron loss by enlargement of the periphery, J. Comp. Neurol. **170**:311, 1976.
6. Prestige, M. C.: Differentiation, degeneration, and the role of the periphery: quantitative consideration. In Schmitt, F. O., ed.: The neurosciences: second study program, New York, 1970, Rockefeller University Press, p. 116.
7. Stoeckel, K., and Thoenen, H.: Retrograde axonal transport of nerve growth factor: specificity and biological importance, Brain Res. **85**:337, 1976.
8. Varon, S. S., and Bunge, R. P.: Trophic mechanisms in the peripheral nervous system, Ann. Rev. Neurosci. **1**:327.
9. Wood, P. M.: Separation of functional Schwann cells and neurons from normal peripheral nerve tissue, Brain Res. **115**:361, 1976.
10. Young, J. Z.: The functional repair of nervous tissue, Physiol. Rev. **22**:318, 1945.

DISCUSSION

Betty Uzman (Shreveport): Have you looked for soluble active factors in either pure Schwann cells in culture or in the Schwann cells that can be obtained in large numbers in degenerated stumps? Can you tell us if it is possible that we could obtain the message for myelin formation in a bottle?

Bunge: Dr. Uzman is referring to the fact that the signal for myelinogenesis resides somehow within the axon, as recent experiments have shown, including those of Dr. Aguayo and his colleagues. Tissue culture axons that you'd expect to be myelinated do myelinate, and those that do not myelinate in the animals don't myelinate in the tissue culture either. But we don't know why that is; we don't have the signal. We do suspect that the signal for mitogenesis that goes from axon to Schwann cell appears to be on the surface of the neurite and is removable by tricks in chemical digestion. Furthermore the signal can be transferred to the Schwann cells after axonal homogenation, but that's all I can say.

Sterling Mudd (Santa Ana): Is there any evidence of a retrograde effect of nerve growth factor?

Bunge: I think what you are asking is has it been demonstrated that nerve growth factor release can guide and attract axons to targets or to sources of NGF.

Mudd: Yes, in other words can you lay to rest controversy over epineurial repair vs. funicular repair?

Bunge: No, I cannot lay that matter to rest. It's controversial as to whether or not nerve growth factor can exert attractive forces on nerves. Some people believe they have shown nerves will preferably go toward sources of NGF, others have not. This is probably as controversial as the question regarding the best type of nerve repair.

Editor: See also Chapter 12 by Diamond and Jackson in this volume for further discussion of the growth of nerve fibers to target organs.

Michael Mitnik: Can insulin substitute for nerve growth factor?

Bunge: Insulin has some peptide sequences similar to nerve growth factor but does not substitute for nerve growth factor in any situation that I know of in terms of its specific action on nerves.

Jewett: Is there any evidence that there's a time course involved such that primary and secondary repairs might differ, that the Schwann cell may ultimately tire of waiting and become unresponsive?

Bunge: Well, the Schwann cell was the "hero" of Cajal, and it is my hero too, so I'm convinced it won't tire! For example, one can prepare beds of Schwann cells in tissue culture and hold them for many months. They do not divide; they wait. As soon as they see an axon, they are ready. They divide and they may even myelinate. So the Schwann cell is tireless, at least in tissue culture.

Niebauer: Is the effectiveness of nerve growth factor related to age in animals?

Bunge: NGF has some demonstrable effects in adult animals, but it is true that antibodies to NGF have their main effect on animals during development and have little effect on mature animals.

McCarrol: Axons can grow across a 2 cm gap in cats. Is nerve growth factor likely to be effective over such a distance?

Bunge: Cajal commented on "trophic factors" that seem to travel only short distances, a matter of a few millimeters at most, perhaps even less. His comment on this is as current today as it was in 1917: after nerve transection Schwann cells migrate out of the nerve only short distances. It must be remembered, however, that in lower vertebrate forms axonal regeneration is much more vigorous; it may become more dependent on Schwann cell support as we ascend the vertebrate animal scale.

Sunderland: Axons have a remarkable capacity to regenerate and to cross, unaided, considerable gaps to reach the distal stump. We first came across this problem when we were attempting to keep muscles denervated for very long periods, in excess of a year. The great problem was to prevent regenerating proximal stump axons from getting to the distal stump. Now what we were doing in the Australian opossum was excising the median and ulnar nerves between the axilla and the elbow. That's quite a considerable gap (all things in life being relative). We knew from the gross behavior of these animals that regenerating axons were getting through. And sure enough when we terminated the experiments and examined the proximal stump, the distal stump, and the intervening tissue, we found that regenerating axons were getting into the distal stump in large numbers—not in small numbers, in large numbers! Now, if you follow the concept of Paul Weiss that the only factors that control the advance of axons between two stumps are physical, then you would say that here you have an ideal situation in which these regenerating axons would track down the brachial artery. To our surprise we found that many of these regenerating axons, which tracked down the brachial artery then shifted, passed through dense scar tissue, and picked up the ulnar stump behind the elbow. Now of course we didn't know, and there was no way in those days of testing, whether they were ulnar fibers that were getting back to an ulnar stump or whether it was just a group of regenerating axons that decided that they'd move in that direction. In other words, they could have been median regenerating axons going back to the ulnar distal stump, but we rather have the feeling that the distal stump is exerting an influence on the path taken by regenerating axons. Another reason for making that

statement is that if you add up all of those factors that complicate regeneration at the suture line, you say to yourself, "How is it that one ever gets any reasonable recovery?" I suspect that there are factors operating that are directing regenerating axons into funiculi and perhaps even into functionally related endoneurial tubes. We can't answer these question now, but the old concept that it was physical factors and physical factors only that influence the growth and passage of axons to the periphery needs to be amended and modified, and I would not be surprised if there is some trophic influence operating that continues to elude us.

Editor: However, "trophic influence" needn't be chemical—it could be electrical, for example. This would be a "phsyical factor" that was not morphological/mechanical.

Rosen: Dr. Sunderland, in the experiments you just mentioned you said there were large numbers of distal fibers. How do you know it wasn't just a few fibers growing down and branching 10 or 20 times rather than a large number of proximal axons going down?

Sunderland: The only data we had were from the proximal stump of the nerve, the intervening tissue, and the distal stump of the nerve. There's no doubt whatsoever that axon branching was contributing to the distal counts just as it does in any repair process. To what extent, of course, it's extremely difficult to say. So clearly you have two factors that influence reinnervation: (1) the parent axon itself, which is regenerating, and (2) the axon sprouts, many of which are surviving and will pass distally.

Rosen: If there is considerable branching, the reinnervation will not be what you'd expect from those large numbers of axons counted distally.

Sunderland: That is a pretty fair comment. One needs to evaluate reinnervation (which we did not) not only in terms of nerve ending relationships but also in terms of the weight of the muscle, its appearance, and the way in which it was functioning.

We're getting into some very interesting areas here. We do need to follow through these points because by extreme axon branching you can overload the parent neuron. With high nerve transections you may overload neurons in two ways: (1) the branching of the axon and (2) possibly a longer axon to sustain. An axon that originally ran a short course to a proximal portion of the limb may enter an endoneurial tube that will take it a long distance out to the periphery.

Then there is the further question of the relationship between axonal caliber and axonal function, which is extremely difficult, generally neglected, and yet deserving of far more attention that it has been given. If a nerve is compressed sufficiently slowly, it can be deformed to a degree where it is very difficult to recognize it as nerve tissue except by histological techniques. An example is a facial nerve deformed by an acoustic neuroma with no disturbance of facial nerve function at the periphery. Here then you have nerve fibers with a greatly modified structure but no peripheral defect. Perhaps the modified fibers are conducting more slowly with adjustments to the central circuitry covering up the deficit.

Another example concerns the original teaching that when endoneurial tubes atrophied in the manner I described in Chapter 3, a regenerating axon entering and growing down such a tube would not have the capacity to reinflate it and this would put some sort of barrier on the maturation of the fiber. It was that concept that led us to look at cutaneous nerves with a view to finding those that contained the largest number of large fibers as a preliminary to investigating their suitability for autografting. This is a good example of bogus biology because we know from very late repairs of peripheral nerves (denervated for 12+ months) that regeneration can proceed as it would following an immediate repair with a remarkable degree of recovery in the proximal musculature despite atrophy of the distal neural tubes to 2 to 3 μ. Now, either the regenerating axon has the capacity to reinflate the endoneurial tube and have its original structural features restored, or a fiber of greatly reduced diameter can function normally.

Editor: In this case, as well as the facial nerve example, it may be that we have clinical "normality" because in the usual activities engaged in by these patients the nerves are not called on to function maximally, as might occur in athletes on the motor side or aesthetes on the sensory side. It would be nice to know if fiber diameters increase when axon activity increases chronically.

6

Experimental nerve grafts

Albert J. Aguayo and Garth M. Bray

Nerve grafts are most commonly used for the repair of extensive nerve injuries where a direct end-to-end suture is not possible.[33] Clinical results and surgical methods of nerve grafting are discussed elsewhere in this volume. This chapter reviews recent studies of the behavior of regenerating axons and Schwann cells in grafted nerves of experimental animals.

METHODS

For the experimental nerve grafts described in this report, a segment of donor nerve (approximately 5 mm in length) is placed between the cut ends of the sciatic or sural nerve of a recipient mouse. Using a dissecting microscope, the grafted segments are secured to the host nerve stumps with 10-0 nylon sutures. For allotransplants, which involve genetically dissimilar animals of the same species, segments of sciatic nerves were obtained from mice of different strains than the host. For xenogenic nerve grafts (transplants between different species), single fascicles of human sural nerves from diagnostic biopsies or limb amputations were used. To prevent rejection of the allo- and xenogenic grafts, antilymphocytic serum (ALS) was prepared by injecting rabbits with a suspension of 10^9 living thymocytes.[19] This antiserum was administered subcutaneously to the host animals in doses of 0.5 ml twice weekly beginning on the day of transplantation. At various intervals after grafting, the host animals were perfused with fixative and the regenerated nerves examined by quantitative phase and electron microscope techniques and, in selected cases, by radioautography.[3]

AXON AND SCHWANN CELL RESPONSES TO NERVE GRAFTING

Transection of a peripheral nerve is followed by axonal degeneration and Schwann cell proliferation in the distal stump of the injured nerve.[34] Using radioautographic techniques to indicate premitotic DNA synthesis, it has been shown that Schwann cell multiplication in the distal stump reaches its highest values 3 days after axonal interruption and continues with decreasing frequency for approximately 2 weeks after injury.[7,11] Reactive and degenerative changes also occur in the proximal stumps of severed nerves; adjacent to the level of transection, axons become swollen and contain accumulations of organelles. Subsequently, regenerative axon sprouts appear at this level.[3,10,12] Schwann cells also proliferate along the last few millimeters of the proximal stump.[20]

In nerve graft experiments axon degeneration and Schwann cell proliferation primarily involve two nerve segments: the graft and the recipient distal stump. However, using Schwann cells identifiable by radioactive labels or cytoplasmic markers, it has been demonstrated that most transplanted Schwann cells multiply but remain confined to the grafted segment[1,2,4,7,14] (Fig. 6-1, a). In regenerated experimental grafts, there are distinct boundaries between Schwann cell populations derived from the host proximal and distal stumps and those from the trans-

Host **Graft** **Host**

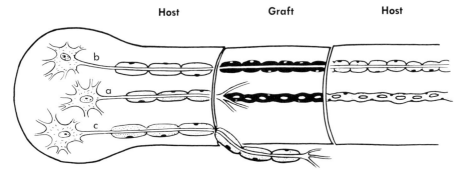

Fig. 6-1. Schematic representation of axon–Schwann cell relationships during degenerative and regenerative phases that follow nerve grafting. *a*, In early stages, axons of fibers in graft and distal (host) segments undergo wallerian degeneration leaving columns of "denervated" Schwann cells. *b*, Axons regenerating from proximal stump are ensheathed by two populations of Schwann cells: those in graft (black) originate from donor nerve, while those in distal stump (white) are host Schwann cells. *c*, Aberrant axons that grow outside perineurium are ensheathed and myelinated by Schwann cells migrating from proximal stump. (Modified from Aguayo, A. J., et al.: Ann. N. Y. Acad. Sci. 1978.)

planted segment.[2,4,7,8] Thus axons regenerating from the proximal stump become ensheathed by transplanted donor Schwann cells in the graft and host Schwann cells in the distal stump (Fig. 6-1, *b*).

Although the mobility of Schwann cells appears to be restricted where there is regeneration-in-continuity, Schwann cell migration must be important for the regrowth of nerves deprived of a distal stump, for the bridging of short nerve gaps,[7] and for the ensheathment of axons that follow an aberrant extrafascicular course or grow between the sheaths of the perineurium or epineurium of injured nerves[1,31] (Fig. 6-1, *c*). In nerve grafts where there is little evidence of Schwann cell migration, it is possible that interactions between the contiguous populations of Schwann cells are responsible for inhibiting the advance of host cells into the graft. This hypothesis is consistent with the observation that Schwann cells do not migrate along anastomosed nerves but will do so along axons devoid of sheath cells.[8]

The persistence of donor cells in nerve grafts permits a novel experimental approach to the study of interactions between axons and Schwann cells. By combining host and donor nerves with different cytological and immunological characteristics, it is possible to create new combinations of axons and Schwann cells and thereby investigate certain biological and immunological aspects relevant to an understanding of peripheral nerve transplantation and regeneration.

EXPERIMENTAL NERVE GRAFTS USED TO STUDY SCHWANN CELL DIFFERENTIATION AND MYELIN FORMATION

In myelinated fibers, one Schwann cell is responsible for the ensheathment and myelination of the segment of a single axon that extends between two consecutive nodes of Ranvier. In unmyelinated fibers, on the other hand, individual Schwann cells ensheath several axons and interdigitate with neighboring Schwann cell processes.[5,17,23] To determine if the structural features that distinguish myelinated and unmyelinated fibers are due to intrinsic Schwann cell properties or if Schwann cell differentiation is controlled by extrinsic influences exerted during growth or regeneration, a 5 mm segment from the unmyelinated cervical sympathetic trunk (CST) of a mature mouse was grafted between the stumps of a transected, richly myelinated sural nerve in the same animal. One month after transplantation, the previously unmyelinated CST segments became myelinated, and there was no radioautographic evidence for the migration of myelin-forming Schwann cells from the host into the graft.[7] Additional studies using CST grafts containing tritiated thymidine-labeled Schwann cells confirmed that Schwann cells from the unmyelinated nerve had been induced to form myelin.[2] These experiments as well as studies in cross-anastomosed myelinated and unmyelinated nerves[7,36,37] support the concept that all Schwann cells are potentially capable of elaborating myelin or the cytoplasmic sheaths of unmyelinated fibers. The axonal properties that are responsible for Schwann cell differentiation remain largely unknown; these properties in peripheral nerve axons appear to exert similar influences on myelin-forming cells from the central nervous system.[9,39]

Thus, after axonal interruption, sheath cells originating from degenerated fibers, either myelinated or unmyelinated, are capable of myelination when contacted by axons regenerating from myelinated nerve fibers. The demonstration of this bipotentiality in Schwann cells makes a match in fiber composition between host and donor nerves unnecessary for nerve grafting. Furthermore, within certain limits there appears to be an adjustment between the numbers of axons and Schwann cells in regenerated experimental grafts; in allografts in mice neither "naked" axons nor large numbers of "denervated" Schwann cells were observed 6 months after grafting, although the original populations of fibers in the host and grafted nerves were dissimilar. The mechanisms involved in this adaptation may include an axon-triggered proliferation of Schwann cells[22,41] or a gradual loss of Schwann cells that fail to become innervated by the regenerating axons.[38]

EXPERIMENTAL XENOTRANSPLANTATION OF PERIPHERAL NERVE

It is a known characteristic of tissue transplantation that the greater the phylogenetic disparity between donor and recipient, the greater the chances of graft rejection. Thus the use of xenografts has had a long and undistinguished history.[29] The advent of various forms of immune suppression, however, has increased the chances for the survival of xenografts. Although the future of xenografts in man must await advances in immunological methodology, there are few restraints on the experimental transplantation of human tissues into animal hosts. Indeed, important advances in the understanding of tumor pathology and in the testing of therapeutic methods have been accomplished by studying human cells grafted into immunologically tolerant animals.[35] Hence, xenografts of human peripheral nerve segments may be used to investigate transplantation requirements and to delineate specific roles of axons and Schwann cells in normal and pathological nerves.

Acceptance of xenografts may be enhanced by using immune suppressed animals or immunologically deficient mutants as hosts. Neonatal thymectomy, corticosteroid therapy, or the administration of cytotoxic drugs such as azathioprine, 6-mercaptopurine, cyclophosphamide,[25] or antilymphocytic serum[19] will render host animals capable of accepting allo- or xenografts. The thymus-deficient mutant mouse known as "nude"[42] or the asplenic-athymic mutant[27] will also accept allo- and xenografts. By using some of these techniques, it has been determined that Schwann cells from human nerve segments transplanted into mice immunosuppressed with antilymphocytic serum[8] or "nude" mice[16] will ensheath and myelinate axons regenerating from the host animal. Soon after the grafting of single fascicles from human nerves into immunologically tolerant mice, the nerve fibers in the graft and also in the distal stumps of recipient nerves undergo changes that are characteristic of wallerian degeneration, but there is no

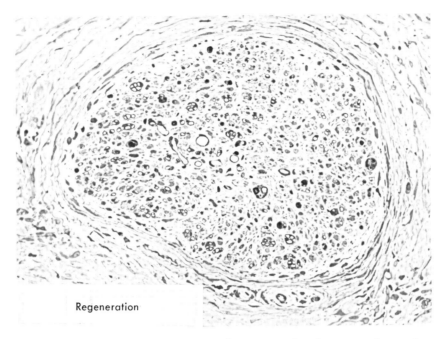

Regeneration

Fig. 6-2. Cross section of midportion of xenograft originating from human sural nerve 2 months after transplantation into sciatic nerve of immune-suppressed mouse. Within graft, mouse axons have been myelinated by human Schwann cells. (Phase micrograph ×230.)

rejection of the human xenograft. Two months after grafting, axons have regenerated from the proximal stump, through the graft (Fig. 6-2) and into the distal stump with many myelinated fibers at both these levels.

When the thickness of the myelin sheath in regenerated xenografts was assessed in electron micrographs, it was determined that myelination in the distal stump approximated normal values by 2 months after grafting, but equivalent myelination of mouse axons by the grafted human Schwann cells was only accomplished by 6 months.[9] The differences between rates of myelination of mouse axons by human and mouse Schwann cells may be due to peculiar axon–Schwann cell interactions in the xenograft, true species-related differences in the speed of myelination, or to experimental conditions.

Because normal human and mouse Schwann cells are morphologically identical, it has been necessary to prove that the Schwann cells within the grafted segment of these regenerated nerves actually originated

from the human nerve and not from cells migrating from the stumps of the recipient mouse nerve. The origin of Schwann cells in the xenograft was determined by discontinuing immunosuppression of the host animal at variable intervals after the transplantation of the human nerve segments. In addition, 2 weeks after the discontinuation of ALS, host mice received an intravenous dose of 10^8 lymphoid cells obtained from the spleen and lymph nodes of syngeneic mice hyperimmunized against human tissue by intraperitoneal injection of 10^8 human leukocytes twice weekly for 3 consecutive weeks.[32] This immune cell transfer was used to abrogate xenograft acceptance in the recipient animal. Although discontinuation of ALS is followed by xenograft rejection, the additional transfer of immune cells permitted a more accurate timing of the rejection, which was advantageous for the sequential study of the underlying cellular events. The earliest signs of xenograft rejection, observed 8 days after immune cell transfer (between 3 and 4 weeks after stopping ALS), consisted of mononuclear cell accumulations in the grafted segments (Fig. 6-3). In later stages, Schwann cells of myelinated and unmyelinated fibers were surrounded, penetrated, and eventually replaced by mononuclear cells[8] (Fig. 6-4). Perineural fibroblasts were also rejected in the graft. During the acute phase of rejection, some axons became totally denuded of Schwann cells and were surrounded only by basal lamina. The basal lamina, presumably because of its weak antigenicity, appeared to have escaped the immune response. Schwann cells and fibroblasts in the proximal and distal stumps of the grafted nerve were not rejected. Aberrant fibers growing outside the perineurium of the grafted fascicle remained intact, indicating that these axons were ensheathed by host Schwann cells. During graft rejection, many fibers in the distal stump remained myelinated, an indication that the continuity of their axons was preserved. However, some axons were damaged, presumably within the graft, because a variable number of fibers underwent walle-

rian degeneration in the distal stump of the nerves containing the rejected xenograft. Axonal damage in rejected grafts may represent a secondary "bystander" effect of the immune response.[21] Damage to axons during xenograft rejection varied from extensive to minimal in the different animals examined.

The method used for the identification of the exact origin of Schwann cells in the grafted segment of regenerated xenografts also helped to document morphological features of a cell-mediated immune response directed against sheath cells (Schwann cells of both myelinated and unmyelinated fibers as well as fibroblasts) rather than one that primarily affects myelin, as occurs in most allergic neuropathies.[40] This study would not have been possible during primary rejection of nerve grafts, because in such instances, the immunological response is directed toward all cellular components, sheath cells and axons alike, within the graft.[15,24] In animals permitted to survive the period of xenograft rejection for over 2 months, segments of nerve at the site of the original graft were

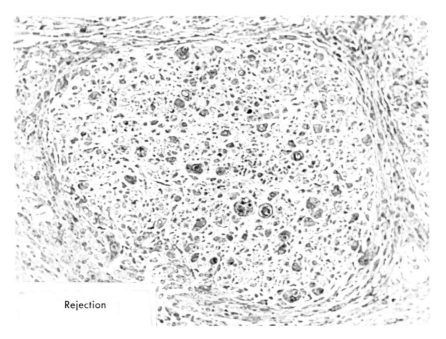

Rejection

Fig. 6-3. Rejection of regenerated, 6-week-old xenograft is characterized by intense infiltration of perineurial and intrafascicular portions of graft. (Phase micrograph ×230.)

again myelinated. In these animals, which had recovered their immunological competence, it appears that the mouse axons were reensheathed by host Schwann cells that must have migrated from the recipient nerve stumps. This Schwann cell migration may have been facilitated and guided by the axons and basal lamina that survived rejection. Thus, in these immune-suppressed experimental animals, the grafts containing xenogenic Schwann cells and connective tissue may have served as temporary agents to facilitate axonal regrowth and the bridging of nerve gaps. These experimental findings suggest that the immune suppression necessary for allogenic or xenogenic nerve grafts may only be a temporary requirement.

ADDITIONAL APPLICATIONS OF EXPERIMENTAL NERVE GRAFTS

Nerve grafts not only provide support and guidance for the regeneration of nerve fibers but, as demonstrated in these studies using experimental animals, they also serve as useful systems in which to investigate various aspects of the interrelationships between axons and Schwann cells. In addition, the persistence of donor cells in the regenerated

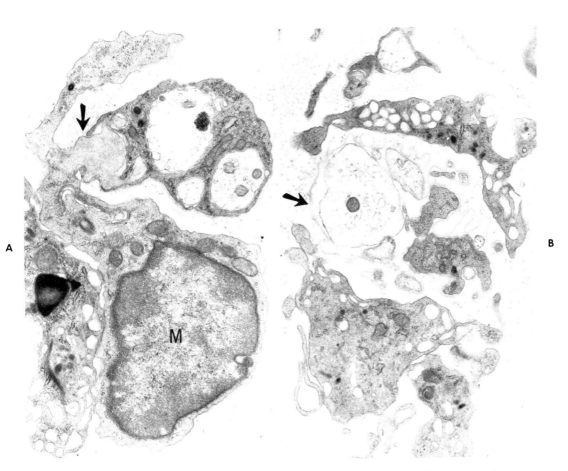

Fig. 6-4. Details of rejection of xenograft in Fig. 6-3. **A,** Cytoplasmic process from mononuclear cell, *M,* has penetrated basal lamina of an unmyelinated fiber (arrow.) **B,** After Schwann cell rejection, there are several macrophage processes on both sides of residual basal lamina that surrounds "naked" axons. (Electron micrograph ×16,000.) (Reproduced from Aguayo, A. J., et al.: Nature **268:**755, 1977.)

grafted nerves of experimental animals has permitted in vivo studies of the mechanisms involved in the pathogenesis of certain genetically determined neuropathies in man[8,9] and in two mutant mice.[1,4] Experimental transplantation of neuronal tissue,[18,26,28,43] the recent demonstration of the feasibility of grafting CNS glia from optic nerves into peripheral nerves,[6,39] as well as advances in histocompatability typing[30] and in the application of immunological methods to the study of Schwann cells[13] are promising steps for the future understanding and application of neural transplantation.

ACKNOWLEDGMENTS

We thank the Medical Research Council, Multiple Sclerosis Society, Muscular Dystrophy Association of Canada, and the Dysautonomia Foundation of America for their generous support. We also thank M. Attiwell, J. Trecarten, and S. Harrington for their valuable technical assistance.

REFERENCES

1. Aguayo, A. J., Bray, G. M., and Perkins, S. C.: Axon-Schwann cell relationships in neuropathies of mutant mice, Ann. N. Y. Acad. Sci. **317:**512, 1979.
2. Aguayo, A. J., Charron, L. C., and Bray, G. M.: Potential of Schwann cells from unmyelinated nerves to produce myelin—a quantitative ultrastructural and radioautographic study, J. Neurocytol. **5:**565, 1976.
3. Aguayo, A. J., Peyronnard, J. M., and Bray, G. M.: A quantitative ultrastructural study of regeneration from isolated proximal stumps of transected unmyelinated nerves, J. Neuropathol. Exp. Neurol. **32:**256, 1973.
4. Aguayo, A. J., et al.: Abnormal myelination in transplanted Trembler mouse Schwann cells, Nature **265:**73, 1977.
5. Aguayo, A. J., et al.: Three dimensional analysis of unmyelinated fibers in normal and pathologic autonomic nerves, J. Neuropathol. Exp. Neurol. **35:**136, 1976.
6. Aguayo, A. J., et al.: Ensheathment and myelination of regenerating CNS fibers by transplanted optic nerve glia, Neurosci. Lett. **9:**97, 1978.
7. Aguayo, A. J., et al.: Multipotentiality of Schwann cells in cross-anastomosed and grafted myelinated and unmyelinated nerves, Brain Res. **104:**1, 1976.
8. Aguayo, A. J., et al.: Myelination of mouse axons by Schwann cells transplanted from normal and abnormal human nerves, Nature **268:**753, 1977.
9. Aguayo, A. J., et al.: Human and animal neuropathies studied in experimental nerve transplants. In Canal, N., and Pozza, G., eds.: Periph-

eral neuropathies, Amsterdam, 1978, Elsevier/North-Holland Biomedical Press.
10. Blumcke, S., Niedorf, H. R., and Rode, J.: Axoplasmic alterations in the proximal and distal stumps of transected nerves, Acta Neuropathol. **7:**44, 1966.
11. Bradley, W. G., and Asbury, A. K.: Duration of synthesis phase in neurolemma cells in mouse sciatic nerve degeneration, Exp. Neurol. **26:**275, 1970.
12. Bray, G. M., Peyronnard, J. M., and Aguayo, A. J.: Reactions of unmyelinated nerve fibers to injury—an ultrastructural study, Brain Res. **42:**297, 1972.
13. Brockes, J. P., Fields, K. L., and Raff, M. C.: A surface antigenic marker for rat Schwann cells, Nature **266:**364, 1977.
14. Charron, L., Aguayo, A. J., and Bray, G. M.: Schwann cell kinetics in experimental nerve grafts, Can. J. Neurol. Sci. **3:**143, 1976.
15. DasGupta, T. K.: Mechanism of rejection of peripheral nerve allografts, Surg. Gynecol. Obstet. **125:**1050, 1967.
16. Dyck, P. J., Lais, A. C., and Low, P. A.: Nerve xenografts to assess cellular expression of the abnormality of myelination in inherited neuropathy and Friedreich ataxia, Neurology **28:**261, 1978.
17. Eames, R. A., and Gamble, H. J.: Schwann cell relationships in normal human cutaneous nerves, J. Anat. **106:**417, 1970.
18. Katzman, R., Broida, R., and Raine, C. S.: Reinnervation, myelination and organization of iris tissue implanted into the rat midbrain—an ultrastructural study, Brain Res. **138:**423, 1977.
19. Levey, R. H., and Medawar, P. B.: Nature and mode of action of antilymphocytic antiserum, Proc. Natl. Acad. Sci. USA **56:**1130, 1966.
20. Lubinska, L.: Demyelination and remyelination in the proximal parts of regenerating nerve fibers, J. Comp. Neurol. **117:**275, 1961.
21. Madrid, R. C., and Wisniewski, H. M.: Axonal degeneration in demyelinating disorders, J. Neurocytol. **6:**103, 1977.
22. McCarthy, K., and Partlow, L.: Neuronal stimulation of ^{3}H-thymidine incorporation by primary cultures of highly purified non-neuronal cells, Brain Res. **114:**415, 1976.
23. Ochoa, J., and Mair, W. G. P.: The normal sural nerve in man. I. Ultrastructure and numbers of fibers and cells, Acta Neuropathol. **13:**197, 1969.
24. Pollard, J. D., and Fitzpatrick, L.: An ultrastructural comparison of peripheral nerve allografts and autografts, Acta Neuropathol. **23:**152, 1973.
25. Pollard, J. D., and McLeod, J. G.: An assessment of immunosuppressive agents in experimental nerve transplantation, Surg. Gynecol. Obstet. **132:**839, 1971.
26. Rosenstein, J. M., and Brightman, M. W.: Intact cerebral ventricle as a site for tissue transplantation, Nature **276:**83, 1978.
27. Searle, A. G.: Hereditary absence of spleen in the mouse, Nature **184:**1419, 1959.

28. Seiger, A., and Olson, L.: Quantitation of fiber growth in transplanted central monoamine neurons, Cell Tissue Res. **179**:285, 1977.

29. Shons, A. R., Morberg, A. W., and Najarian, J. S.: Xenotransplantation. In Najarian, J. S., and Simmons, R. L., eds.: Transplantation, Philadelphia, 1972, Lea & Febiger, p. 729.

30. Singh, R., Medrelse, K., and Stefanko, S.: Role of tissue typing on preserved nerve allografts in dogs, J. Neurol. Neurosurg. Psychiatry **40**:865, 1977.

31. Spencer, P. S.: Light and electron microscope observations on localized peripheral nerve injuries, Ph. D. Thesis, University of London, 1971.

32. Steinmuller, D.: Cross species transplantation in embryonic and neonatal animals, Transplant. Proc. **2**:438, 1970.

33. Sunderland, S.: Nerve grafting. In Nerves and nerve injuries, Edinburgh, 1968, Churchill-Livingstone, p. 687.

34. Thomas, P. K. Nerve injury. In Bellairs, R., and Gray, E. G., eds.: Essays on the nervous system, Oxford, 1974, Clarendon Press, p. 44.

35. Unterharnscheidt, F. J.: Routine tissue culture of CNS tumours and animal implantation. In Homburger, F., ed.: Recent advances in brain tumour research—progress in experimental tumour research, vol. 17, Basel, 1972, S. Karger, p. 111.

36. Weinberg, H. J., and Spencer, P. S.: Studies on the control of myelinogenesis. I. Myelination of regenerating axons after entry in a foreign unmyelinated nerve, J. Neuroctyol. **4**:395, 1975.

37. Weinberg, H. J., and Spencer, P. S.: Studies on the control of myelinogenesis. II. Evidence for neuronal regulation of myelin production, Brain Res. **113**:363, 1976.

38. Weinberg, H. J., and Spencer, P. S.: Fate of Schwann cells deprived of axonal contact, Neurology **28**:355, 1978.

39. Weinberg, E. L., and Spencer, P. S.: Studies on the control of myelinogenesis. III. Signaling of oligodendrocytes myelination by regenerating peripheral axons, Brain Res. **162**:273, 1979.

40. Wisniewski, H., Prineas, J., and Raine, C. S.: An ultrastructural study of experimental demyelination and remyelination. I. Acute experimental allergic encephalo-myelitis in the peripheral nervous system, Lab. Invest. **21**:105, 1969.

41. Wood, P., and Bunge, R.: Evidence that sensory axons are mitogenic for Schwann cells, Nature **256**:662, 1975.

42. Wortis, H. H.: Immunological responses of "nude" mice, Clin. Exp. Immunol. **8**:305, 1971.

43. Zalewski, A. A., Goshgarian, H. G., and Silvers, M.: The fate of neurons and neurilemmal cells in allografts of ganglia in the spinal cord of normal and immunologically tolerant rats, Exp. Neurol. **59**:322, 1978.

DISCUSSION

Editor: Can you speculate on the time course of the process by which "denervated" Schwann cells disappear? Is there any indication of when this might become irreversible or more difficult to reverse?

Answer: The sequence of histologic events that occur in chronically denervated distal stumps has been studied in transected tibial nerves by Weinberg and Spencer.* These investigators studied changes by light and electron microscopy from 3 to 58 weeks after nerve section and ligation of the proximal stump. In early stages the Schwann cells that were deprived of axonal contact remained arranged in columns that were progressively encircled by fibroblasts and later by cells of perineurial type. The "denervated" Schwann cell columns underwent gradual shrinkage and eventually disappeared to be replaced by connective tissue. The eventual disappearance of the Schwann cells and the proliferation of connective tissue must undoubtedly impair the regrowth of axons and hinder the reinnervation of target tissues.

Editor: Do you think it may be possible to use cells that have been cultured in vitro for nerve repair?

Answer: Recently, rat Schwann cells grown in tissue culture preparations, rather than those derived from whole nerve grafts, have been successfully used for experimental transplantation. For this purpose, Holtzmann rat Schwann cells, cultured and separated from neurites, were transplanted into a reservoir created by suturing a 5 mm segment of a blood vessel between the stumps of sciatic nerves of immune-suppressed mice and studied from 3 to 18 weeks later. By cell rejection techniques it was demonstrated that axons from the host mouse had been ensheathed and myelinated by rat Schwann cells in the grafted segment of the regenerated nerves of these animals.†

---

*Weinberg, H. J., and Spencer, P. S.: J. Neurocytol. 7:555, 1978.

†Aguayo, A. J., et al.: Neurology **29**:589, 1979.

7

Calcium requirement for axoplasmic transport and the role of the perineurial sheath

Sidney Ochs

In recent years it has been generally accepted that various materials manufactured by the neuron cell bodies are carried outward in the axons, a process called axoplasmic transport.[10,14,22,31] Some of the materials are required to maintain the form and function of the fiber. The classical picture of wallerian degeneration seen when nerve fibers are separated from their cell bodies is due to the loss of key material(s) normally carried down the axon and thence into the Schwann cells.[24] It is now considered a possibility that several neurological and muscular diseases may have their etiology in a defect in the supply of some of the materials carried down into the fibers by axoplasmic transport.[26,33]

In our studies of axoplasmic transport, a labeled amino acid, typically ^{3}H-leucine, is used as a marker.[29] The isotope is injected into the L7 dorsal root ganglion of the cat, where the ^{3}H-leucine is taken up by the nerve cell bodies. It is rapidly incorporated into a wide range of proteins and polypeptides that are then moved down the nerve fibers of these neurons. The rate and characteristics of the process of transport are shown by removing the sciatic nerve at different times after injection of the precursor, cutting the nerve into equal small pieces and determining the radioactivity in each. A characteristic downflow pattern is found and from it the rate of transport evaluated by the change with time in the position of the front of the crest of transported radioactivity

(Fig. 7-1). The transport rate found in a large number of animals is close to 410 mm/day with the same fast rate present in nerves taken from mammals of different sizes. It is also the same regardless of nerve fiber diameter or the function of the fiber.[29]

TRANSPORT FILAMENT MODEL

A basic problem is the mechanism underlying axoplasmic transport. In this brief review, we will describe some new advances regarding the transport mechanism, particularly with respect to our recent finding that Ca^{2+} is needed to maintain transport.[34,35] Several years ago we found that axoplasmic transport can be carried on in vitro with the same outflow pattern and at the same fast rate as is the case in the animal.[32] This was shown by allowing several hours of downflow in cats after L7 dorsal root ganglia injection with ^{3}H-leucine. The sciatic nerves were then removed from the animals, placed in an oxygenated media, either in a chamber exposed to a moist atmosphere of 95% O_2 + 5% CO_2 or in Ringer's solution vigorously bubbled with this gas mixture. Comparing the downflow in vitro and in vivo showed no apparent differences between them.

Using the in vitro system, we found that O_2 was required for the maintenance of transport.[30] High-energy phosphate ($\sim$P) levels (the combined levels of ATP and creatine phosphate) fell to a critical level of half control levels (1.2 μM/gm) after approximately

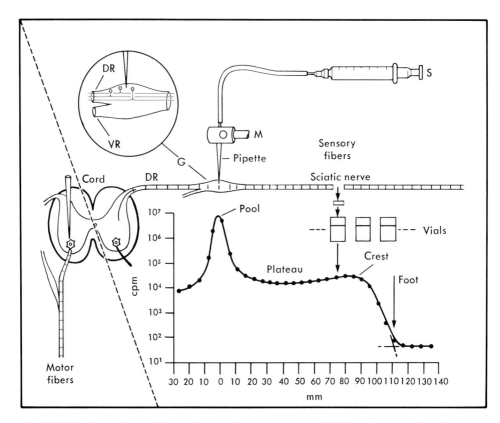

Fig. 7-1. Injection and sampling technique showing transport. L7 dorsal root ganglion shown in insert contains T-shaped neurons with one branch ascending in dorsal root *DR*, and other descending into sciatic nerve. Pipette is passed into ganglion and ³H-leucine is injected. After incorporation of precursor, downflow of labeled components in fibers is sampled at various times by sacrificing animal and sectioning nerve into 5 mm pieces. Each segment is placed in vial, solubilized, scintillation fluid added, and activity counted. Outflow pattern is displayed on ordinate using log scale in counts per minute (cpm). Abscissa gives segments in millimeters from center of ganglion taken as zero. After 6.5 hours of downflow, high level of activity is seen remaining in ganglion region with more distally, plateau rising to crest before abruptly falling at front of crest to baseline levels. Left-hand side of cord shows injection of precursor into region of L7 motoneuron cell bodies with similar treatment of ventral root, *VR*, and sciatic nerve and an outflow of same rate found in motor fibers.

15 to 20 minutes of anoxia at the time when axoplasmic transport and electrical responses were both seen to fail.[30] Various metabolic blocking agents such as cyanide, dinitrophenol, and azide were also able to block transport quickly within this same time of 15 to 20 minutes. Those studies showed that oxidative phosphorylation produces the necessary supply of ATP needed to energize the transport mechanism. Another indication of dependence of axoplasmic transport on energy supply was the high Q_{10} found for transport.[32]

Taking into account the dependence of transport on an ATP supply and the body of evidence implicating the microtubules of the axons in transport, the block of axoplasmic transport with mitotic blocking agents such as colchicine and the vinca alkaloids,[6,18,25] a model was proposed based on analogy to muscle.[28] In this model, a hypothetical transport filament to which the various components transported are bound, is considered to be moved down along the microtubules, and possibly also neurofilaments, by means of the cross-bridges or cross-arms. These structures are seen in electron micrographs projecting at intervals from both microtubules and neurofilaments. Recently, it was shown that microtubule-associated proteins (MAP's) could be removed from a tubulin preparation. When microtubules were reassembled from tubulin with MAP present, side arms were seen on the microtubules; when reassembled without MAP's present, microtubules with smooth walls were found.[40]

As one of the pieces of evidence in accord with the model, the presence of Ca-Mg-ATPase at high levels was found in peripheral nerves.[17] This enzyme could utilize the ~P of ATP for transport. An enzyme with closely similar properties was also found in giant fibers.[20] However, there appeared to be a conflict between the model and the numerous in vitro experiments we made, which showed that eliminating Ca^{2+} or Mg^{2+}, or both, from the medium had no effect on the course or rate of transport. This was shown not only in our laboratory but also in the studies carried out in other laboratories.[9,12] On the other hand, a blocking effect of oxalate when present in the medium in high concentrations suggested that a reduction of Ca^{2+} was effective in accord with the role postulated for the ion.[28] The reason for the apparent insensitivity of axoplasmic transport to a lack of Ca^{2+} in the medium was traced to the relative impermeability of the perineurial sheath of the nerve. This sheath acts to maintain relatively normal ionic medium in the fluid of the endoneurial compartment in which it and the fibers are contained by the perineurium. With the aid of desheathed nerve preparation we found that Ca^{2+} is in fact necessary for axoplasmic transport.[34, 35]

PERINEURIUM

The anatomy of the various sheaths present around nerve trunks and their individual bundles, fasciculi or funiculi, have recently been much clarified by the use of electron microscopy.[23,45] Around the smaller nerve bundles, we can distinguish three different layers. The outer layer is the relatively loose and bulky epineurium containing connective tissue elements. These include collagenous fibrils that run circumferentially, longitudinally, and spirally around the fasciculus with fibroblasts, macrophages, and mast cells present throughout the epineurium. The middle layer, the perineurium, is the layer of greatest functional importance. It is composed of a number of concentric layers of flat cells with tight junctions between them that may number from 1 to as many as 12, the perineurial thickness depending on the diameter of the fasciculus.[44]

A basement membrane is also characteristically present on each side of the individual perineurial layers. There is some question as to whether the flat cells of the perineurium should be considered as epithelial cells because a basement membrane is found on both surfaces. Perhaps they should be classed as special perineurial cells, possibly related to the Schwann cells.[23] While the epineurium has at times been identified as the permeability barrier,[5] the perineurium with its tight junctions is now recognized as the barrier site.[39] Ions penetrate slowly through the perineurium,[11,19,36] while the permeability to substances such as O_2, CO_2, and lipid-soluble materials is high.

Within the perineurial sheath of the funiculus is the endoneurial space containing the nerve fibers. Some reticular fibers, a small number of fibroblasts, and endoneurial fluid are present in this compartment. The composition of the endoneurial fluid, which, as we shall show, is important in maintaining nerve function, is maintained by action of the endothelial cells of the capillaries within the perineurium and the low permeability of the perineurium. Possibly an active contribution to a regulation of constitutents is also carried out by the perineurial cells.

In the larger nerve trunks a number of fasciculi are bound together within the epineurium.[43] The course of the funiculi within a large nerve is complex, with nerve fibers passing back and forth between the various fasciculi, as has been fully described by Sunderland[43] (see Chapter 3). This variability of funicular pattern creates a problem in desheathing suitably long lengths of nerve in order to study axoplasmic transport in vitro for periods of 4 to 6 hours. Fortunately, the peroneal nerve of the cat consists, for the most part, of a single funiculus of suitably long length.

DESHEATHING PROCESS AND PREPARATION FOR TRANSPORT STUDY

The epineurium binding the peroneal and the tibial branches of the sciatic nerve of the cat is readily separated up to a point some 30 mm from the center of the L7 dorsal root ganglion. Fortunately, in the cat the peroneal nerve is, with only small exceptions, covered by a single perineurial sheath. To desheath the peroneal nerve, a small broken piece of razor blade is used to make a longitudinal section of the perineurium at a distance of 35 mm below the center of the L7 dorsal root ganglion. The cut is extended down the nerve with fine scissors and the perineurial sheath grasped with a fine forcep and stripped from the nerve down to the point where branching occurs, a distance usually of about 135 mm from the center of the ganglion (Fig. 7-2).

The experimental plan followed was to inject the L7 dorsal root ganglia of anesthetized cats with ^{3}H-leucine and let the labeled incorporated materials be transported down into the fibers passing into the tibial and peroneal nerves for a period of 2 hours. Then the sciatic nerves are taken from the animals and the peroneal branch desheathed. The tibial nerve is a much more complicated structure with numerous branches, making desheathing over a long length difficult. We have therefore chosen to leave the tibial nerve sheathed to serve as a control.

To observe the effect on transport of the removal or addition of various ions to the media, the nerve with its desheathed peroneal nerve and sheathed tibial nerve branches is put into incubation media of various compositions for some 4 to 6 hours. The desheathed and sheathed branches were each cut into equal small sections and the outflow pattern of activity in each of the two branches determined.

LOW Ca^{2+} INCUBATION MEDIA

Using Ringer's solution as the incubation medium, downflow in the desheathed branch and sheathed branch was seen to be similar (Fig. 7-3). The differences between the plateau heights of the sheathed tibial and desheathed peroneal nerve branches seen in Fig. 7-3 are not significant. The plateau may vary somewhat from experiment to experiment. The main point is that the fronts of the advancing crests have moved to approximately the same distance in the two branches, showing that the same fast rate of transport is present in the desheathed as it is in the sheathed nerves. The usual pattern was also seen when an isotonic NaCl solution with 5 mM Ca^{2+} added was used as the incubation medium.

When, in similar experiments, Ca^{2+} was

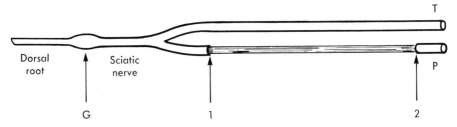

Fig. 7-2. Desheathed peroneal and sheathed tibial branches of sciatic nerve. In this diagram peroneal nerve, *P*, is shown desheathed from point 35 mm distal from center of L7 dorsal root ganglion, *G*, indicated by arrow *1*, down to 135 mm as shown by arrow *2*. Tibial nerve, *T*, is left sheathed. Peroneal nerve is usually contained in single funiculus. Therefore all nerve fibers ordinarily within sheath (shown in this figure by horizontal stripes) are exposed to medium.

deleted from the incubation medium, that is, when an isotonic NaCl medium was used, a different pattern was found (Fig. 7-4). The sheathed tibial nerve branch shows the usual shape and rate of transport, but in the desheathed peroneal nerve a damming up of activity is seen above the sheathed region and then a steep decline of outflow, ending in a block of transport. The decline in axoplasmic transport appears early, within about 20 to 30 minutes after incubation in the Ca^{2+}-free medium. It should be noted that the usual pattern of axoplasmic transport is maintained in the sheathed tibial nerve in conformity to our earlier studies showing that Ca^{2+} deletion had little effect on sheathed nerves.

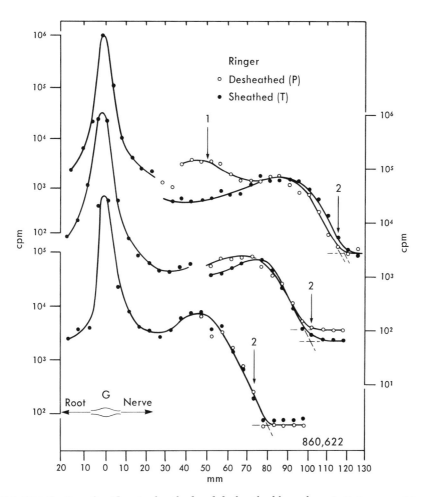

Fig. 7-3. Distribution of outflow in sheathed and desheathed branches. Activity present in dorsal root ganglia and peroneal desheathed, ○, and sheathed tibial, ●, nerves are shown for sciatic nerves of three cats taken 4.5, 6, and 7 hours after injection of ^{3}H-leucine into L7 dorsal root ganglia, G. Activity present in 5 mm segments of ganglia and nerves is given on ordinate in logarithmic divisions on partial scales. Ordinate scale for lowest nerve (4.5 hr) is at bottom left, at right for middle nerve (6 hr), and a partial scale at top left for uppermost nerve (7 hr). Approximate location of upper region where desheathing had been started is indicated by arrow *1*. In all cases fronts of outflow in sheathed and desheathed branches are closely similar (arrow *2*). Some variation in plateau regions is seen in upper nerves but this is not a constant feature.

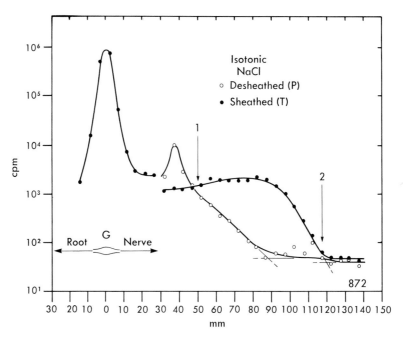

Fig. 7-4. Transport in Ca-free medium–isotonic NaCl. Following injection of L7 ganglion with ^{3}H-leucine and 2 hours of downflow in animal, sciatic nerve is removed, peroneal branch desheathed, and nerve placed in in vitro medium containing Ca-free isotonic NaCl. Points representing labeled materials are determined as indicated in Fig. 7-1. Above arrow, *1*, where peroneal nerve, ○, was desheathed, peak of dammed activity is seen followed by steep descent of outflow to baseline at close to 85 mm from ganglion where transport was blocked. Crest in tibial nerve, ●, shows normal outflow down to arrow *2* at expected distance of fast axoplasmic transport.

If different amounts of Ca^{2+} ranging from 3 to 5 mM are added to an isotonic NaCl solution, transport in the desheathed nerve has the normal shape and rate as that seen in the sheathed nerve branch (Fig. 7-5). However, this range of concentration is higher than that usual for Ca^{2+} in the extracellular fluid where a concentration of 1.5 to 2 mM Ca^{2+} is usually present. When this lower level of Ca^{2+} was present in the incubation medium, the crest was somewhat sloped, indicating a less than optimal outflow. On addition of 4 mM K^+ to the medium, a concentration of K^+ close to that found in the extracellular fluid, a normal outflow pattern and rate of transport was found with Ca^{2+} in the range of 0.75 to 2 mM.

Addition of buffer to the incubation medium does not apparently matter very much nor the buffer used—whether a phosphate, carbonate, or a tris buffer. For that matter, the medium may be left unbuffered. Transport is not very sensitive to variations of pH, most likely because the fibers have an internal buffering. Sodium does not appear to be essential for transport. If the NaCl of the medium is replaced with an isotonic sucrose medium, axoplasmic transport is maintained when Ca^{2+} is also present in the incubation medium.

Magnesium showed a small effect in the same direction as Ca^{2+}. With 5 mM Mg^{2+} present in an isotonic NaCl or sucrose medium a block occurs. However, the time of block is somewhat prolonged as compared

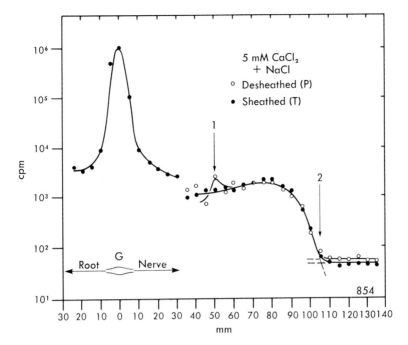

Fig. 7-5. Transport in 5 mM Ca-medium. After 2 hours of downflow in vivo, peroneal nerve, ○, was desheathed, tibial nerve, ●, left sheathed, and nerve placed in in vitro medium of 5 mM CaCl₂ and 140 mM NaCl for additional 4 hours. Outflow as determined in Figs. 7-3 and 7-4 shows similar rate of transport indicated by arrow *2* of crests of transported material in both nerves. Above arrow *1* indicating upper end of desheathed region, small degree of damming of activity is seen. Subsequent shape of outflow in both sheathed and desheathed branches was then closely comparable in shape.

to the block seen in a Ca²⁺-free medium.[34,35] Magnesium thus cannot maintain transport as does Ca²⁺.

HIGHER CONCENTRATIONS OF CALCIUM

When Ca²⁺ in concentrations above 35 mM is present in the incubation medium, a block of transport is also seen. With 50 mM Ca²⁺ present, the block effect on transport was clearly apparent (Fig. 7-6) and it occurred earlier than with 35 mM Ca²⁺. At very high concentrations of Ca²⁺, 95 to 100 mM, the block was much steeper and it occurred still more rapidly. With the collaboration of Dr. Jersild we have looked at these nerves, and in electron micrographs we found much alteration in the myelin sheaths, shrinkage of the axons, and a loss of microtubules and disruption of other organelles.

The implications of the morphological changes and transport block seen with high concentrations of Ca²⁺ present in the incubation medium is that regulatory processes for Ca²⁺ present in the fiber are able to maintain Ca²⁺ within some narrow range optimal for transport. When high amounts of Ca²⁺ are present in the medium, a sufficiently high level can enter the desheathed nerve fibers and overcome that regulation. Schlaepfer[37] has shown that Ca²⁺ can cause a loss of microtubules in axons when small pieces of nerve several millimeters long were immersed in media containing only several mM of Ca²⁺. In this procedure, Ca²⁺ can readily enter the fibers via their cut ends. In the desheathed nerve preparation the route for Ca²⁺ entry is through the membrane where normally only a small amount enters. The amount entering can be enhanced with A23187, an ionophore

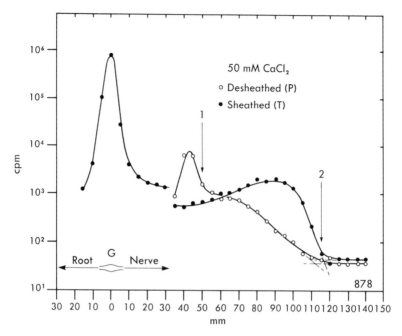

Fig. 7-6. Block of transport with high levels of Ca^{2+}. Using same experimental methods given in Fig. 7-5, with 50 mM Ca^{2+} present in solution (made isotonic with NaCl), damming of activity was seen above upper level of desheathing (arrow *1*) with decline in outflow distally. Sheathed nerve shows usual pattern of outflow and distance expected of fast axoplasmic transport (arrow *2*).

that predominately carried Ca^{2+} across the membrane. Schlaepfer[38] has shown that A23187 causes a disappearance of microtubules and neurofilaments from the fibers of desheathed rat nerves immersed in media containing 2 mM of Ca^{2+}. These changes did not occur in nerves with A23187 when Ca^{2+} was not present in the incubation medium, suggesting that the morphological changes seen in nerves treated with A23187 are due to a much increased level of Ca^{2+} inside the fibers, a level greater than the concentration of 10^{-7} M usually considered present in cells. We shall discuss this in a later section dealing with a new model of axoplasmic transport, one that includes Ca^{2+} and its intra-axonal regulation.

CALCIUM-BINDING PROTEIN

When ^{45}Ca is injected into the L7 dorsal root ganglion of the cat for uptake by the cell bodies, the same pattern of outflow of labeled activity seen with labeled proteins was found

and at the same fast rate of close to 410 mm/day.[15,16,35] While a plateau and a crest are present in the Ca^{2+}-labeled outflow curves, a much higher level of background activity was characteristically found. The higher background is due to a leakage of the injected Ca^{2+} into the circulation because the uptake mechanism for Ca^{2+} by the cell bodies is less active than it is for amino acids. With only a small amount of Ca^{2+} entering the cells, the remainder passes into the circulation to be locally taken up by the nerve sheaths. In the in vitro frog preparation, where the ganglia were loaded with ^{45}Ca and without circulation present, a large outflow pattern typical of fast transport was found.[12] It had the same fast rate as that of the mammalian nerve when the temperature was scaled to the higher temperature of the mammal and the Q_{10} taken into account.

In our studies of Ca^{2+} transport the transported Ca^{2+} is found carried down in association with a 15,000 mol wt protein, a protein

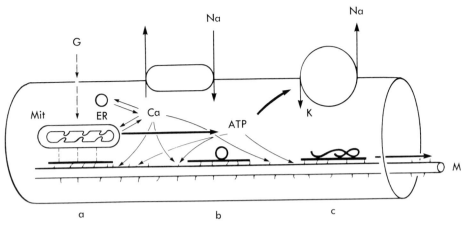

Fig. 7-7. New transport filament hypothesis. Glucose, *G*, enters fiber and, after glycolysis, oxidative phosphorylation in mitochondrion, *Mit*, gives rise to ATP. ~P of ATP supplies energy to sodium pump controlling level of Na$^+$ and K$^+$ in fiber and to cross-bridges activating movement of transport filaments along microtubules. Transport filaments are shown as black bars to which various components transported are bound and carried down fiber by cross-bridge activity. Components transported include mitochondria, *a*, attaching temporarily as indicated by dashed lines; soluble protein, *b*, shown in folded or globular configuration; polypeptides and small particulates, *c*. Thus a wide range of various components are transported at same fast rate of transport. Mg-Ca-ATPase found in nerve presumably utilizes ATP as source of energy. In addition, Ca^{2+} is shown present in fiber where it participates in movement of transport filaments, most likely by affecting CaBP (calmodulin) carried on transport filaments. Calcium level is regulated by mitochondria; endoplasmic reticulum, *ER;* and a Ca-Na exchange or Ca^{2+} pump in membrane.

identified as a calcium-binding protein (CaBP).[16] Sephadex G100 or G200 columns were used to separate higher molecular weight peak I and lower molecular weight peak II columns from high-speed supernatant fractions and Biogel A5m columns to further separate peak I into several subpeaks. Peak Ic contained a 15,000 mol wt protein fraction having properties similar to those found for CaBP obtained from other tissues. The CaBP found in brain synaptosomes has a similar molecular weight and a dissociation constant close to 6.6×10^{-5}.[15]

A NEW MODEL OF AXOPLASMIC TRANSPORT

The model of transport shown in Fig. 7-7 was modified to take into account our new findings with respect to Ca^{2+}. The Ca^{2+} in the nerve fiber is considered to be regulated at some low level as it is in the case of the squid giant axon and other cells where a concentra-

tion of about 10^{-7} M has been reported[8]; several mechanisms are required to regulate the overall level of Ca^{2+} in the fibers. Although only a small amount of Ca^{2+} continually enters the fibers at rest and a small increased entry of Ca^{2+} occurs during an action potential,[1] eventually it would accummulate without a process of Ca^{2+} removal.

A Ca^{2+}-pump or a Ca^{2+}-Na$^+$ exchange carrier is present in the membrane to remove Ca^{2+}.[1] A possible requirement for ATP by the Ca^{2+}-Na$^+$ exchange carrier in the squid axons membrane is not a settled matter. The Ca^{2+} could be removed from the cell in exchange for Na$^+$ entering the fiber as a passive process, with the Na$^+$ that enters eventually pumped out by the sodium pump. Possibly ATP is directly required as an energy source for the Na$^+$-Ca^{2+} exchange mechanism.[7] Another possibility is that ATP is needed as the nucleotide to promote Ca^{2+} exchange.[2,3,27]

Within cells, the level of Ca^{2+} is regulated also by the mitochondria. In the mitochondrion the supply of ATP and uptake of Ca^{2+} are interrelated.[4,21] We have found that nerves incubated in a low Ca^{2+} medium show some decrease in their level of $\sim$P—not enough to stop the transport on that account but enough to indicate that ATP production has been affected.[30]

The endoplasmic reticulum may also act to sequester and regulate the level of Ca^{2+} in the axoplasm. In some preliminary experiments carried out with Chan and Jersild, pyroantimonate staining of nerves for Ca^{2+} indicated dark-staining granules present inside the endoplasmic reticulum and the mitochondria in electron micrographs. A similar finding was recently reported for giant axons using an oxalate method.[13]

Another possible regulation of Ca^{2+} in nerve fibers may be afforded by the CaBP described in the preceding section. As noted above, the CaBP appears to be carried down the fibers at the fast rate. We can consider that the CaBP could be part of the transport filament and act as a local regulatory protein similar to other calmodulins. It responds to the low level of Ca^{2+} to in turn activate the ATPase. Thus the transport filament could control the utilization for ATP for movement of the transport filament by carrying calmodulin as well as the various components bound to it.

Depletion of Ca^{2+} by its removal from the medium and thence the fibers can thus inactivate the transport mechanism. An excess of Ca^{2+} entering the fibers could also overload the Ca^{2+} regulatory mechanisms and block transport by interfering with ATP utilization. Still higher levels could cause morphological changes as well, including microtubule disaggregation.

SOME SPECULATIONS ON THE NERVE SHEATH IN RELATION TO NERVE REPAIR

The effect on axoplasmic transport of a removal of Ca^{2+} from the media in which the desheathed preparation is incubated had a surprisingly early onset, the outflow slope beginning to decrement within 15 to 20 minutes. This suggests that the Ca^{2+} regulatory processes are likely to be very active in the fibers of mammalian nerve. Damage to the perineurial sheath as a result of disease or trauma could, by altering Ca^{2+} levels around the fibers, indirectly cause a block of transport. This in turn would lead to degeneration and, if maintained, prevent nerve regeneration. It has been shown that even a small incision of the perineurium leads to morphological signs of damage in the fibers.[41,42] Clinical experience also suggests the importance of the perineurium; an aim in nerve repair being to close the sheaths to promote the healing and regeneration of the fibers.

Study of the perineurium for its role in regulation of the composition of the endoneurial compartment has so far received relatively little attention. Most information relating to ionic regulation within the nervous system has been directed to the brain.[36] Further study of a possible contribution of the perineurium to the regulation of the composition of the fluid components of the endoneurium and in turn the normal maintenance of axoplasmic transport may very well be important for development of procedures to restore nerve function after trauma and in the management of other neuropathies.

ACKNOWLEDGMENTS

I am grateful to my colleagues, Dr. Z. Iqbal, Dr. R. Worth, and Shew-Yin Chan, who integrally participated in these studies, and to the able technical help of Mr. Larry Smith and Ms. Jenny Gallagher. Thanks are also due to the Illustrations Department. The support of the NIH grant PHS R01 NS 8706-09 and the NSF grant BNS 75 03868-A03 were instrumental in the pursuit of these studies.

REFERENCES

1. Baker, P. F.: Transport and metabolism of calcium ions in nerve, Prog. Biophys. Mol. Biol. **24**:177, 1972.
2. Baker, P. F.: The regulation of intracellular calcium, Symp. Soc. Exp. Biol. **30**:67, 1976.
3. Blaustein, M. P.: The interrelationship between sodium and calcium fluxes across cell membranes, Rev. Phsyiol. Biochem. Pharmacol. **70**:33, 1974.

4. Carafoli, E., and Crompton, M.: Calcium ions and mitochondria, Symp. Soc. Exp. Biol. **30**:89, 1976.

5. Crescitelli, F.: Nerve sheath as a barrier to the action of certain substances, Am. J. Physiol. **166**:229, 1951.

6. Dahlström, A.: Influence of colchicine on axoplasmic transport of amine storage granules in rat sympathetic adrenergic nerves, Acta Physiol. Scand. **76**:33A, 1969.

7. DiPolo, R.: The influence of nucleotides on calcium fluxes, Fed. Proc. **35**:2579, 1976.

8. Duncan, C. J., ed.: Calcium in biological systems. Symposium 30, Society Experimental Biology, Cambridge, 1976, Cambridge University Press.

9. Edström, A.: Ionic requirements for rapid axonal transport in vitro in frog sciatic nerves, Acta Physiol. Scand. **93**:104, 1975.

10. Grafstein, B.: Axonal transport: the intracellular traffic of the neuron. In Kandel, E. R., ed.: Handbook of physiology. Section 1: the nervous system. Vol. 1: cellular biology of neurons, Part 1, Washington, D.C., 1977, The American Physiological Society, Chap. 19, p. 691.

11. Gray, E. G.: The fine structure of nerve, Comp. Biochem. Physiol. **36**:419, 1970.

12. Hammerschlag, R., Dravid, A. R., and Chiu, A. Y.: Mechanism of axonal transport: a proposed role for calcium ions, Science **188**:273, 1975.

13. Henkart, M., Reese, T. S., and Brinley, F. J.: Oxalate produces precipitates in endoplasmic reticulum of Ca-loaded squid axons, Biophys. J. **21**:187a, 1978.

14. Heslop, J. P.: Axonal flow and fast transport in nerves, Adv. Comp. Physiol. Biochem. **6**:75, 1975.

15. Iqbal, Z., and Ochs, S.: Calcium binding protein in brain synaptosomes, Soc. Neurosci. Abst. **1**:47, 1976.

16. Iqbal, Z., and Ochs, S.: Fast axoplasmic transport of a calcium-binding protein in mammalian nerve, J. Neurochem. **31**:409, 1978.

17. Khan, M. A., and Ochs, S.: Magnesium or calcium activated ATPase in mammalian nerve, Brain Res. **81**:413, 1974.

18. Kreutzberg, G. W.: Neuronal dynamics and axonal flow. IV. Blockage of intra-axonal enzyme transport by colchicine, Proc. Natl. Acad. Sci. U.S.A. **62**:722, 1969.

19. Krnjević, K.: The distribution of Na and K in cat nerves, J. Physiol. **128**:473, 1955.

20. Lasek, R.: Personal communication.

21. Lehninger, A. L.: Biochemistry, ed. 2, New York, 1975, Worth Publishers, Inc.

22. Livett, B. G.: Axonal transport and neuronal dynamics: contributions to the study of neuronal connectivity, Int. Rev. Physiol. **10**:37, 1976.

23. Low, F. N.: The perineurium and connective tissue of peripheral nerve. In Landon, D. N., ed.: The peripheral nerve, New York, 1976, John Wiley & Sons, Inc., p. 159.

24. Lubińska, L.: Early course of Wallerian degeneration in myelinated fibres of the rat phrenic nerve, Brain Res. **130**:47, 1977.

25. McClure, W. O.: Effect of drugs upon axoplasmic transport, Adv. Pharmacol. Chemother. **10**:185, 1972.

26. McComas, A. J., et al.: Sick motor neurones and dystrophy: a reappraisal. In Rowland, L. P., ed.: Pathogenesis of human muscular dystrophies, Amsterdam, 1977, Excerpta Medica, p. 180.

27. Mullins, L. J.: A mechanism for Na/Ca transport, J. Gen. Physiol. **70**:681, 1977.

28. Ochs, S.: Fast transport of materials in mammalian nerve fibers, Science **176**:252, 1972.

29. Ochs, S.: Rate of fast axoplasmic transport in mammalian nerve fibres, J. Physiol. **227**:627, 1972.

30. Ochs, S.: Energy metabolism and supply of ~P to the fast axoplasmic transport mechanism in nerve, Fed. Proc. **33**:1049, 1974.

31. Ochs, S.: Axoplasmic transport. In Siegel, G. J. et al., eds.: Basic neurochemistry, ed. 2, Boston, 1976, Little, Brown & Co., p. 429.

32. Ochs, S., and Smith, C.: Low temperature slowing and cold-block of fast axoplasmic transport in mammalian nerves in vitro, J. Neurobiol. **6**:85, 1975.

33. Ochs, S., and Worth, R. M.: Axoplasmic transport in normal and pathological systems. In Waxman, S., ed.: Physiology and pathobiology of axons, New York, 1978, Raven Press.

34. Ochs, S., Worth, R. M., and Chan, S. Y.: Calcium requirement for axoplasmic transport in mammalian nerve, Nature **270**:748, 1977.

35. Ochs, S., et al.: Calcium requirement for axoplasmic transport and its deregulation in relation to elements of the transport filament model. In Roberts, S., Lajtha, A., and Gispen, W. H., eds.: Mechanisms, regulation and special function of protein synthesis in the brain, Amsterdam, 1977, Elsevier, p. 129.

36. Rapoport, S. I.: Blood-brain barrier in physiology and medicine, New York, 1976, Raven Press.

37. Schlaepfer, W. W.: Calcium-induced degeneration of axoplasm in isolated segments of rat peripheral nerve, Brain Res. **69**:203, 1974.

38. Schlaepfer, W. W.: Structural alterations of peripheral nerve induced by the calcium ionophore A23187, Brain Res. **136**:1, 1977.

39. Shanthaveerappa, T. R., and Bourne, G. H.: The 'perineural epithelium', a metabolically active, continuous, protoplasmic cell barrier surrounding peripheral nerve fasciculi, J. Anat. (Lond) **96**:527, 1962.

40. Sloboda, R. D., et al.: Microtubule-associated proteins (MAPs) and the assembly of microtubules in vitro. In Goldman, R., Pollard, T., and Rosenbaum, J., eds.: Cell motility. Book C: Microtubules and related proteins, New York, 1976, Cold Spring Harbor Laboratory, p. 1171.

41. Spencer, P. S., et al.: The perineurial window—a new model of focal demyelination and remyelination, Brain Res. **96**:323, 1975.

42. Sunderland, S.: The effect of rupture of the perineurium on the contained nerve-fibres, Brain **69:**149, 1946.

43. Sunderland, S.: Nerves and nerve injuries, London, 1968, Livingstone.

44. Sunderland, S., and Bradley, K. C.: The perineurium of peripheral nerves, Anat. Rec. **113:** 125, 1952.

45. Thomas, P. K., and Olsson, Y.: Microscopic anatomy and function of the connective tissue components of peripheral nerve. In Dyck, P. J., Thomas, P. K., and Lamberts, E. H., eds.: Peripheral neuropathy, vol. 1, Philadelphia, 1975, W. B. Saunders Co., Chap. 9, p. 168.

DISCUSSION

Jewett: Would you describe the role of fast axonal transport in axonal growth?

Ochs: The rate of transport that we determine by this technique is regular, at 410 mm/day or roughly 17 mm/hr. The rate of regeneration varies in clinical material and in experimental material but is some several millimeters or so a day. The rate of transport then should be looked on as a much faster supply of materials, which are going down to the fiber and to the growth cone. This is a very active region of the growing nerve fiber, most likely acted on by tropic materials from the environment as indicated by Cajal, a directive influence of some kind on the wandering growth cone moving incessantly in response to the tropic signal in the environment. Behind it is the enlarging fine unmyelinated fiber, the growing fiber. We are dealing with a supply line that is supported by a much faster transport than the longitudinal growth itself. Thus a number of mechanisms are involved, those maintaining the growth cone and those acting to enlarge and increase the length of the growing fiber.

Jewett: When a large fiber with many microtubules having a constant rate of transport enters a small endoneurial tube, does that mean that the axonal growth is going to be greater from then on?

Ochs: No. The relation of transport to microtubules, however, raises some interesting considerations. If we go back to embryogenesis of the ganglion neurons, these are at first bipolar cells with fibrillary material passing out each pole. The fibers themselves are very thin. Later, as growth continues, we have a situation in which fibrillary material passes both centrally and peripherally from the cell body. The dorsal root cell maintains an orientation so that this fibrillary material is going to be directed both into the central nervous system where its terminals are transmitters and to the sensory ends where there are receptors. As was subsequently shown, this fibrillary material consists of microtubules and neurofilaments. Some 3 to 5 times more material is moving down the sensory branch compared to the dorsal root branch even though the numbers of microtubules and neurofilaments are similar in each branch. Thus it is possible for more material to move down a given set of microtubules than the other. In the case of regeneration, the growing fibers are probably small enough to enter old nerve tubes. If the tubes they are going to are too small for that fiber, there is likely to be a reduction in the size of the fibers in the restricted region.

Tupper: What is the correlation between the axoplasmic transfer of axonal material and the oozing of material one sees at the cut end of the nerve at surgery?

Ochs: The subject of oozing of material from the ends of cut nerves is very old. In the 17th and the 18th centuries, material oozing out from cut nerves was taken as evidence for a constant movement of fluid down the hollow nerve tubes. All I can say is that this phenomenon probably indicates that there is some internal pressure present within the fiber, but this oozing is not related to the actual mechanism of material transport in the axon.

8

Effects of graded compression on axonal transport and nerve barriers

J. Sjöstrand, B. Rydevik, G. Lundborg, and W. G. McLean

Trauma to a nerve trunk may affect all tissue components of the trunk, that is, nerve fibers, connective tissue, and intraneural microvessels. These various structures react to trauma in different ways; nerve fibers may react to the injury by demyelination, for example, as discussed by Ochoa in this volume, or by degeneration.

Within the nerve fibers there is a continuous transport of macromolecules and organelles both from the cell body to the synaptic terminals and in a retrograde direction as reviewed by Ochs in this volume. This axonal transport may be partially or completely blocked by local ischemia or compression.[1,4,10,11,16]

Normal nerve function requires a continuous supply of oxygen by the intraneural microcirculation, and impairment of intraneural blood flow may cause varying degrees of deterioration of nerve function.[6,17]

Furthermore, trauma to a nerve trunk may induce increased permeability of the intraneural microvessels leading to intraneural edema formation (see reviews by Lundborg[7] and Olsson[14]).

The endothelium of the *intrafascicular* capillaries normally constitutes a *blood-nerve barrier*[12,23] analogous to the blood-brain barrier of the central nervous system. The nerve fascicles are surrounded by a *perineurial sheath*, which acts as a diffusion *barrier* against a number of substances, for example, proteins.[8,15,22] The local environment of the nerve fibers in the intrafascicular space is normally controlled by the joint action of the blood-nerve barrier and the perineurial barrier.[7,15]

Derangement of one or both of these barriers might have serious consequences for nerve function as seen after experimental ischemic, mechanical, and chemical trauma.[6,12,13,20]

To elucidate the pathophysiology of acute nerve compression we have studied the alterations in axonal transport, intraneural microcirculation, and nerve barriers produced by experimental compression injury to peripheral nerves. A compression apparatus consisting of a small Plexiglas chamber containing a pair of rubber membranes was used (for details see Rydevik and Lundborg[18]). The two halves of the chamber were apposed around vagus or tibial nerves in rabbits, and the membranes were inflated to controlled pressure (50, 200, or 400 mm Hg).

AXONAL TRANSPORT

The fast axonal transport of ^{3}H-labeled proteins along the cervical vagus nerve was measured as described previously,[9] and the effect of local, graded compression was studied. In acute experiments (that is, without recovery from compression) vagus nerves were compressed 2 hours after labeling of the nodose ganglion with ^{3}H-leucine; in others, recovery from compression of up to 14 days was allowed before the ganglia were labeled. In all experiments 4 hours were allowed for the synthesis of protein in the cell body in the nodose ganglion, transport along the cervical vagus nerve, and time for radioactive pro-

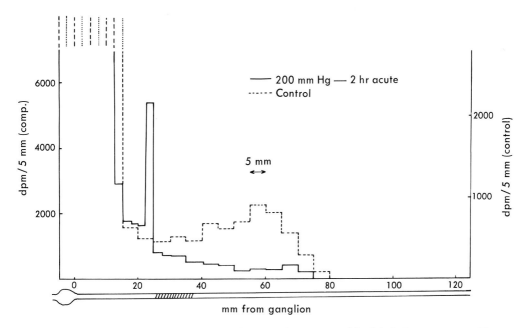

Fig. 8-1. Effect of nerve compression on fast axonal transport of ^{3}H-labeled proteins in rabbit vagus nerves. Profiles demonstrate distribution of ^{3}H-labeled material along vagus nerves 4 hours after injection of ^{3}H-leucine into nodose ganglia in untreated nerve (interrupted line) and nerve subjected to pressure of 200 mm Hg for 2 hours (solid line) within indicated zone. Total block of axonal transport can be seen in compressed nerve.

teins to accumulate in the case of transport block caused by the local compression.

The profile of the distribution of labeled proteins in the vagus nerve 4 hours after the injection into the nodose ganglion is illustrated in Fig. 8-1. In untreated nerves a wave front of labeled proteins was seen in agreement with previous studies.[9]

In nerves that had been subjected to local compression, an acute accumulation of labeled proteins was found in the region of compression (Fig. 8-1). A pressure as low as 50 mm Hg for 2 hours disrupts axonal transport and causes an accumulation of rapidly transported proteins proximal to the compression site; however, this is reversible within 1 day. The higher pressures tested, that is, 200 mm Hg and 400 mm Hg, applied for 2 hours, induced a corresponding block (Fig. 8-1) that was more pronounced in these nerves. Reversal of transport blockade occur-

red in most cases within 3 days after compression at 200 mm Hg for 2 hours and within 7 days after compression at 400 mm Hg for 2 hours.[21] Thus, time required for recovery of normal transport was correlated to the magnitude of the pressure applied and recovered transport was mostly found within the first week after compression.

Some effects of elevated pressure on axonal transport have been reported previously[1,11] with recovery of fast transport after restoration of normal pressures. The precise mechanism by which nerve compression may block axonal transport has not been demonstrated. It is clear from the work reported here that axonal transport can recover from blockade caused by ischemia and/or compression without nerve degeneration and subsequent nerve regeneration. In our results the rate of recovery of transport was dependent on the severity of compression.

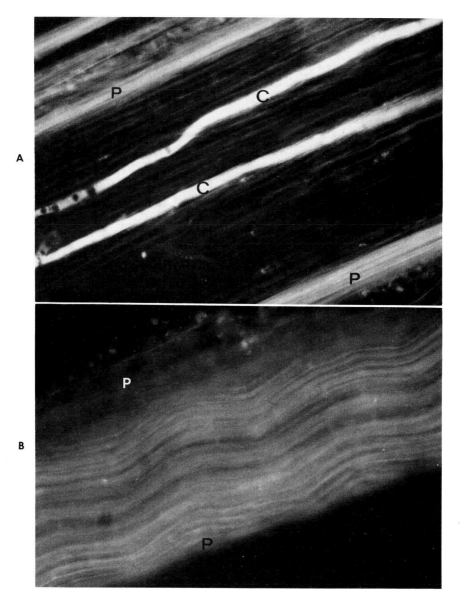

Fig. 8-2. Fluorescence microscopic examination of longitudinal sections of rabbit tibial nerve. Evans-blue-albumin (EBA) has been injected 30 minutes prior to removal of specimens. **A,** Control nerve. One fascicle is shown. Red-fluorescent EBA-complex (here white) has perfused intrafascicular (endoneurial) capillaries, *c*. Dye is strictly confined to lumina of these vessels, which contrasts distinctly to green nerve tissue (here greyish black). Perineurium, *p*, surrounds fascicle. **B,** Tibial nerve following compression by 400 mm Hg during 2 hours. Specimen taken from *edge* of compressed segment. Trauma has induced increased permeability of intrafascicular capillaries leading to formation of intrafascicular edema. This is demonstrated by diffuse orange-red fluorescence (here white) among nerve fibers.

INTRANEURAL MICROCIRCULATION AND NERVE BARRIERS

Complete ischemia is followed by blocked impulse conduction in the nerve within 30 to 90 minutes.[2,3,6] However, if ischemia time does not exceed 6 hours, nerve function generally recovers when intraneural blood flow is reestablished.[6]

In experiments where a tourniquet was insufflated around the thigh of rabbits, alterations in nerve function after release of the pressure were correlated to intraneural edema formation.[6] The nerves studied were the tibial nerve (situated distal to the cuff and thus subjected to ischemia only) and the sciatic nerve (subjected also to compression of the cuff). It was found that there was a parallelism between the establishment of *intrafascicular edema* and persistent *loss of nerve function*, which occurred after 8 hours ischemia of the tibial nerve and after 4 hours cuff compression of the sciatic nerve.

In recent experimental investigations[18] the mechanisms behind edema formation in peripheral nerves following acute, graded compression, applied by the previously mentioned compression chamber, have been analyzed. The results show that a slight trauma induced in a rabbit's tibial nerve (for example, 50 mm Hg during 2 hours) caused an epineurial edema, which was prevented from reaching the nerve fibers in the fascicles by the perineurial barrier. Compression of higher pressure levels (for example, 200 and 400 mm Hg during 2 hours) or prolonged duration induced breakdown of the blood-nerve barrier, leading to intrafascicular edema formation (Fig. 8-2), which generally was most prominent at the edges of the compressed nerve segment. The perineural barrier was, however, remarkably resistant to compression trauma.

An intrafascicular edema may increase the intrafascicular pressure,[5] leading to further impairment of the intrafascicular microcirculation. The edema also alters the local environment of the axons by deranging the ionic balance. Moreover, a long-standing edema may become invaded by fibroblasts and transferred to an intrafascicular fibrotic scar.[19]

In summary, compression trauma induced in peripheral nerve trunks may affect nerve fibers as well as intraneural microvessels. Factors like intraneural edema formation and disturbances in axonal transport may contribute to the reversible or irreversible functional deterioration sometimes seen after such lesions.

REFERENCES

1. Andersson, D. R., and Hendrickson, A.: Effect of intraocular pressure on rapid axoplasmic transport in monkey optic nerve, Invest. Ophthalmol. **13**:771, 1974.
2. Gerard, R. W.: The response of nerve to oxygen lack, Am. J. Physiol. **92**:498, 1930.
3. Lehmann, J. E.: The effects of asphyxia on mammalian nerve fibers, Am. J. Physiol. **119**:11, 1937.
4. Levy, N. S.: The effects of elevated intraocular pressure on slow axonal protein flow, Invest. Ophthalmol. **13**:691, 1974.
5. Low, P. A., and Dyck, P. J.: Increased endoneurial fluid pressure in experimental lead neuropathy, Nature **269**:427, 1977.
6. Lundborg, G.: Ischemic nerve injury. Experimental studies on intraneural microvascular pathophysiology and nerve function in a limb subjected to temporary circulatory arrest, Scand. J. Plast. Reconstr. Surg. Suppl. **6**, 1970.
7. Lundborg, G.: Structure and function of the intraneural microvessels as related to trauma, edema formation and nerve function, J. Bone Joint Surg. **57A**:938, 1975.
8. Martin, K. H.: Untersuchungen über die perineurale Diffusionsbarriäre an gefriertrockneten Nerven, Z. Zellforsch. Mikr. Anat. **64**:404, 1964.
9. McLean, W. G., Frizell, M., and Sjöstrand, J.: Slow axonal transport of proteins in sensory fibers of rabbit vagus nerve, J. Neurochem. **26**:1213, 1976.
10. Minckler, D. S., Tso, M. O. M., and Zimmerman, L. E.: A light microscopic autoradiographic study of axoplasmic transport in the optic nerve head during ocular hypotony, increased intraocular pressure, and papilledema, Am. J. Ophthalmol. **82**:741, 1976.
11. Ochs, S.: Energy metabolism and supply of ~P to the fast axoplasmic transport mechanism in nerve. Fed. Proc. **33**:1049, 1974.
12. Olsson, Y.: Studies on vascular permeability in peripheral nerves. I. Distribution of circulating fluorescent serum albumin in normal, crushed and sectioned rat sciatic nerve, Acta Neuropathol. **7**:1, 1966.
13. Olsson, Y.: Studies on vascular permeability in peripheral nerves. 3. Permeability changes of vasa nervorum and exudation of serum albumin in INH-induced neuropathy of the rat, Acta Neuropathol. **11**:103, 1968.
14. Olsson, Y.: Vascular permeability in the peripheral nervous system. In Dyck, P. J., Thomas, P. K.,

Lambert, E. H., eds.: Peripheral neuropathy, Philadelphia, 1975, N. B. Saunders Co., pp. 190-200.

15. Olsson, Y., Kristensson, K., and Klatzo, I.: Permeability of blood vessels and connective tissue sheaths in the peripheral nervous system to exogenous proteins, Acta Neuropathol. Suppl. **V:**61, 1971.

16. Quigley, H. A., and Anderson, D. R.: The dynamics and location of axonal transport blockade by acute intraocular pressure elevation in primate optic nerve, Invest. Ophthalmol. **15:**606, 1976.

17. Roberts, J. T. The effects of occlusive arterial diseases of the extremities on the blood supply of nerves. Experimental and clinical studies on the role of vasa nervorum, Am. Heart J. **35:**369, 1948.

18. Rydevik, B., and Lundborg, G.: Permeability of intraneural microvessels and perineurium in acute, graded experimental nerve compression, Scand. J. Plast. Reconstr. Surg. **11:**179, 1977.

19. Rydevik, B., Lundborg, G., and Nordborg, C.: In-traneural tissue reactions induced by internal neurolysis, Scand. J. Plast. Reconstr. Surg. **10:**3, 1976.

20. Rydevik, B., et al.: Effects of chymopapain on nerve tissue. An experimental study on the structure and function of peripheral nerve tissue in rabbits after local application of chymopapain, Spine **1:**137, 1976.

21. Rydevik, B., et al.: Blockage of axonal transport induced by acute, graded compression of the rabbit vagus nerve. In press.

22. Shanta, T. R., and Bourne, G. H.: The perineurial epithelium—a new concept. In Bourne, G. H., ed.: Structure and function of nervous tissue, vol. 1, Structure, London, 1969, Academic Press, Inc., pp. 379-459.

23. Waksman, B. H.: Experimental study of diphtheritic polyneuritis in the rabbit and guinea pig. III. The blood-nerve barrier in the rabbit, J. Neuropathol. Exp. Neurol. **20:**35, 1961.

9

The use of axonally transported radioactive proteins as markers of axonal regeneration following crush or suture

David S. Forman

Axonal transport, which Dr. Ochs has described in this volume, has an important role in nerve regeneration. This physiological process can also be exploited as an experimental tool for studying axonal regeneration. Labeling axons with transported radioactive proteins has become a widespread technique for tracing neuroanatomical pathways in the central nervous system.[5] Dr. Richard Berenberg and I[6,7] and others[2,3,8,12] have used this approach in peripheral nerves in order to measure the rate of outgrowth and other properties of the regeneration process. In our experiments we produced a second degree nerve injury by crushing rat sciatic nerves for 90 seconds with plastic covered jeweler's forceps. In other experiments the nerves were sectioned and rejoined with 2 or 3 epineurial sutures using 10-0 nylon. From 2 days to a month after the injury, a radioactive amino acid ([3H]proline) was microinjected stereotactically into the region of the lumbar spinal cord containing the motoneurons that supply the sciatic nerve.[8,10] The rats were killed 24 hours later, and the distribution of radioactivity along the nerve was determined by liquid scintillation counting. Axonally transported radioactive proteins marked the locations of the regenerating motor axons. Typical results are illustrated in Fig. 9-1. From the patterns of radioactivity we were able to deduce the location of the tips of the most rapidly growing axons. In the crushed nerves these axons moved down the nerves at a rate of 4.4 (± 0.2 SE) mm/day after a delay at the scar of 2.1 (± 0.2) days. In the crushed nerves there was also a peak of radioactivity (region 4 in Fig. 9-1, A) that represents the ends of slower axons that grow at a rate of 3.0 (± 0.2) mm/day after a delay of 3.2 (± 0.3) days.[7] In the sutured nerves the delay was longer; the outgrowth was slower (Fig. 9-1, B), and more radioactivity was found at the site of the lesion (Fig. 9-1, B, region 1), reflecting axons that were trapped at the scar. Measurements of the rate of growth in the sutured nerves are still in progress.

We applied this method to study the clinically significant problem of whether thyroid hormone treatment can accelerate axonal outgrowth. Kiernan and co-workers have reported that daily injections of triiodothyronine (T_3) dramatically enhanced the rate of axonal growth in regenerating rat sciatic nerves.[4,9,11] However, in our own laboratory we found that T_3 had no effect on the outgrowth of the fastest sensory axons, although there was a small improvement in the recovery of motor function.[1] We used the axonal transport technique to test whether the improved motor recovery was due to accelerated growth of motor axons and found that 25 μg/kg/day of T_3 had no detectable effect on the growth rate, as reflected in the labeling patterns, in either crushed or sutured nerves. Since the small improvement in the return of motor function is not due to accelerated axonal growth, we are trying to

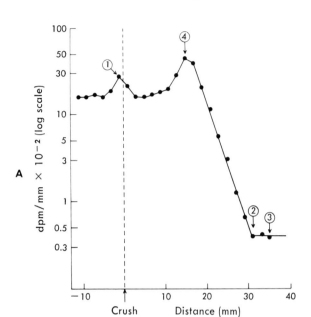
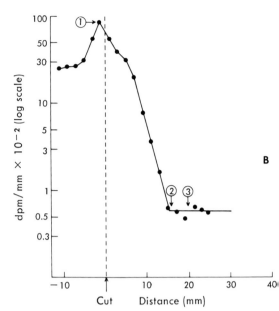

Fig. 9-1. Distribution of axonally transported radioactive proteins in regenerating rat sciatic nerve 8 days after nerve injury. **A,** Nerve crushed without significant damage to endoneurium (second degree injury). **B,** Nerve sectioned and rejoined by epineurial sutures. Tritiated proline was microinjected into lumbar spinal cord[8,10] 24 hours before animals were killed. Nerves were cut into 2 mm segments and radioactivity measured by liquid scintillation counting. Methods are described in detail elsewhere.[7] This labeling pattern does not show first arrival of wave of rapidly transported radioactive proteins, as discussed in Chapter 7, which arrive in this region after a few hours.[8] Instead, it represents radioactivity from that wave that was deposited in axon and remains there 24 hours after injection. Important details of radioactivity distribution include the following: *1,* Peak of radioactivity at region of injury caused by accumulation of radioactivity in ends of axons that have not regenerated into distal stump. *2,* Most distal axonally transported radioactivity, which therefore marks location of tips of axons that grew most rapidly. *3,* Low constant level of radioactivity in this region is not caused by axonal transport; rather, it is produced by labeled precursor that was carried to nerve in bloodstream and incorporated into non-neural cells. *4,* Crushed nerve only: this peak of radioactivity shows location of ends of large number of axons that grow down nerve together.

determine what other mechanism might be responsible. Our conclusion is that T_3 does not speed up axonal outgrowth and that the effect on return of motor function is small. Therefore the results of our animal experiments to date do not lend support to the idea that clinical trials of thyroid hormone therapy in humans with nerve injuries would be worthwhile. The method we used to reach this conclusion, tracing the regenerating axons with axonally transported radioactivity,

can be applied to a broad range of other experimental questions concerning the regeneration of injured nerves.

REFERENCES

1. Berenberg, R. A., et al.: Recovery of peripheral nerve function after axotomy: effect of triiodothyronine, Exp. Neurol. **57:**349, 1977.
2. Black, M. M., and Lasek, R. J.: The use of axonal transport to measure axonal regeneration in rat ventral motor neurons, Anat. Rec. **184:**360, 1976.
3. Black, M. M., and Lasek, R. J.: Axonal regeneration

in immature and adult rats, Neurosci. Abstr. **2:**820, 1976.

4. Cockett, S. A., and Kiernan, J. A.: Acceleration of peripheral nervous regeneration in the rat by exogenous triiodothyronine, Exp. Neurol. **39:**389, 1973.

5. Cowan, W. M., and Cuénod, M., eds.: The use of axonal transport for studies of neuronal connectivity, New York, 1975, Elsevier.

6. Forman, D. S., and Berenberg, R. A.: Regeneration in the rat sciatic nerve studied with axonally transported radioactive proteins, Neurosci. Abstr. **3:**425, 1977.

7. Forman, D. S., and Berenberg, R. A.: Regeneration of motor axons in the rat sciatic nerve studied by labeling with axonally transported radioactive proteins, Brain Res. **156:**213, 1978.

8. Griffin, J. W., Price, D. B., and Drachman, D. B.: Fast axonal transport in motor nerve regeneration, J. Neurobiol. **7:**355, 1976.

9. Kiernan, J. A., and Heinicke, E.: Estimation of lengths of regenerated axons in the nerve, Exp. Neurol. **56:**431, 1977.

10. Lasek, R. J.: Axoplasmic transport of labeled proteins in rat ventral motor neurons, Exp. Neurol. **21:**41, 1968.

11. McIsaac, G., and Kiernan, J. A.: Accelerated recovery from peripheral nerve injury in experimental hyperthyroidism, Exp. Neurol. **48:**88, 1975.

12. McQuarrie, I. G.: The effect of a conditioning lesion on the regeneration of motor axons, Brain Res. **152:**597, 1978.

DISCUSSION

Editor: Does the difference between the fastest axons that grow at a rate of 4.4 mm/day and the slower axons in the peak that move 3 mm/day continue to hold throughout the length of the nerve after crushing?

Forman: Yes. The fastest fibers advance at a constant rate of 4.4 mm/day throughout the length of the nerve. The slower fibers not only begin to grow later but continue down the nerve at the slower speed of 3.0 mm/day.* This seems to suggest that each regenerating axon grows at a characteristic constant velocity that is not the same for all axons.

Editor: Is there any way you can determine whether the slower fiber peak in the crushed nerves (3 mm/day) are smaller diameter fibers than those that grow more rapidly?

Forman: It should be possible using electron microscopic autoradiography.* However, we do not have that information.

---

*Forman and Berenberg: Neurosci. Abstr. **3**:425, 1977; Forman and Berenberg: Brain Res. **156**:213, 1978.

*Griffin, Price, and Drachman: J. Neurobiol. **7**:355, 1976.

10

Metabolic consequences of axotomy and regrowth

Thomas B. Ducker

Injury to a peripheral nerve (axon) involves removal of a large portion of the nerve cell volume; however, the biochemical machinery required for repair remains largely intact because it is localized in the soma or cell body. Because of their unique geometry, nerve cells must synthesize large amounts of structural material and transport these materials over relatively long distances. If the central cell body were the height of an average man, its axon would be 1 or 2 inches in diameter and would extend more than 2 miles. The energy expenditure needed to synthesize structural materials as well as factors associated with neurotransmission and transport these over long distances becomes very large and requires markedly enlarged and metabolically hyperactive cell bodies. The mature nerve cell is among the most metabolically active cell types in our bodies.[34] With axonal injury, or disease, even higher metabolic activity occurs and profound changes take place in the structure as well as the biochemical and physiological properties of the cell body. Some of these changes may be viewed as particularly appropriate for the repair process. After axonal injury, chromatolysis, nuclear eccentricity, nucleolar enlargement, and cell swelling are the most conspicuous morphological changes seen during the retrograde response.[19] For peripheral axons, these changes have been associated with a reorganization and enhanced formation of cytoplasmic ribonucleic acid (RNA) to a more active state directed toward the reconstitution of lost axoplasm and recovery of peripheral connections.[2,27,36]

Increases in RNA synthesis, as expected, have been associated with enhanced cytoplasmic protein synthesis as demonstrated by the incorporation of radioactive amino acid precursors.[3,7,8,9,36] The changes in protein synthesis are complex and appear to involve a reordering of the various types of proteins synthesized by the injured neuron. Materials required for transmitter function are decreased, while materials required for regeneration of the axon are elevated. For example, in adrenergic neurons decreases in dopamine-B-hydroxylase, Dopa decarboxylase, monamine oxidase, and tyrosine hydroxylase activities occur after axotomy.[6,17,30,31] Similar decreases in acetylcholinesterase and choline acetyltransferase have been reported in axotomized cholinergic neurons.[15,19] In contrast, the activity of glucose-6-phosphate dehydrogenase, a key enzyme by which glucose is converted to precursors required for the biosynthesis of nucleic acids and lipids, is significantly elevated in axotomized neurons.[13,14,37]

A number of histochemical and biochemical studies have demonstrated that the activity of glucose-6-phosphate dehydrogenase is increased in axotomized nerve cell bodies. Spinal anterior horn cells, facial nucleus neurons, and sympathetic ganglion cells, all of which direct axons to peripheral structures, show such changes in the pentose phosphate pathway.[12,16,18,29,32] Increases in this activity are not observed in neuronal perikarya whose axons undergo wallerian degeneration.[22] In extended studies of metabolic changes in the axotomized rat superior cervical ganglion, strong evidence has been obtained that increases in glucose-6-phosphate dehydrogenase occurring shortly after axotomy are associated with increased metabolism of glucose via the anabolic pentose pathway.[13,14] This increase occurs in the absence of any gross alteration in the major energy-yielding reactions such as ATP utilization and oxygen consumption.

Enhanced metabolism via the pentose pathway may have special significance in injured peripheral neurons because two functions of this pathway are to generate NADPH for reductive biosynthetic reactions and to form ribose phosphate required for nucleic acid and ribonucleotide biosynthesis. Studies carried out on non-neuronal tissue provide strong evidence that the formation of NADPH by the pentose pathway is intimately related to the biosynthesis of fatty acids.[1] A similar relationship may exist in regenerating neural tissue because significant increases in lipid synthesis begin with the first week after axonal injury.[13,14,25]

The regenerative process in nerve cell bodies is complicated by the simultaneous occurrence of extensive hydrolytic activity during the period of enhanced biosynthetic activity. A marked increase in acid phosphatase and a corresponding increase in the internal complexity and number of lysome-like dense bodies has been frequently noted in axotomized nerve cells.[21,33] Matthews and Raisman[21] have suggested that the increased hydrolytic activity is related to a digestion of transmitter storage granules in axotomized nerve cells. It is not known whether these changes are a necessary prerequisite for axonal sprouting and regeneration.

The regenerative capacity of neurons varies with age. Axonal outgrowth from proximal stumps of transected nerves appears to be more rapid, and reconnection with denervated end-organs occurs more rapidly in younger animals than in older animals.[11,26]

Pertinent histological and temporal characteristics of the retrograde response of various classes of neurons in young animals have been recently reviewed by Brodal.[4] Data concerning biochemical differences between young and mature axotomized nerve cells are minimal, and it is not clear what mechanisms account for the greater regenerative capacity of neural tissue from immature animals. Nerve cells from very young mammals tend to degenerate when axonal lesions are introduced at or during the first few days after birth.[10] These differences reflect but one aspect of the major biological problem of the nature and control of cellular differentiation, which is itself poorly understood.[24] Nevertheless, these findings have important practical implications for the physician.

The glial cells form the supportive structure of the central nervous system and are thought to help regulate metabolic events external to the neuronal membrane. They invest the neurons in such a way that sugars, amino acids, and other solutes freely circulating in the extracellular space are made available for the nerve cell's metabolism.[35] Neuroglia also have comparatively high resting-membrane potentials and a high internal potassium level, which may serve to distribute potassium ions to aid and/or create surface potentials in active axons.[5,28]

Glial cells in close association with axotomized neuronal perikarya undergo alterations that influence metabolic changes accompanying neuronal regeneration. A proliferation of microglia close to axotomized perikarya occurs shortly after axotomy; in some cases this change is associated with displacement of synaptic boutons from the perikarya and dendrites of axotomized nerve cells. Activation of metabolism in glia surrounding injured neurons is suggested by hypertrophy of astrocytes in the vicinity of axotomized nerve cell bodies.[20] Literature dealing with glial responses during anterograde and retrograde neuronal responses has been recently reviewed.[4] Relevant to defining those events that take place in glial elements and nerve cells, Watson[37] has shown that in contrast to neuronal responses the onset of metabolic changes in astrocytes surrounding axotomized nerve cells in the hypoglossal nucleus is independent of the level at which the hypoglossal nerve is injured.

When analyzing studies dealing with nerve regeneration in experimental animals, it is important to consider phylogeny. Although regeneration of spinal cord is currently impossible in man, certain lizards regrow segments of spinal cord when the tail is cut off. Rats and dogs can have their nerves severed and not reanastomosed, yet their regenerative efforts are so strong that nerve continuity is restored and motor and sensory return will occur. Monkeys at times will do the same. The nerves of adult baboons and chimpanzees behave more like those of man.

REFERENCES

1. Banquer, N. Z., et al.: The activity of the pentose phosphate pathway in isolated liver cells, Biochem. Biophys. Res. Commun. **52**:263, 1973.
2. Brattgard, S. O., Edstrom, J. E., and Hyden, H.: The chemical changes in regenerating neurons, J. Neurochem. **1**:316, 1957.
3. Brattgard, S. O., Edstrom, J. E., and Hyden, H.: The productive capacity of the neuron in retrograde, Exp. Cell Res. **5**:185, 1958.
4. Brodal, A.: Anterograde and retrograde degeneration of neurons in the central nervous system. In Haymaker, W., and Adams, R. D., eds.: Histology and histopathology of the nervous system, Springfield, Ill., Charles C Thomas, Publisher.
5. Bunge, R. P.: Structure and function of neuroglia: some recent observations. In Schnitt, R. O., ed.: The neurosciences (second study program), New York, 1970, The Rockefeller Press, pp. 782-796.
6. Cheah, T. B., and Geffen, L. B.: Effects of axonal injury on norepinephrine, tyrosine hydroxylase and monoamine oxidase levels in sympathetic ganglia, J. Neurobiol. **4**:443, 1973.
7. Engh, C. A., et al.: Perikaryal synthetic function following reversible and irreversible peripheral axon injuries as shown by radioautography, J. Comp. Neurol. **142**:465, 1971.
8. Francoeur, J., and Olszewski, J.: Axonal reaction and axoplasmic flow as studied by radioautography, Neurology (Minneap.) **18**:178, 1968.
9. Grafstein, B., and Murray, M.: Transport of protein in gold fish optic nerve during regeneration, Exp. Neurol. **25**:494, 1969.
10. Grant, G.: Neuronal changes central to the site of axon transection. A method for the identification of retrograde changes in perikarya, dendrites and axons by silver impregnation. In Nauta, W. J. H.,

and Ebbesson, S. O. E., eds.: Contemporary research methods in neuroanatomy, New York, 1970, Springer-Verlag, pp. 173-185.
11. Guth, L.: Regeneration in the mammalian peripheral nervous system, Physiol. Rev. **36**:441, 1956.
12. Harkonen, M.: Carboxylic esterases, oxidative enzymes and catecholamines in the superior cervical ganglion of the rat and the effect of pre- and postganglionic nerve division, Acta Physiol. Scand. **63** Suppl 237:1, 1964.
13. Harkonen, M. H. A., and Kauffman, F. A.: Metabolic alterations in the axotomized superior cervical ganglion of the rat. I. Energy metabolism, Brain Res. **65**:127, 1974.
14. Harkonen, M. H. A., and Kauffman, F. A.: Metabolic alterations in the axotomized superior cervical ganglion of the rat. II. The pentose phosphate pathway, Brain Res. **65**:141, 1974.
15. Hebb, C. O., and Waites, G. M. H.: Choline acetylase in antero- and retrograde degeneration of a cholinergic nerve, J. Physiol. **132**:667, 1956.
16. Hirsch, H. E., and Obenchain, T.: Acid phosphatase activity in individual neurons during chromatolysis: a quantitative histochemical study, J. Histochem. Cytochem. **18**:828, 1970.
17. Kopin, I. J., and Silberstein, S. D.: Axons of sympathetic neurons: transport of enzymes in vivo and properties of axonal sprouts in vitro, Pharmacol. Rev. **24**:245, 1972.
18. Kreuzberg, G. W.: Changes of coenzyme (TPN diaphorase and TPN linked dehydrogenases) during axonal reaction of the nerve cell, Nature **199**:393, 1963.
19. Lieberman, A. R.: The axon reaction: a review of the principal features of perikaryal responses to axon injury, Int. Rev. Neurobiol. **14**:49, 1971.
20. Lieberman, A. R.: Some factors affecting retrograde neuronal responses to axonal lesions. In Bellairs, R. and Gray, E. G., eds.: Essays on the nervous system, Oxford, 1974, Clarendon Press, pp. 71-105.
21. Matthews, M. R., and Raisman, G.: A light and electron microscopic study of the cellular response to axonal injury in the superior cervical ganglion of the rat, Proc. R. Soc. Lond. [Biol.] **181**:43, 1972.
22. McCaman, R. E., and Robbins, E.: Quantitative biochemical studies of Wallerian degeneration in the peripheral and central nervous systems. II. Twelve enzymes, J. Neurochem. **5**:32, 1959.
23. McQuarrie, I. G., and Grafstein, B.: Axon outgrowth enhanced by a previous nerve injury, Arch. Neurol. **29**:53, 1973.
24. McQuarrie, I. G., and Grafstein, B.: Axonal regeneration in the rat sciatic nerve: effect of a conditioning lesion and of dbcAMP.
25. Miani, N.: Metabolic and chemical changes in regenerating neurons. III. The rate of incorporation of radioactive phosphate into individual phospholipids of the nerve cell perikaryon of the C-8 spinal ganglion in vitro, J. Neurochem. **9**:537, 1962.
26. Moyer, E. K., Kimmel, D. L., and Winborne,

L. W.: Regeneration of sensory spinal nerve roots in young and senile rat, J. Comp. Neurol. **98:**283, 1953.

27. Murray, M.: ³H-uridine incorporation by regenerating retinal ganglion cells of goldfish, Exp. Neurol. **39:**489, 1973.

28. Murray, M., and Grafstein, B.: Changes in the morphology and amino acid incorporation in regeneration goldfish opitc neurons, Exp. Neurol. **23:**544, 1969.

29. Nandy, K.: Histochemical study on chromatolytic neurons, Arch. Neurol. **18:**425, 1968.

30. Reis, D. J., and Ross, R. A.: Dynamic changes in brain dopamine B-hydroxylase activity during anterograde and retrograde reactions to injury of central noradrenergic axon, Brain Res. **57:**307, 1973.

31. Reis, D. J., Ross, R. A., and Joh, T. H.: Some aspects of the reaction of central and peripheral noradrenergic neurons to injury. In Fuxe, K., Olson, L., and Zotterman, Y., eds.: Dynamics of degeneration and growth in neurons (Wenner-Cren Symposium XII) Oxford, 1974, Pergamon Press.

32. Robbins, E.: Kissane, J. M., and Lowe, I. P.: Quantitative biochemical studies of chromatolysis. In Folch-Pi, J., ed.: Chemical pathology of the nervous system, Oxford, 1961, Pergamon Press, pp. 244-247.

33. Sumner, B. E. H.: The effects of injury on two hydrolases in the hypoglossal nucleus, with quantitative data on N-acetyl-B glucosaminidase, Brain Res. **68:**157, 1974.

34. Turner, R. S.: Chromatolysis and recovery of efferent neurons, J. Comp. Neurol. **79:**73, 1943.

35. Varon, S.: Neurons and glia in neural cultures, Exp. Neurol. **48:**93, 1975.

36. Watson, W. E.: An autoradiographic study of the incorporation of nucleuc acid precursors by neurons and glia during nerve regeneration, J. Physiol. Lond. **180:**741, 1965.

37. Watson, W. E.: Observations on the nucleolar and total cell body nucleic acid of injured nerve cells, J. Physiol. Lond. **196:**655, 1968.

DISCUSSION

Rosen: When a nerve is cut or crushed, how is the surviving number of nerve cell bodies that you find in the dorsal root ganglions and in the anterior horn determined?

Ducker: This is purely from my own observation, looking at the cords and then looking at the dorsal root ganglion. They have not been counted in a scientific way; that is yet to be done.

Rosen: Is neural survival related to the nerve size, fiber size, or the distance?

Ducker: We do not know the exact answer to that. We do know that in part it is dependent on proximal/distal location and probably the age of the animal as well. Let us take the extremes. A proximal lesion in the elderly person is going to have some central cell neuronal death, wheras a distal lesion in the foot in a young person will not have any as far as I can see. It is also dependent on other factors such as how well it is able to respond metabolically. I do not know if survival is related to cell volume or whether it is a function of fiber diameter. I am looking at anterior horn cells, which are usually large A fibers.

Sunderland: I think we are forced into the area of speculation in this regard. It is true that the more proximal the lesion the more severe the retrograde effect and the greater the neuronal fallout. Another factor, of course, is the severity of the injury. An avulsion injury can involve close to 100% neuronal death, such as has been found in facial nerve avulsion. But I think that there could well be mechanical effects transmitted directly to the neurons. I remember being told that with avulsion of ventral nerve roots the anterior horn neurons are often pulled out with them. This may occur, on occasion, but quite clearly the more proximal the lesion, the more axoplasm you are amputating from the nerve cell, and this could well be a very important factor.

Jewett: Are there any guesses as to whether a second, later injury to the axon affects the chromatolytic process, such as may occur in a late repair?

Ducker: I have observed, I think, that a primed cell could regenerate faster, because it actually had the machinery available, at least it could start out faster. This is beautifully followed up by McQuarrie and Grafstein from whom I quote: "after the sciatic nerve had been crushed at the level of the mid-thigh the rate of outgrowth of the regenerating axon was measured. The standard crush lesion or test lesion elicited axonal outgrowth at a rate of 4.3 mm/day with an initial delay of approximately 1.6 days. A conditioning lesion of the tibial nerve at the ankle made 2 weeks before the crush lesion at the back of the leg, caused an increase of 23% in the outgrowth rate, and it had a P value of less than .02, with no appreciable change in the initial delay."

So there are a few things you can do to prime the cell, which I think goes along with these metabolic changes. The other clinical fact, skipping back a minute, is that the system can be delayed by violent injuries too, and I think this influenced the result in peripheral nerve surgery in the various wars where we saw tremendous damage to the extremities. In the early repair, by the work of Bebe and Woodall, writing up our own experience of World War II veterans from this country, of the 3565 nerve repairs we showed a lot of the early repairs; better than 50% of them failed because, I think, the metabolic machinery simply was not ready to perform. This led to the rule that we always wait 3 weeks before repair. On the other hand if you have a nice clean cut in a distal injury, the machinery isn't so hard pressed that you should not do the repair immediately, and this is why hand surgery is one field, and brachial plexus surgery is another. Also, the type of brachial plexus injury, where you're trying to innervate the shoulder or to innervate the forearm will influence the timing of repair. So we do some clean-cut brachial plexuses right off the bat, too. However, the type of brachial plexus injury and whether you're trying to innervate the shoulder or the forearm will also influence the timing of repair.

Sunderland: I would like to comment just briefly on this lesion, because I think it is relevant to this question of the optimal time for the repair of the severed nerve, all other factors being taken into consideration. Watson in England has shown that with repeated severance of the nerve you continually get a retrograde effect, so that you go on repeating the process. Your first lesion produces a retrograde response, and if you produce a lesion some weeks later, you again get a retrograde response, and so on. I think that is interesting. This work of McQuarrie is also interesting, but I am a little bit worried about it. If I remember that paper correctly, there were certain fundamental weaknesses. For example, the number of animals studied in each time period was very small (only two), and I think that is an inadequate study. A second point is that when you work on a 23% or a 25% acceleration of axons, that is very nice if the rate were 100 mm/day and you are increasing it by 25%. But, you see, if you take 4 mm/day and you increase it by 23%, it is a very small increase in rate and this could be well within the range of normal variation, because the rate of regeneration does vary from individual to individual. I feel that they ought to take another look at this problem. It is a very interesting concept and it did arise out of Dr. Ducker's original suggestion that factors at a cellular

level were optimal at 2 or 3 weeks after injury for regeneration.

Bunge: I would like to comment that I think there is an alternate explanation for the degree of chromatolytic response in proportion to the degree of amputation of axon. Our common concepts about that may be entirely wrong. Perhaps the reason that there is more chromatolytic response and more neuronal loss when an axotomy occurs close to the cell body is because the neuron is deprived of more of its necessary trophic factors from the periphery, which come both from Schwann cells along the course of the nerve and from target cells as commonly assumed.

Ochoa: In support of the hypothesis that Dr. Bunge has presented, the chromatolytic response can be prevented by the addition of nerve growth factor. Just one point about the differences in the response of C fibers, unmyelinated fibers, and thicker fibers. I think Lewis in 1974 and Bray and myself have shown that C fibers degenerate backwards much more than thick fibers. So there may be a difference in the way these two fiber types respond to the same injury.

Ochs: I am glad to hear these comments because there was quite a dispute in the literature as to what the possible reason for chromatolysis might be. Among them one was a speeding up of the metabolic rate at the cell body level. I think the best explanation, that I can live very comfortably with, is something that Richard Bunge just said. By retrograde flow, which has rates somewhere around a half or maybe even three fourths or more of the anterograde rate, there is some substance that is needed to regulate and perhaps repress the level of cell body metabolism. And when that is missing, there is some kind of a derepression, and then the cell goes through its typical process of chromatolysis.

11

Functional specificity and somatotopic organization during peripheral nerve regeneration

K. W. Horch and P. R. Burgess

CLASSES OF CUTANEOUS SENSATION AND CUTANEOUS RECEPTORS

The division of cutaneous sensations into touch (or pressure), temperature, and pain modalities clearly identifies each as a separate entity but may give a misleading impression of receptor uniformity within each modality. Cutaneous sensibility is subserved by over a dozen different types of receptors, and restoration of this function after peripheral nerve lesion requires that these receptors once again relay information to the central nervous system in an appropriate manner. It is our intent here to briefly outline some of what is known about the physiological basis for cutaneous sensation and to present certain of our recent findings on the properties and spatial organization of cutaneous receptors after nerve regeneration.

Paralleling the three major classes of cutaneous sensation are three major classes of cutaneous receptors.[5,14] Activation of cutaneous nociceptors, which respond specifically to stimuli that are threatening or overtly damaging to the skin, results in a sensation of pain. Changing skin temperature excites either cold or warm thermoreceptors, producing a sensation of cold or warmth. Touch, light pressure, and tickle are sensations arising from activity in cutaneous mechanoreceptors, of which there are a number of specific types.[16] Table 11-1 presents a list of most of the known cutaneous receptors and some of their properties.

Each afferent neuron in a cutaneous nerve is specified not only with respect to the receptor function it performs but also as to where on the skin its receptors are located. Information carried by the neurons is routed centrally and interpreted by the central nervous system in accordance with these functional and somatotopic specifications. Presumably, recovery of function after nerve lesion will be enhanced if the neurons not only regenerate back to the skin but form there functionally and somatotopically appropriate connections. We will consider these concepts in more detail by focusing on the sense of touch and the cutaneous mechanoreceptors that subserve it.

Sense of touch

As shown in Table 11-1, different types of cutaneous mechanoreceptors are selective for different types of stimuli. For instance, hair receptors respond to the movement of single hairs, but field receptors normally do not. Pacinian corpuscles are tuned to high-frequency vibratory stimuli by virtue of their sensitivity to the acceleration components of mechanical events, while Ruffini endings respond well to slow or maintained stretch of the skin. Any given object contacting the skin will thus activate a particular set of cutaneous mechanoreceptors, the responses of which

Table 11-1. Types of cutaneous receptors and some of their important characteristics

Class	Type	Axon size	Adequate stimulus	Receptor structure
Nociceptor	Mechano	Aδ, C	Threatening or damaging deformation of skin	Free nerve endings?
	Thermo-mechano	Aδ, C	Above and noxious heat or cold	Free nerve endings?
	Polymodal	C	Mechanical or thermal damage and irritant chemicals	Free nerve endings?
Thermo-receptor	Warm	C	Skin temperature above 30° C*	Free nerve endings?
	Cold	Aδ, C	Skin temperature below 35° C*	Intraepithelial free nerve endings
Mechano-receptor	PC	Aα	Accelerating displacements of skin and deeper tissue†	Pacinian corpuscle
	G1 hair	Aα	Rapid movement of hair shaft†	Endings around hair follicles
	G2 hair	Aα	Displacement of hair shaft from rest position‡	Endings around hair follicles
	F1 field	Aα	Rapid movement of skin§	Krause end bulb,
	F2 field	Aα	Indentation of skin‡	Meissner's corpuscles, and structurally similar receptors
	T1	Aα	Indentation of touch spot	Merkel cell—neurite complex
	T2	Aα	Skin stretch	Ruffini ending
	D mechano	Aδ	Movement of hair or skin†	?
	C mechano	C	Lingering deformation of skin	?

*Response depends on acclimation temperature and rate of warming or cooling.
†In any direction.
‡Responds to slow movements, but soon ceases responding when movement is stopped.
§Indentation or retraction from an indented position.

will convey information about the size, location, and movement of the stimulus to the central nervous system. Different stimuli produce different patterns of receptor activation, and this provides the sole basis for sensory discrimination between them. The somatotopic organization of the receptors is probably as important as their functional specificity. Somatotopy is maintained to the level of the sensory cortex and is necessary for stimulus localization, two-point discrimination, and detection of the direction of stimulus movement across the skin.

Within a cutaneous nerve the neurons are mixed with respect to functional modality and only coarsely organized somatotopically. If a nerve were to be transected and the regrowing axonal sprouts innervated the distal stump at random, the majority of them would be led back to receptor structures that are inappropriate both in terms of function and location. If this condition persisted, ordinary tactile stimuli would produce a "kaleidoscope" of neural activity that the central nervous system would be hard pressed to analyze correctly.

Fortunately, both after crush (axonotmesis or second degree injury) and transection

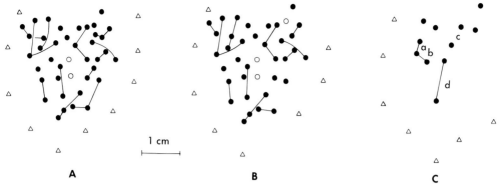

Fig. 11-1. Maps made of location of Merkel cell (T1) receptors (Haarscheiben) and their innervation patterns on thigh of cat. Symbols; △, reference tattoo marks; ●, T1 receptors innervated by single T1 neurons from posterior femoral cutaneous nerve (PFCN); 0, T1 receptors innervated by more than one T1 neuron from PFCN; ●—●, T1 receptors innervated by same neuron. **A,** Map made on first examination of animal. Because of nature of technique used to map innervation pattern, it is not known what other T1 receptors the two multiply innervated receptors may have shared innervation with. Some 20 to 22 different T1 neurons innervated area of skin shown. Immediately after making map **A,** PFCN was thoroughly crushed. **B,** Map made of same area 3 months later. Although there were a few minor changes, locations of receptors and their connections (innervation patterns) are strikingly similar to those seen originally. Maps made in control animals, in which no nerve lesion was made, showed a similar degree of variability, reflecting either limits in accuracy of mapping procedure or changes occurring naturally in receptor population. Number of fibers present matched that seen in **A.** Subsequent experiments have shown that this replication of pattern is due to T1 fibers following their old Schwann tubes back to skin. PFCN was then cut, and map **C** was made 7 months later. In this case, number of T1 fibers is only 40% of that seen in **A** and **B,** and new patterns of connections are seen. Analysis of data from a number of cats showed that one was about equally likely to find connections corresponding to ones originally present, *a;* or new connections in which Merkel cell receptors originally innervated by two different fibers are now innervated by the same fiber, *b;* or lost connections, where the reverse had occurred, *c.* In addition, this figure illustrates a connection, *d,* about which no judgment can be made since it is with what used to be a multiply innervated receptor and hence could not be mapped originally. Note absence of such multiply innervated receptors after nerve transection. If sufficient time (more than 1½ years) is allowed for recovery, number of receptors increases by additional appearance of receptors in locations generally not corresponding to old receptor locations. In **C** nearly all receptors are found in locations corresponding to receptor sites in **A.**

(neurotmesis or fifth degree injury) lesions of cutaneous nerves, the primary afferent neurons maintain their functional specificity. Most regenerating fibers that reestablish functional connections in the skin do so by reinnervating or reforming the same type of receptor that they originally innervated.[4,15] Since the receptor properties (after sufficient time has elapsed) are largely normal, the regenerated axons are correctly labeled as to their functional properties.

After nerve transection the somatotopic organization of axons is not properly restored.[20] This is shown by observations of incorrect localization after recovery from such injuries in man,[11,13] by disruption of cortical "maps" in primates,[23] and by our own data in cats that show sensory fibers do not preferentially reinnervate the correct fascicle in the distal stump of a cutaneous nerve, much less the correct endoneurial tubes. In contrast, the somatotopic pattern is restored after crush injuries because the axons follow their old Schwann tubes in the distal stump back to the same receptor sites they had originally innervated (Fig. 11-1). Such guidance has long been hypothesized,[24,26,30] but until now it was not supported by any experimental evidence.[1] Our data provide direct evidence that specific conduit guidance of regrowing crushed sensory fibers does occur.[17]

After cutaneous nerve crush, essentially all the sensory neurons reform peripheral connection in the skin, but after nerve section there is typically some deficit in the number of fibers and receptors seen (Fig. 11-1). The extent to which this deficit is important in determining the degree of functional recovery is not known. Experimental evidence indicates that clean nerve transections produce a permanent deficit in the number of fibers and receptors, which may be less than that seen in man as a result of aging[7,8,12,32] (see also Chapter 15). Thus the reduction in innervation density, per se, does not appear adequate to produce the sensory impairments observed after nerve transection.[11,18] It is also not clear what role collateral sprouting of fibers from neighboring, nondenervated regions play in the restoration of tactile sensation[10] (see also Chapter 12). Our own data suggest that such sprouting is a local phenomenon and likely to be important only near the perimeters of denervated areas[6] (see also Fig. 11-1).

It seems that the preservation of somatotopy after nerve crush and its loss after section can explain much of the difference in recovery seen after these two types of lesions.[22,27] If so, one need ask to what extent can the central nervous system compensate for somatotopically inappropriate peripheral connections? Presently available evidence indicates limited plasticity in this regard,[21,28] although it has recently been suggested that gross changes in the central connections to motor neurons can occur following peripheral nerve damage[3] (however, see Kimura, Rodnitzdy, and Okawara[19]). Both sensory and motor neurons are reported to show reversible alterations in their aborizations in the spinal cord after peripheral axotomy.[9,29] Moreover, some experimental studies of cutaneous nerve section in humans have

shown that once tactile function has returned (that is, the ability to appreciate a nonpainful component of light pressure or touch), localization can be remarkably accurate.[2,25,31] This is true even in the presence of incorrectly referred sensations. These observations suggest that the central nervous system may have the capacity for local reorganization, thus correcting for relatively minor somatotopic disorganizations. Large-scale disturbances, such as might follow transection of the median nerve, appear to be beyond the ability of the central nervous system compensation.

SUMMARY

In summary, cutaneous innervation consists of a somatotopically organized network of functionally specific receptor types. Nerve crush is followed by good recovery because the somatotopic and functional pattern is effectively restored during regeneration. Good recovery after nerve section is less frequent, in spite of the maintenance of functional specificity, because of the loss of somatotopic specificity and, perhaps, a reduction in the innervation density. Surgical procedures may materially improve the latter but seem unlikely to completely restore the former except on a coarse scale determined by the degree to which regrowing fibers can be induced to enter appropriate fascicles in the distal stump. Therefore factors like motivation, persistence, and trainability may be as important as the number of regenerated fibers in determining the degree to which function can be restored after nerve division, particularly if experience promotes local reorganization of somatosensory pathways.

REFERENCES

1. Bernstein, J. J., and Guth, L.: Nonselectivity in establishment of neuromuscular connections following nerve regeneration in the rat, Exp. Neurol. **4**:262, 1961.
2. Boring, E. G.: Cutaneous sensation after nervedivision, Q. J. Exp. Physiol. **10**:1, 1916.
3. Bratzlavsky, M., and vander Eecken, H.: Altered synaptic organization in facial nucleus following facial nerve regeneration: an electro-physiological study in man, Ann. Neurol. **2**:71, 1977.
4. Burgess, P. R., and Horch, K. W.: Specific regener-

ation of cutaneous fibers in the cat, J. Neurophysiol. **36**:101, 1973.

5. Burgess, P. R., and Perl, E. R.: Cutaneous mechanoreceptors and nociceptors. In Iggo, A., ed.: Handbook of sensory physiology, New York, 1973, Springer-Verlag, Inc., pp. 29-78.

6. Burgess, P. R., et al.: Patterning in the regeneration of type I cutaneous receptors, J. Physiol. **236**:57, 1974.

7. Cauna, N.: The effects of aging on the receptor organs of the human dermis. In Montagna, W., ed.: Advances in biology of skin, vol. VI. Aging, New York, 1965, Pergamon Press, pp. 63-96.

8. Corbin, K. B., and Gardner, E. D.: Decrease in number of myelinated fibers in human spinal roots with age, Anat. Rec. **68**:63, 1937.

9. Csillik, B., and Knyihár, E.: Degenerative atrophy and regenerative proliferation in the rat spinal cord, Z. mikrosk. ant. Forsch. **89**:1099, 1975.

10. Edds, M. V. Jr.: Collateral nerve regeneration, Q. Rev. Biol. **28**:260, 1953.

11. Ford, F. R., and Woodhall, B.: Phenomena due to misdirection of regenerating fibers of cranial, spinal and autonomic nerves, Arch. Surg. **36**:480, 1938.

12. Gutmann, E., and Sanders, F. K.: Recovery of fibre numbers and diameters in the regeneration of peripheral nerves, J. Physiol. **101**:489, 1943.

13. Hawkins, G. L.: Faulty sensory localization in nerve regeneration. An index of functional recovery following suture, J. Neurosurg. **5**:11, 1948.

14. Hensel, H.: Cutaneous thermoreceptors. In Iggo, A., ed.: Handbook of sensory physiology, vol. 2, New York, 1973, Springer-Verlag, Inc., pp. 79-110.

15. Horch, K. W.: Ascending collaterals of cutaneous neurons in the fasciculus gracilis of the cat during peripheral nerve regeneration, Brain Res. **117**:19, 1976.

16. Horch, K. W., Tuckett, R. P., and Burgess, P. R.: A key to the classification of cutaneous mechanoreceptors, J. Invest. Dermatol. **69**:75, 1977.

17. Horch, K.: Guidance of regrowing sensory axons after cutaneous nerve lesions in the cat, J. Neurophysiol. **42**, 1979.

18. Jabaley, M. E., et al.: Comparison of histologic and functional recovery after peripheral nerve repair, J. Hand Surg. **1**:119, 1976.

19. Kimura, J., Rodnitzdy, R. L., and Okawara, S. H.: Electrophysiologic analysis of aberrant regeneration after facial nerve paralysis, Neurology **25**:989, 1975.

20. Langley, J. N.: On the regeneration of pre-ganglionic and of post-ganglionic visceral nerve fibres, J. Physiol. **22**:215, 1897.

21. Mendell, L. M., and Scott, J. G.: The effect of peripheral nerve cross-union on connections of single Ia fibers to motoneurons, Exp. Brain Res. **22**:221, 1975.

22. Osborne, W. A., and Kilvington, B.: The arrangement of nerve fibers in a regenerated nerve trunk, J. Physiol. **38**:276, 1909.

23. Paul, R. L. Goodman, H., and Merzenich, M.: Alterations in mechanoreceptor input to Brodmann's areas 1 and 3 of the postcentral hand area of *Macaca mulatta* after nerve section and regeneration, Brain Res. **39**:1, 1972.

24. Ramón y Cajal, S.: Degeneration and regeneration of the nervous system, vol. 1 (translated by R. M. May), New York, 1968, Hafner.

25. Rivers, W. H., R., and Head, H.: A human experiment in nerve division, Brain **31**:323, 1908.

26. Seddon, H. J.: Peripheral nerve injuries, Glasgow Med. J. **21**(89):61, 1943.

27. Sharpey-Schafer, E.: The effects of denervation of a cutaneous area, Q. J. Exp. Physiol. **19**:85, 1929.

28. Sperry, R. W.: The problem of central nervous reorganization after nerve regeneration and muscle transposition, Q. Rev. Biol. **20**:311, 1945.

29. Sumner, B. E. H., and Watson, W. E.: Retraction and expansion of the dendritic tree of motor neurones of adult rats induced *in vivo*, Nature **233**:273, 1971.

30. Sunderland, S.: Nerves and nerve injuries, Baltimore, 1968, The Williams & Wilkins Co.

31. Trotter, W., and Davies, H. M.: Experimental studies in the innervation of the skin, J. Physiol. **38**:137, 1909.

32. Winkelmann, R. K.: Nerve changes in aging skin. In Montagna, W., ed.: Advances in biology of skin, vol. VI. Aging, New York, 1965, Pergamon Press, pp. 51-61.

DISCUSSION

Jewett: Do you have any data on proximal vs. distal nerve lesions? A cut that was farther proximal might be expected to innervate a wider area compared with a distal lesion.

Horch: We do not have any real data on that. The nerve that I prefer to use, the femoral cutaneous nerve in the cat, is rather short from the point where it emerges from the sciatic notch, so all of these are what would be classified as distal cuts.

Anonymous: Cajal has a beautiful drawing that worries me showing a cut axon with about 25 or 50 sprouts growing out of the end of it. Our scanning electron microscope grant has not come through yet, so I cannot see these, but I have implicit faith in basic research, and I think they are there. I worry about them, and I want to know what his information about fiber specificity means for all of these 25 sprouts, $1^1/_2$ or 2 years after a nerve cut or laceration.

Horch: My feeling would be that those sprouts that get back to the skin all form the same class of functional connections. We have not really looked in great detail, but at least when you look at cats 2 or 3 years after nerve cuts, you do not find very many, if any, split fields. Most of the fields seem to be sort of contiguous, which would argue that if multiple sprouts do survive, get back to the skin, and form functional connections, they do so all in the same neighborhood. Alternatively, as a lot of people, including J. Z. Young, have hypothesized, a single sprout may get back before the others, make functional connections, become dominant, and then the other sprouts essentially atrophy (or become relatively inactive). Perhaps they can be activated with very strong mechanical stimuli, but they are not normally activated under standard physiologically important cutaneous stimuli.

Julia Terzis (Nova Scotia): Is there evidence that tactile domes regenerate?

Horch: What I am going to do is hedge a little on that issue and say that it is conceivable that where these new domes appear, there are sitting, lurking in the skin, latent Merkel cells. Occasionally, if you do serial sections in mammalian skin, you find isolated Merkel cells. So it is conceivable that new Merkel cell receptors are occurring in places where there was a single isolated Merkel cell or perhaps (invisible to us) a precursor group of Merkel cells that the nerve turned on. We have not been able to rule that out yet.

Niebauer: If you take a piece of skin in which the nerves have been cut so that the receptors have degenerated, and then transplant it to a new location, what happens?

Horch: Well, we have not done that experiment directly, but some investigators have done experiments, especially in animals other than mammals, where they retransplant skin from one area to another, looking at the question of whether it is the nerve or the skin that specifies the receptive structures. In some cases it turns out that the skin determines what the receptive structure is going to be. In the case of pacinian corpuscles, they do not degenerate: so if you transplanted skin with pacinian corpuscles in it, they would be innervated by whatever neurons came back to that skin.

Orgel: I would like to add some morphological observations that we made several years ago in rabbits by using methylene blue preparations. We transferred some skin from one portion of the rabbit, the scrotum specifically, to the ear, which can be shown to be two very different types of skin, and we were unable to show that the skin transferred to the ear was able to reform any corpuscular endings about the hair follicles. This was also shown around 1970 in a study from England by skin transfer in the human where forearm skin was transferred to the fingertip.

Rosen: How much selection is there for large myelinated fibers over the small myelinated fibers when you do single unit studies?

Robert Dykes (Halifax): I cannot answer that question in quantitative terms, but it is certainly true that the large fibers are selected over the small fibers by dissection techniques. It is also quite true that dissection techniques usually do not isolate unmyelinated fibers.

Ochoa: This is a rather unfair question for animal experimenters, but what happens to function when a particular receptor is innervated by the wrong type of nerve fiber?

Horch: Actually I am not too pessimistic about being able to answer that question. About 150 years ago, the concept of specific nerve energy was put forth, by Müller, and brilliantly confirmed by von Frey and others. The idea is that a particular nerve element, by virtue of its central connections, is assigned a specific interpretation by the brain; so if, for instance, you stimulate a cold spot in your skin and you can do this either with a stiff von Frey hair or with an electrical stimulus, the sensation you get is one of cold. It is independent of the actual stimulus modalities used and is determined by the nature and connections of the neuron activated. Similarly if you press on your eye, the pressure will indirectly activate ganglion cells, which you see as light; although the actual physical stimulus is pressure. I would therefore suspect, in view of the absence of any evidence for sensory reorganization in the adult mammal, that if you had inappropriate terminal connections, the brain would interpret the activity coming in on the neurons on the basis of what they used to be originally connected to. So that if you had a thermoreceptor fiber innervating a mechanoreceptor, mechanical stimuli might in fact activate that neuron, but you would feel it as a sensation of warmth or cold.

Michael Jabalay (Jackson, Miss.): I understand what you say about functional specificity but we also need to consider if incorrect connections occur. I would like to point out a study that was reported in *Science* about 3 or 4 years ago, from the group at the University of Miami, where the hypogastric nerve, which goes to the bladder in the cat, was crossed to the anterior mesenteric nerve, which goes to the mesentery. The mesentery contains pacinian corpuscles, while the bladder does not. After regrowth had occurred, a number of the pacinian corpuscles responded to stimulation suggesting that fibers that had originally not gone to pacinian corpuscles were capable of being stimulated from receptors foreign to them.

Horch: My view is one that has been put forward by others studying development and it is that if given the choice, neurons prefer to go back and perform the same functions they had originally. However, if put into a forced situation where they cannot choose their old original territory, they are capable of innervating "foreign" structures and having in this sense functional properties unlike what they would normally have. But this occurs as far as we know only in situations where you have done cross-nerve union and the neurons are not given a choice anymore.

Graham Lister (Louisville): We may be seeing something of this in more recent work that is being done clinically in transferring tissue from the foot to the hand. We know from a series of studies done by Jim May in Dr. Brown's laboratory that the normal two-point discrimination on the foot in the first web space is 11 mm, but when that skin is transferred to the hand and attached to a digital nerve or a median nerve in the hand, we are getting two-point discrimination of significantly less tham 11 mm.

Dykes: I can speak to that, and that is a very interesting situation. I have examined such patients where skin of the other foot serves as a control within that particular patient.

The skin originally provided directional information and two-point thresholds that were appropriate for a foot, but that were not as good as a hand. When that skin tissue was transferred to a digital nerve, there was detection of directional information, which was much in excess of what had been observed in that same piece of skin on the foot. This was obviously regeneration of a sutured nerve. This observation raises a large number of questions: What happened to the peripheral organization? Has the receptor density increased? Could it be that the parts of the somatic sensory cortex that are now functionally connected to this skin region are better able to handle information from those receptors and to process that information in a way that gives better two-point discrimination? So there are several kinds of questions, centrally as well as peripherally, that must be answered before we know what's going on. Even without answers to these questions, we must decide that one has to pay attention to the types of tissue transferred. It appears to me that this anecdotal observation is very important for future developments in free tissue grafts because this means first that hairy skin cannot replace the function of glabrous skin, and second it means that the limitations that we see in the donor site may not necessarily be the limitations of that tissue when transferred to another site. These are very important problems for both the basic scientist and the clinician.

Bennet O'Brien (Melbourne): Regarding tissue transplantation from the foot, it has been implied that there is consistent upgrading of sensibility in transplants from the foot to the hand. That has not been my observation in these cases; it is not a consistent finding. I can think of many cases in which sensibility has been worse in the finger than it was originally in the foot. We are about to review in the next month or so the long-term results in more than 25 of these foot transplants and I think then we will have a much better idea of what the pattern is.

Lister: This is just a response to Dr. O'Brien. The important cases are not the ones where the two-point discrimination is less after you transfer the skin; there are many explanations for that. The important thing is that there are cases in existence where skin was transferred and the two-point discrimination was indubitably improved. These are the cases that need explanation.

Cameron Dale (New York): Concerning this increased two-point discrimination that has been mentioned, I have noticed this in situations, for example, where the nerve has not been divided, but where one has done a sensitized cross-finger flap using the dorsal branch of the radial nerve. In a number of situations the sensitivity has increased and the two-point discrimination has increased from a little bit above 1 cm to less than 5 mm, and this occurred where the nerve was not damaged at all, at least as far as one can know. The story of the computer upstairs must surely be a very relevant one.

Tupper: It has long been known that abdominal pedicle skin that has very poor normal two-point discrimination will improve its two-point discrimination immensely by being transferred to the hand, in an area with a greater cerebral tactile representation.

Ochoa: Is there any difference in the recovery of the functional specificity between the nerve sections and crushed nerves?

Horch: If you combine my observations with those of Dr. Dykes, it seems that following nerve crush, fibers probably recover their normal or nearly normal properties sooner than they do after a nerve section. I know that in the case of nerve cut, fibers can be back to the skin, functionally operational, and classifiable by 6 months, yet they are not normal—they are just not right. The gestalt you get, even without doing any complicated mechanical stimulation, just stimulating by hand, is that they are sluggish. They are not performing normally. The fibers tire easily and their receptive fields may not be normal. Recovery periods of 2 or 3 years are needed before these responses are really vigorous, and they still may never fully recover the original properties after a cut. In contrast, after distal crush, if you waited a year or so, you probably would have skin that you would be very hard pressed to distinguish from normal skin, physiologically. We did this in a couple of cases. We just looked at crushed nerves and decided that we could not tell them from normal so there was no sense in proceeding with further work on them.

Aguayo: To stress what Dr. Horch has just said, I think that it is very important that we keep the conclusions that come from transection experiments and those from crush experiments separated, because I think that they are completely different experimental models.

Sunderland: It may be pertinent at this time to discuss the question of classification of nerve injuries. In the early 1940's Seddon produced a classification of nerve injuries that was a very useful one: neurapraxia, axonotmesis, and neurotmesis. I never liked those terms; it took me a very long time to make sure what was what, so to speak, but at the same time we were thinking in terms of a similar classification based on the histological structure of nerve fibers and nerve trunks. This classification covers more than Seddon covered in his classification, although his initial attempt was a definite advance and a great help. Now there are, in terms of the histological structure of the nerve trunk, five degrees of nerve injury (and you can add a sixth that represents a combination of 1, 2, 3, or 4). The first degree injury is one that produces a conduction block and nothing else in the nerve fiber. Conduction is blocked, conduction continues as far as the block, below it, but not across it. Reference has already been made to this type of injury. It is the simplest type of injury. After a quiescent period, the block is cleared and function is fully restored. The second degree injury, which is a little more severe, is the injury that ruptures the axon but does not rup-

ture the endoneurial tube. This is an intrafunicular injury; it is an axonal injury, and it leads to wallerian degeneration. However, in this case the architecture of the nerve trunk and the nerve fibers is fully retained right out to the periphery, to the final termination. After a little longer quiescent period, axon regeneration commences, with the axon tip confined to the endoneurial tube that originally contained it. This means that the pattern of reinnervation is precisely, in every detail, the pattern of the original innervation. These cases show a complete functional recovery in every respect. I would be very surprised if after a simple crush injury you did not get complete recovery. Now the third degree injury is yet more severe; there is rupture not only of the axon but also the endoneurial wall. Here we are dealing with a true intrafunicular injury, the funiculus is in continuity; this is the type of injury we see with stretch lesions and some compression lesions. In this case the regenerating axon tip, when it appears at the terminal of the endoneurial tube, can now escape into the intervening tissue and find its way into another endoneurial tube. Whether or not this is likely to be functionally useful will depend on the fiber composition of the funiculus. For example, if all of the fibers in the funiculus are sensory, then of course that sensory process will enter a sensory tube, and though it will not go back to its original end-organ, it will go back at least to a cutaneous region and may well function. On the other hand, if a sensory process enters a motor endoneurial tube, that represents a dead loss. So we now have the question of a confusion of regeneration despite the fact that the funiculi are in continuity. Finally you take it a step further to the fourth degree injury in which there has been rupture of the funiculus and now you have only loose tissue holding the nerve ends together. This has all of the problems of the third degree injury just discussed with greater likelihood of incorrect regrowth. The fifth degree injury is present if the nerve ends are apart with complete separation with a gap between them. Now you can have a combination of degrees 1, 2, 3, and 4, but of course, you cannot combine 5 with any of the others since it represents a complete transection. So I think that in some of the lesions that we have been discussing, we area dealing with a confirmation of the classical second degree injury, namely that in which the crush disrupts the axon at the site of injury leading to wallerian degeneration that is followed inevitably by regeneration in the axon, which goes back to where it originally went and does precisely what it originally did. In these cases, we expect function to be complete in every respect. However, in the case of a transection, or in the case of a third degree injury (which represents a rupture of the system within the funiculus) we must also consider axon sprouting. Two or more sprouts can enter one endoneurial tube. Present belief is that the axon sprout that first establishes a functional relationship with the periphery takes over the endoneurial tube, and all other sprouts within that single tube then degenerate. However, if the multiple sprouts from that axon enter other endoneurial tubes, they will survive and go on and reinnervate the periphery. You can then have a situation where you are overloading the parent neuron. These differences must be kept in mind when comparing crush experiments with those done with nerve transections.

Ochs: Perhaps I might add a comment to recommend that a localized freeze be used as a minimal technique of disruption when one wants a second degree lesion.

Ochoa: Is there any evidence that decreased function seen after nerve section could be due to the unsatisfied distal endoneurial tube or oversprouting of axons?

Horch: Of course, one needs a reasonable number of fibers reinnervating the skin in order to get reasonable function. Part of the functional deficit is likely to be due to a lack of fibers forming functional connections, but what I have been struck by in our work, and what some other people have told me they are finding too, is that the deficit in fibers doesn't seem to be quite as great as one would expect on the basis of the deficit in function. It seems to be more than just simply a lack of fibers getting back.

Sunderland: I think Dr. Horch has directed our attention to a very significant feature in nerve regeneration. We do not want to confuse imperfect reinnervation with incomplete reinnervation. They are two very different things. Of course you can have reinnervation that is both incomplete and imperfect, but they are two different mechanisms with potentially different results.

Dykes: The anecdotal observation about improved two-point discrimination in the hand, with skin transferred from the foot, is relevant here. In these cases disorganization must have come about in suturing the nerve, since there could be no possible matching of endoneurial tubes, and so on. Yet, there was very good two-point discrimination, the ability to localize, and there was a detection of direction of movement. These processes must depend on the spatial relationships among the receptors, which somehow either must have been properly reorganized, or there must have been some central reorganization.

12

Regeneration and collateral sprouting of peripheral nerves

Jack Diamond and Patrick C. Jackson

Aside from adaptive processes operating within the central nervous system, there are at least two peripheral mechanisms that contribute to the recovery of function after nerve lesions. The first mechanism is the progressive proximodistal regeneration of the central portions of the lesioned fibers; in theory this mechanism might exactly restore the innervation of the deprived target tissue. The second mechanism (sometimes called "denervation sprouting") involves nerve fibers that escaped damage; these fibers can extend their peripheral field of innervation by collateral sprouting at the target tissue.[7] In either event the degree of functional recovery is related to the extent to which the affected target tissue becomes successfully reinnervated. In our work we have been especially concerned with how functional nerve sprouting at target tissues is regulated; the results say little about the difficulties that nerves lesioned at a distance may experience in regenerating toward these tissues. However, it would seem clear that ultimately the terminals both of regenerating and of intact sprouting nerves must achieve an appropriate functional relationship with the target, possibly with specific target sites, and then effectively cease further growth.[11] Our results throw light on these problems and, of special interest to the problems of nerve repairs, indicate that regenerating nerves and undamaged sprouting fibers may not be governed to the same extent by territorial "rules." Some unexpected findings indicate

that cutaneous nerve sprouting in the mammal may be subject to constraints that are not apparent in lower vertebrates. A tentative suggestion has emerged of a possible neurosurgical intervention that might be of therapeutic value in conditions in which skin sensation is lost after nerve lesions.

Nerves regenerating across the site of a lesion will usually regrow along the peripheral portion of the nerve trunk whether or not there is target tissue available, and the latter may play no role either in the initiation of regeneration or in its progress. In contrast, the sprouting of remaining undamaged nerves at a target that has been only partially denervated appears to depend on a sprouting stimulus from the target tissue itself.[1]

A model preparation for the investigation of nerve sprouting

The preparation we used to investigate the regulation of nerve sprouting was the peripheral innervation of the salamander hindlimb.[1] (Recent results from the mammal are described below.) The mechanosensory nerves of the salamander skin supply the "touch spots" that we defined from an analysis of a systematic survey of the distribution of sensory thresholds; we recorded the afferent impulses evoked by stimulating the skin with an electromechanical prodder of 10 μ tip diameter.[2] The mechanoreceptors in salamander skin were found to be all rapidly adapting (Fig. 12-1). By a correlative physio-

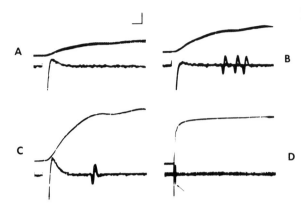

Fig. 12-1. Response of rapidly adapting mechanoreceptors in salamander skin. Top trace of each pair shows photocell output that monitors prodder movement. Bottom trace shows extracellular recording from nerve trunk approximately 3 cm from skin. **A,** Applied stimulus was subthreshold; three traces are superimposed. **B,** Stimulus intensity was increased to just threshold. Three traces are superimposed, and one spike occurred in each. Variation in latencies of spike is typical with a just-threshold stimulus. **C,** Response to suprathreshold stimulus, which elicited one spike of constant latency; three traces are superimposed. **D,** Single sweep with same stimulus as in **C**; sweep speed was slowed to show that these rapidly adapting mechanoreceptors respond to suprathreshold sustained stimulus with single spike (arrow). Horizontal calibration is 2 ms in **A, B,** and **C,** and 50 ms in **D.** Vertical calibration is 7 μm for prodder movement and 20 μV for extracellular records. (From Parducz, et al.: Neuroscience 2:511, 1977.)

logical and morphological investigation, we showed that each touch spot is composed of nerve endings in intimate association with a single specialized cell at the base of the epidermis, the Merkel cell[15] (Fig. 12-2). Each touch spot, and thus each Merkel cell, is rarely, if ever, supplied by more than one axon.[2] In addition, using two stimulators in an occlusion technique, we showed that the "receptive field" of a mechanosensory axon overlapped only slightly with those of neighboring axons; the Merkel cells supplied by each axon therefore form a discrete colony comprising from 4 to 100 such cells, and presumably this number reflects the extent of branching of any one axon.

This relatively simple nerve-target situation would seem a favorable one for the investigation of the peripheral consequences of nerve lesions and of the neuron-target interactions that might be involved in the regulation of nerve sprouting.

The Merkel cell as a nerve target

One question of special importance follows from this description of the mechanosensory innervation of salamander skin. During development, do the Merkel cells differentiate under the influence of the arriving nerves, or do they appear independently of nerves and provide true targets for those axons destined to have a mechanosensory function?

There are inevitable uncertainties in know-

Fig. 12-2. Merkel cells in salamander skin. **A,** Light micrograph of skin. Merkel cells were always found near basal layer of epidermis. One circled here was identified by electron microscopic examination of adjacent section that is shown in **B.** V, Blood vessels; G, secretory glands. **B,** Electronmicrograph of skin. Merkel cell, M, from **A** above and its associated nerve endings, NE, are located near basal lamina, BL. It can be distinguished from other epidermal cells, E, by presence of dense-cored granules in its cytoplasm. D indicates dermis. **C,** Higher power view of another Merkel cell and nerve endings, former showing dense-cored granules and latter clear vesicles and mitochondria. (From Diamond, J. In Schmitt, F. O., and Worden, F. G., eds.: The neurosciences: fourth study program, Cambridge, 1979, The M.I.T. Press.)

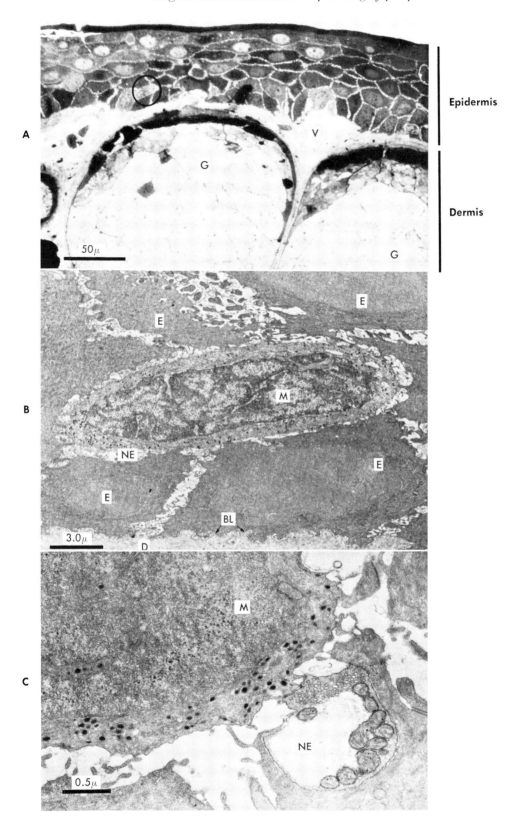

Fig. 12-2. For legend see opposite page.

ing exactly when nerves first arrive at target tissues during embryonic development. However in the salamander we were able to take advantage of a related situation that offered the opportunity to investigate a possible target nature of the Merkel cell. After skin is removed from a limb, new skin regenerates, and this occurs even if the limb is totally denervated. A significant result emerged from the electron microscopic examination of such regenerated skin; it contained typical Merkel cells in about normal numbers, but of course without any associated nerve endings. When nerves were allowed to innervate such new skin after regenerating from the site of a nerve lesion, these Merkel cells then became innervated.[4] Once again the location of the Merkel cells correlated with those of the physiologically identified touch spots[17] (Fig. 12-3). We have not found nerve endings with a similar relationship to other cells in either normal or regenerated epidermis. In the latter, as in normal skin, only one axon appears to supply each touch spot, and thus one Merkel cell. It seems then that in regenerated skin, the Merkel cell displays the character of a true

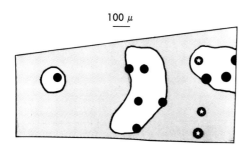

100 μ

Fig. 12-3. Correlation of "touch-spots" and Merkel cell locations in regenerated salamander skin after its innervation. Relationship between low-threshold regions (white areas) determined in physiological studies and Merkel cells (black spots) whose distribution was obtained by electron microscopic examination of same piece of skin. Correlation between Merkel cells and sensitive areas was highly significant (P < 0.001, Chi-square test). Merkel cells marked with asterisk did not show associated nerve endings.

"target"; it becomes selectively innervated by the ingrowing mechanosensory nerves even though the ratio of Merkel cells to other epidermal cells is only about 1:1000.[15]

There are now a number of reports in the literature suggesting that specific target sites, including Merkel cells, can be distinguished in embryos (and, in certain abnormal circumstances, in older animals) before clear indications of their nerves are present.[5] Taken together, the evidence points in many situations to the existence of specific targets that can develop before their nerves arrive. It should be noted however that in other preparations characteristic target specializations may be induced by the nerves.[5]

THE TARGET AND THE SPROUTING STIMULUS

Removal of part of the nerve supply to the skin of a salamander causes an immediate drop in the number of touch spots. However, after an initial delay of 5 to 7 days, the number begins to increase, and within 3 to 4 weeks the original density of touch spots is restored. As detected physiologically, this sprouting of the remaining mechanosensory axons then appears to cease.[3] (We showed that the recovery was not due to regeneration of cut axons.) We have now shown that Merkel cells survive denervation; their number in denervated skin appears quite normal, and these cells retain their characteristic morphology except of course for the absence of associated nerve endings.[4] When denervated skin becomes reinnervated by regenerating axons and partially denervated skin by the collateral sprouts of remaining undamaged fibers, the denervated Merkel cells become innervated; this is correlated with the appearance of new touch spots.[16] We conclude that denervated Merkel cells exhibit the same target character as that of the Merkel cells that appear in regenerated skin. A simple hypothesis that encompasses all these findings is that nerve-free Merkel cells constitute a source of a stimulus that causes nearby axons to sprout; these sprouts eventually reach and innervate the available Merkel cells. This explanation accounts for the quantitative restoration of physiological touch spots in totally or partially denervated skin[3,16] and their development in newly regenerated skin[4] when nerves are available.

The evidence that target tissues are the sources of sprouting stimuli that act on nerves is now fairly strong, and indeed one such agent, nerve growth factor (NGF), has been convincingly identified.[12] In salamander skin, the Merkel cells seem excellent candidates for the role of providing a sprouting stimulus, and the resultant concentration gradient could assure directional growth of nerves toward these cells. It is however quite possible that the nerves grow randomly, the terminals ceasing growth when they successfully contact, "recognize," and form an association with an available Merkel cell. Such neuron-target interactions would be fairly local in their effectiveness and unlikely to explain how regenerating nerves that begin their growth at a distance from the target tissue actually reach it. (It is worth recalling however that during embryogenesis prospective target tissues are relatively close to the developing neuraxis.) Nevertheless, when regenerating nerves arrive in the vicinity of the target tissue, our results indicate that they too, like the collateral sprouts of uninjured axons, come under the influence of the local "stimulus"; they associate with denervated Merkel cells in apparently the same way, and the appropriate distribution of sensory endings is thus determined for both types of "growing" nerves at the level of the target tissue itself.[16]

The role of the nerve in regulating sprouting

Since a physiological touch spot in all the situations we have described is supplied by the endings of only one axon, we may presume that the target character of the Merkel cell is "switched off" by the first nerve that contacts it; the endings of other axons are thus no longer attracted to that Merkel cell or do not "recognize" it if they do encounter it. However, after section of its nerve the Merkel cell rapidly reattains its target character, so we may assume that the nerve exerts a

continual restraining influence in this regard. We speculated that this ability of the nerve continually to offset the sprouting effect of the target would itself depend on the continued availability at the endings of some factor(s) and that this would most likely be provided by axoplasmic transport.[1] If this hypothesis were correct, a reduction of axoplasmic transport, even in an otherwise normally functioning nerve, might be expected eventually to result in sprouting of other neighboring axons. We examined this possibility by bathing a selected nerve in an appropriate dose of colchicine, which we showed reduced neuronal transport.[1,10] In the most successful experiments there was no change in either impulse conduction, sensory threshold, or distribution of the touch spots associated with the treated nerve; in these circumstances, neighboring nerves reacted as if the colchicine-treated ones had been sectioned, and untreated axons sprouted and hyperinnervated the skin.[1,3] There were preliminary indications that individual touch spots became hyperinnervated, although we have not yet excluded the possibility that new touch spots (and new Merkel cells) appear under these conditions. All-in-all, the evidence supports the hypothesis that fast axoplasmic transport in a nerve brings to the endings some factor(s) that is needed to maintain a "neutralizing" influence of the nerve on the target cell and is responsible ultimately for the loss of effectiveness of the sprouting stimulus.

These findings, we suggest, obviate the need to invoke "products of degeneration" as the source of a sprouting stimulus that acts on undamaged axons adjacent to lesioned ones. The scheme proposed is attractive in its single explanation of the sprouting that occurs both during primary development and in conditions of partial denervation or colchicine treatment.[7] Moreover, the proposed mechanism offers a possible means of achieving alterations in the density of endings within axonal fields during adaptive situations in the mature organism, which would be of special importance in the central nervous system.

SPROUTING IN MAMMALIAN SKIN

How generally applicable are the findings from the salamander? When we did similar experiments in the mammal, we obtained a surprising result. After section of nerves supplying skin either in the adult rabbit or in the adult rat, we found no evidence that remaining cutaneous nerves enlarged their low-threshold mechanosensory fields into the adjacent denervated regions (for example, Fig. 12-4). Nociceptive fields similarly appeared not to have enlarged in the few experiments in which they were measured. These results are in contrast to an earlier report suggesting that in the rabbit, collateral sprouting after adjacent denervation did occur.[19] In the following we mention an explanation that might explain the discrepancy, at least in part.

The young animal

When we turned to the newborn animal the situation proved to be quite different, and we obtained results that were consistent with our findings in the salamander. We used rat pups of various postnatal ages. We selected for experimentation the dermatomes of the trunk, particularly in the region of the dorsal midline where the skin is supplied by the easily accessible dorsal cutaneous nerves.

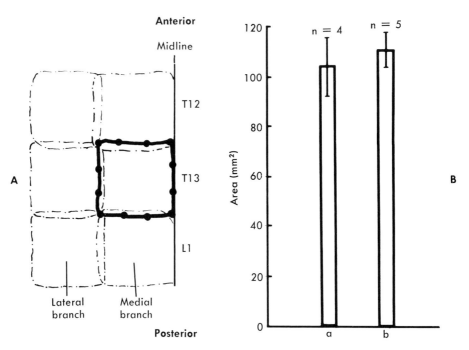

Fig. 12-4. A, Cutaneous mechanosensory fields in the dorsal midline region of rat. To left of midline low-threshold mechanosensory fields of dorsal cutaneous nerves (DCN's) originating from T12, T13, and L1 roots are outlined. Each DCN divides into medial and lateral branch, supplying corresponding subfields, which are illustrated. Medial DCN-T13 field is defined by heavy line joining tattooed dots. This field becomes "island" of innervation referred to in text, when following nerves are sectioned: both right and left DCN's of T12 and L1; right DCN of T13; and *lateral* branch of left DCN of T13. **B,** Lack of sprouting in mature rats. Histograms show areas of low-threshold mechanosensory field of *medial* branch of DCN of T13 for two groups of 30-day-old animals (see also **A**). No denervations had been done on animals of control group, *a;* those of group *b* had been operated on 10 days earlier and denervated as described in **A** to produce innervated "island." Similar results were obtained when rats were denervated at any age greater than 20 days, and for postoperative periods up to 90 days or more. Normal enlargement of such innervated "islands" during growth of animal was unaffected by denervation of skin surrounding them.

After partial denervation of skin, a single remaining area of low-threshold mechanosensitivity was mapped physiologically by a fine bristle while recording the afferent impulses from the intact nerve. In all but the youngest animals the border of the field so defined were marked by tattooing, thus outlining a mechanosensory "island" surrounded by a "sea" of denervated skin (Fig. 12-4, *A*). In mature rats these islands of touch innervation did not change over periods of many months (Fig. 12-4, *B*). However, when the partial denervation was performed before 20 days of age, the remaining field enlarged during the following few days well beyond the normal area increase that occurred as the animals grew in size (Fig. 12-5). This physiological indication of collateral sprouting was almost never observed if the initial operation was done after 20 days of age. Moreover, the sprouting (that is, the "extra" enlargement of the field) seemed to cease at about 20 days of age, irrespective of when it was brought about. Thus there may be a "critical period" for denervation sprouting of low-threshold mechanosensory nerves in the mammal. In the rat this period ends at about 20 days postnatal life. Although after that time nerve fields normally enlarge in proportion to the increase in skin area as the animal grows, there is no *extra* sprouting of low-threshold nerves in response to adjacent denervation. Whether the disappearance of the phenomenon in the maturing animal depends on a failure of the target to produce an appropriate sprouting stimulus when it is deprived of its innervation or whether these nerves have lost their capacity to respond to such a stimulus has not yet been determined.

The available evidence, despite sporadic reports to the contrary (for example, Livingston[13] but also see Gutman[8]), suggests that in humans too collateral sprouting of remaining cutaneous nerves after partial lesions may not occur to any significant extent. Sensory recovery, when it occurs, is likely to depend on "central" mechanisms or on the regeneration of damaged nerve fibers (see other chapters in this book).

NERVE FIELDS AND "DOMAINS"

How do peripheral nerve fields become established, and are these fields modifiable after nerve lesions? What we have dealt with so far throws light on how the sprouting of mechanosensory nerves is regulated at the level of the target tissue, at least in the skin of the salamander; in the mammal some of the mechanisms involved appear to operate only during early postnatal life.[6] The *regeneration* of a nerve after it is lesioned may be triggered by some signal set off by the lesion itself; in

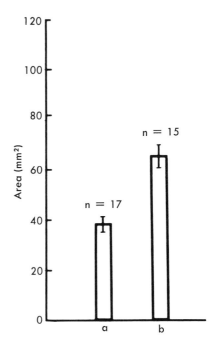

Fig. 12-5. Mechanosensory nerve sprouting in young rats. Similar experiments to those illustrated in Fig. 12-4 were performed in animals in which mapping of low-threshold mechanosensory fields for both control group, *a*, and experimental group, *b*, was done at 20 days of age. Experimental group had been denervated at 10 days of age so as to leave "island" of innervation supplied by medial DCN of T13. Increase in area of "island" in experimental group reflects collateral sprouting evoked by surrounding denervation. In these experiments tattooing of fields was not done at time of initial operation to eliminate possibility of damage to remaining intact nerve. However at 10 days of age areas of *medial* DCN of T13 fields would have been in region of 15 to 20 mm².

any event much of its progress seems to be independent of the target tissue. Taken together, the phenomena we have described might help explain how peripheral nerve *fields* develop. The "classical" view[9] is that somatic nerves grow out from a central neuraxis (which has become segmented) toward the adjacent developing somites; these are penetrated by sensory nerves that establish "territories," often exclusively, in the overlying integument. As the animal grows, the changing shape and disposition of the peripheral tissues, organs, and limbs leads to corresponding alterations in the observed pattern of the sensory fields. In the region of the trunk however the "serial banding" of the dermatomes (the sensory fields corresponding to the individual dorsal roots) is relatively well preserved. Although there is often an overlap at the borders of adjacent dermatomes, their contours are relatively smooth,[18] which is perhaps curious when account is taken of the absence of any surface or histological features that might distinguish the skin of one dermatome from that of its neighbor.

Is there "territorial integrity?"

In the salamander we showed that a *regenerating* nerve readily formed a sensory field in skin of a "foreign" dermatome when the regenerating nerve was appropriately redirected.[7] Furthermore, when regenerating mechanosensory nerves were allowed equal access to both their original skin and that of another denervated dermatome, they showed no obvious preference for the denervated Merkel cells they originally innervated over the denervated Merkel cells in the adjacent dermatome.[16] The results clearly indicated that regenerating nerves show little if any discrimination for skin of one region compared to another. It appeared that the nerves that arrived first at a region of denervation were responsible for "keeping out" those arriving later; according to our hypothesis, this occurred because the earlier arriving nerves occupied all the available Merkel cells, causing the disappearance of the sprouting stimulus as we have described

previously. Thus it is understandable from our findings why adjacent nerves may not invade each other's territory during development. The classical view of the formation of peripheral fields is also supported, at least at the level of the target tissue; dermatomes could indeed be an inevitable consequence of the spatial organization of discrete bundles of nerve fibers growing directly to the skin. The symmetry and relative smoothness of the borders of the fields would be a remarkable, but not impossible, outcome of such development.

Other mechanisms regulating fields

A suggestion that some other mechanism could be involved in preserving the shapes of dermatomal fields came from unexpected observations in both salamanders[7] and rats. If, in a salamander hindlimb, only *one* of the three spinal nerves supplying it was left intact, the subsequent invasion of the adjacent denervated skin by sprouting of the remaining undamaged nerve was confined to a small strip along the frontier between the adjacent dermatomes. Sprouting then appeared to cease, at least for a significant length of time. There seemed to be some sort of hindrance to the sprouting of intact nerves into a "foreign" dermatome. When, however, a dermatome was *partially* denervated, the remaining intact fibers sprouted to occupy the denervated Merkel cells *within* the dermatome. Intact sprouting nerves thus seemed to be restricted in some way to their parent dermatome, in contrast to regenerating nerves (at least redirected ones), which, as mentioned above, recognize no barrier to their invading of "foreign" territory.

An intriguing result came from similar experiments in salamanders in which an additional maneuver was performed; skin flaps were excised and then replaced after 180-degree rotation. The nerves that invaded these flaps reestablished the frontier between adjacent dermatomes along a line defined by the original location of the frontier *on the limb* (not the misplaced line on the rotated patch of skin), that is, with reference to the limb coordinates; it was as though the skin had not been manipulated at all (Fig. 12-6). These and related experiments[7] suggested that the spatial organization of the dermatomes is determined by a mechanism that does not reside in the skin itself; indeed, in this respect the skin seems to act merely as a "receiving" surface. However, as we showed,[14] the nerves invaded the rotated skin flaps from their edges and did *not* simply project upward from the underlying tissue. The nerves behaved as though they recognized and preferred to occupy "domains" of body space. Sprouting of a nerve occurred readily into skin within its allotted domain but not into skin (even skin it had originally innervated) when it was relocated outside the domain boundary.[5,14]

"Domains" in the mammal

We have now extended our investigations to include the neonatal rat. The results are in some respects even more striking than those in the salamander. In a 10-day-old rat (that is, within the critical period we have described previously) we partially denervated one dermatome in combination with total denervation of the adjacent regions of the dermatomes rostral and caudal to it (see Fig. 12-4, *A*). The resultant enlargement of the remaining low-threshold mechanosensory subfield was clearly "directional"; the sprouting occurred almost entirely mediolaterally into the denervated area of the parent dermatome, and little, if any, extension of the field occurred into the denervated and contiguous skin of the adjacent dermatomes (Figs. 12-5 and 12-7). The corollary to these findings came from experiments in which an entire dermatome was left with its innervation intact, but that of the adjacent dermatomes was eliminated by section of their dorsal cutaneous nerves. Even though the operations were performed well within the critical period, no subsequent low-threshold mechanosensory nerve sprouting into the denervated skin on either side of the still innervated dermatome could be detected (Figs. 12-5 and 12-8). There are no morphological features indicating where the skin of one dermatome merges with that of its neighbors, but *the nerves* behave as though they recognize the boundary and respect it.

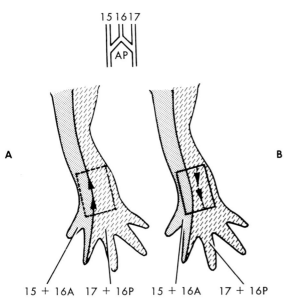

Fig. 12-6. Evidence for nerve domains from skin rotation experiments in salamanders. Hindlimbs **A** and **B** show mechanosensory fields of spinal nerves 15, 16, and 17 in same animal, **A** being control limb and **B** the experimental one. **A,** Control limb. Broken line indicates original position and arrows indicate original orientation of skin, which in experimental limb **B** was rotated and grafted. **B,** Experimental limb. Skin flap was rotated 180 degrees 6 weeks earlier. Note that after graft became reinnervated, *15* to *17* boundary in it was reestablished according to original location of this boundary *with respect to limb coordinates; 15 to 17* line bore no relation to its original position as defined on skin itself, which is indicated by arrowed line within graft. Note that subfields of *16* (*16A* and *16P*) overlap and coincide exactly with fields of *15* and *17*, respectively. Nerves that grew into graft in general extended from edges toward middle, and frequently fibers of *15* and *16A* must have reached border before those of *17* and *16P* had become established there. (From Diamond, J. In Schmitt, F. O., and Worden, F. G., eds.: The neurosciences: fourth study program, Cambridge, 1979, The M. I. T. Press.)

Regenerating nerves

What is the behavior of *regenerating* nerves in the rat? Here the situation differs

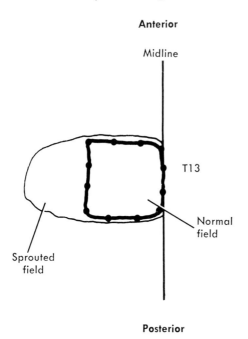

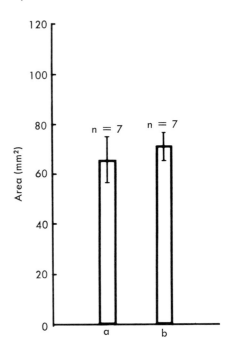

Fig. 12-7. Spatially restricted sprouting of low-threshold mechanosensory nerve within "critical period." Characteristic pattern of enlargement of *medial* DCN of T13 field after surrounding denervation performed at 10 days of age. Heavily outlined field with dots is typical of medial DCN of T13 field of 20-day-old animals in control group of Fig. 12-5. Enlarged field shown by thin outline is that of animal in experimental group; mechanosensory nerve sprouting that occurred was restricted almost entirely to "parent" dermatome, that of T13 (see Fig. 12-4).

Fig. 12-8. Failure of mechanosensory nerves to sprout outside their "domain" within critical period. In this investigation *entire* DCN of T13 low-threshold mechanosensory field, that is, medial *plus* lateral, was mapped at 20 days of age, both for control group of animals, *a*, and experimental group, *b*. However in animals of latter group DCN's of T10, T11, T12, L1, L2, and L3 on both sides and that of T13 on right had been cut 10 days earlier. There was no significant extension of remaining "dermatomal" field of T13 into denervated skin of adjacent dermatomes. (Compare Fig. 12-5; note too that enlarged DCN *sub*field [medial] of experimental group in Fig. 12-5 had value approximately equal to that of *combined* medial and lateral DCN fields measured in this experiment [65 to 70 mm^2]; this is additional evidence that in experiments of Fig. 12-5 and 12-7 sprouting medial branch of DCN of T13 had occupied available area originally supplied by *lateral* branch but had failed to extend significantly into denervated dermatomes cranial and caudal to it.)

dramatically from that for intact nerves. There is no critical period for regeneration; this process occurs in the adult much as it does in the neonate. Of special interest however is the result obtained when a single remaining nerve regenerates into a relatively large region of denervated skin. A partial denervation of back skin was performed (in a *post*critical–period animal) that left only one nerve branch supplying a portion of a single dermatome intact, as in the experiments described previously; however, this remaining nerve was then crushed at its entry into the skin. This was followed by regeneration of the nerve. The regenerating fibers first grew

to fill their original field, *but they then continued to grow outside it and established mechanosensory function in the denervated skin of the adjacent dermatomes* in addition to that of their parent dermatome (Fig. 12-9; see also the neonatal sprouting shown in

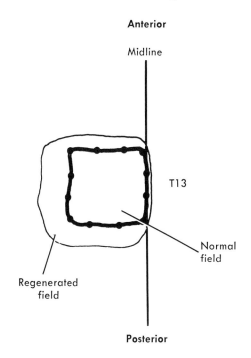

Anterior

Midline

T13

Normal field

Regenerated field

Posterior

Fig. 12-9. Invasion of "foreign" skin by regenerating nerve in mature rat. Typical result obtained in 68-day-old animal, in which mechanosensory field of medial branch of DCN of T13 would be approximately that indicated by heavy outline (about 160 mm²). However, 28 days earlier, (well beyond end of "critical period" for sprouting) denervation was done to leave this field as "island" of innervation (see Fig. 12-4); however, in addition, *remaining medial branch of DCN of T13 was crushed at its entry to the skin.* Regenerating nerve grew back to its original field and then invaded skin of adjacent dermatomes to produce mechanosensory area shown by thin outline.

Fig. 12-7). Frontiers were not recognized, any more than a critical period, by these *regenerating* nerves.

CONCLUSIONS AND A TENTATIVE SUGGESTION

We propose that nerves remaining after partial denervation, regenerating nerves, and almost certainly those first arriving during development sprout locally at their target tissue under the influence of a sprouting stimulus provided by the target itself.[7] The nerve endings probably associate with spe-cific target sites and then provide a continuous influence that reduces the effectiveness of the sprouting stimulus, so that sprouting eventually ceases. Section of nerves, or reduction of axoplasmic transport in them (at least in some systems), removes part of the constraint imposed by the nerves and thus restores the effectiveness of the sprouting stimulus with subsequent collateral sprouting of the untreated or undamaged fibers.[1,3] However, there are important differences between normal intact nerves and regenerating ones. The former appear to be contained within defined regions that we call "domains," which are probably established during development.[5] Intact nerves will sprout in partially or totally denervated skin located within the borders of their domain but not readily into similar skin outside those borders. It seems that the skin itself does not play a role in maintaining these domains, which are defined with reference to the coordinates of the body. Thus a mechanism separate from that which *evokes* sprouting exists to restrict sprouting to defined areas. However, regenerating nerves do not appear to be susceptible to this spatial control; they will readily extend across dermatomal frontiers into denervated skin of neighboring domains.[6,14]

These findings suggest an interesting possibility. If our results in the rat and the rabbit are applicable to the human, then collateral sprouting of *intact* low-threshold cutaneous nerves will be confined to early life and even then would conform to the limitations imposed by the "domains." Consider a nerve lesion so irreparable as to permit no significant regeneration. In the adult the resultant area of anesthetic skin would almost certainly fail to become invaded by sprouting of adjacent undamaged nerves. However, deliberate surgical intervention to *crush* an adjacent intact cutaneous nerve should be followed by successful regeneration of the crushed fibers. As we have shown, such *regenerating* nerves may be expected to extend without restriction into denervated skin. Furthermore, regeneration occurs at virtually all ages. Of course there could be difficulties in the central interpretation of signals coming from nerves that now occupy areas of the body outside their allotted domains, but this would perhaps be less of a problem than the possession of a permanently nerve-deprived area of skin.

Finally, we wonder if the sprouting of remaining nerves in the adult rabbit described by Weddell, Guttmann, and Gutmann[19] might not have been evoked by their techniques of testing for sensory innervation. The repeated deep pinprick of skin at the edge of an anesthetic area might traumatize the surrounding intact nerve fibers, evoking their *regeneration*, with subsequent invasion of the denervated region.

We are currently extending our investigations to see if other modalities, in particular high-threshold mechanosensory nerves, are subject to similar constraints in sprouting to those that operate on the low-threshold fibers.

SUMMARY

Recovery from nerve lesions is assisted by two peripheral processes, axonal regeneration from the site of the lesion and collateral sprouting of remaining undamaged fibers at the affected target tissue. In the salamander the epidermal Merkel cells are the targets for the cutaneous mechanosensory nerves; when these cells are denervated, other intact mechanosensory nerves are induced to sprout and reinnervate them. However, once it is innervated a Merkel cell loses its target character, and sprouting of functional endings ceases when all of the Merkel cells are occupied. The nerves themselves thus appear to regulate the sprouting stimulus of the target tissue by a continually active influence, and this was shown to depend on axoplasmic transport. The distribution of the endings of *regenerating* nerves (when these reach the skin) is also dependent on the equilibrium between the local sprouting stimulus from the target and the "neutralizing" effect of the nerves themselves. *Mammalian* skin gives different results; collateral sprouting can have a "critical period" confined to neonatal life; for example, in rats older than 20 days of

age, low-threshold mechanosensory nerves that remain intact after a lesion appear not to sprout new functional endings into the denervated skin. Nevertheless nerves *regenerate* after lesions, and such regenerating nerves will functionally innervate deprived skin at *all* ages.

A separate mechanism from that which evokes sprouting appears to regulate the *area* of target tissue that a nerve will supply. The low-threshold axons of segmental nerves will sprout only within certain "domains" of body space whose borders, especially in the mammal (the neonatal rat), usually coincide the dermatomal ones. These borders are recognized and respected by intact nerves, which do not readily invade denervated skin of a "foreign" domain. However, the domain boundaries are not respected by *regenerating* nerves. This finding plus the ability of nerves to *regenerate* at all ages in the mammal suggest a means of encouraging the extension of cutaneous innervation after an irreparable nerve lesion in man. The surgical crushing of a remaining intact nerve would be followed by its regeneration, first into its original field, and *then beyond it* into adjacent deprived skin (even if this were part of a "foreign" domain). In mature rats exactly this procedure was shown by us to be successful in restoring touch sensation to a region of skin permanently deprived of its original nerves.

ACKNOWLEDGMENT

This work was supported by the Medical Research Council of Canada and by the Multiple Sclerosis Society of Canada.

REFERENCES

1. Aguilar, C. E., et al.: Evidence that axoplasmic transport of trophic factors is involved in the regulation of peripheral nerve fields in salamanders, J. Physiol. **234:**449, 1973.
2. Cooper, E., and Diamond, J.: A quantitative study of the mechanosensory innervation of the salamander skin, J. Physiol. **264:**695, 1977.
3. Cooper, E., Diamond, J., and Turner, C.: The effects of nerve section and of colchicine treatment on the density of mechanosensory nerve endings in salamander skin, J. Physiol. **264:**725, 1977.
4. Cooper, E., Scott, S. A., and Diamond, J.: Control of mechanosensory nerve sprouting in salamander

skin. In Cowan, W. M., and Ferrendelli, J. A., eds: Approaches to the cell biology of neurons, Neurosci. Symp. **2:**120, 1977.

5. Diamond, J.: The regulation of nerve sprouting by extrinsic influences. In Schmitt, F. O., and Worden, F. G., eds.: The neurosciences: fourth study program, Cambridge, 1979, The M.I.T. Press.

6. Diamond, J., and Jackson, P.: Do cutaneous nerves sprout in the mammal? J. Physiol. **280:**52, 1978.

7. Diamond, J., et al.: Trophic regulation of nerve sprouting, Science **193:**371, 1976.

8. Guttmann, L.: Median-ulnar nerve communications and carpal tunnel syndrome, J. Neurol. Neurosurg. Psychol. **40:**982, 1977.

9. Hamilton, W. J., and Mossman, H. W.: Human embryology, ed. 4, chapter XIII, Cambridge, 1972, W. Heffer and Sons Ltd.

10. Holmes, M. J., et al.: Neuronal transport in salamander nerves and its blockade by colchicine, Brain Res. **136:**31, 1977.

11. Lasek, R. J., and Hoffman, P. N.: The neuronal cytoskeleton, axonal transport and axonal growth. In Goldman, R., Pollard, T., and Rosenbaum, J., eds.: Cell motility, Cold Spring Harbor Laboratory, 1976.

12. Levi-Montalcini, R., and Angeletti, P. V.: Axoplasmic transport, Prog. Neurobiol. **2:**205, 1974.

13. Livingston, W. K.: Evidence of active invasion of denervated areas by sensory fibers from neighbouring nerves in man, J. Neurosurg. **4:**140, 1947.

14. Macintyre, L., and Diamond, J.: In preparation.

15. Parducz, A., et al.: The Merkel cell and the rapidly adapting mechanoreceptors of the salamander skin, Neuroscience **2:**511, 1977.

16. Scott, S. A., Macintyre, L., and Diamond, J.: In preparation.

17. Scott, S. A., Cooper, E., and Diamond, J.: In preparation.

18. Sherrington, C. S.: Experiments in examination of the peripheral distribution of the fibres of the posterior roots of some spinal nerves, Philos. Trans. R. Soc. Lond. [Biol.] **184:**641, 1893.

19. Weddell, G., Guttmann, L., and Gutmann, E.: The local extension of nerve fibers into denervated areas of skin, J. Neurol. Neurosurg. Psychiatry **4:**206, 1941.

DISCUSSION

Tupper: With a severed distal nerve we rarely see any return of sensation in a significant amount unless the nerve is repaired. This would agree with your rat results where intact nerves do not invade denervated areas. On the other hand, in recent years we've been removing a large number of sural nerves for grafts. There is frequently a large patch of numbness after removal of the sural nerve immediately, and yet over the course of 6 to 7 months this patch shrinks markedly in size when tested by pinpricks. How do we explain this?

Diamond: You didn't record nerve impulses, and there may be other nerves that are involved, especially near the borders of the denervated area; the input from these nerves may become "unmasked" in time, as assessed subjectively. This, of course, is only a speculation. Perhaps Sir Sydney can speak to this?

Sunderland: I would like to comment on the degree of overlap in the distribution of main cutaneous nerves. You know that in the old days of *Gray's Anatomy*, you dissected out the cutaneous distribution of the ulnar and median nerves and you had a nice line running down the palm, with ulnar nerve innervation on the ulnar side and the median nerve innervation on the median side. Well now I suspect that the distribution of our peripheral nerves is far greater than the scalpel and forceps leads us to believe. Because I know that in my advanced years now, if I fully flex my elbow on my chest I can put my ulnar nerve to sleep without any difficulty at all, and its innervation extends as far radially as the entire index finger. Yet I'm sure that if someone dissected out my ulnar nerve, he'd come to the conclusion that it only innervated the classical one and a half or perhaps the two ulnar digits. I think that

there's a much finer microscopical distribution of nerve terminals out in the skin than we've been led to believe.

Jewett: Dr. Diamond, do you suggest that if we do have a denervated area of skin, deliberate damage of the skin might act like a more direct nerve crush to give a chance of further reinnervation?

Diamond: If you want to get sensation back, I believe you've got to somehow damage the nearest nerve to initiate its regeneration. You can do it locally, you don't need to go up in the limb. If you actually even make cuts in the skin towards the edge of the still-innervated field, my guess would be, on the basis of our results, that they would start regenerating and invading the numb area. It would be regeneration from the side; it wouldn't be denervation sprouting, which happens with an intact nerve. But this is only a guess.

Also, let me reiterate my views about pinpricks. Weddell, Guttmann, and Gutmann[*] describe how they push the pin at 1 mm intervals into the skin of the rabbit. What we have found is that if you deliberately damage the skin nerve endings, they regenerate from that point on vigorously, and they can sometimes just go sweeping across the denervated rat skin. I wonder if the actual testing is damaging some fibers, and once they are damaged, they are then *regenerating* fibers. You see, such fibers are not intact normal collateral fibers, they are fibers that, in effect, have been cut and then regenerate We have a lot of evidence, in the salamander too, that you can achieve this very readily by just local damage in the skin. In other words, you must not test by using damaging procedures. Light touch alone would be a better test,

---

[*]Weddell, G., Guttmann, L., and Gutmann, E.: J. Neurol. Neurosurg. Psychiatry 4:206, 1941.

but then you might not get the sensory return!

Editor: One wonders what the pounding of amputation stumps does to peripheral innervation in patients with phantom pains and/or hyperesthesia.

Diamond: From our work we suspect that continuous traumatization of skin would initiate nerve sprouting. Could this cause hypersensitive endings to appear in the skin? Such endings may never differentiate fully because they do not find appropriate target sites.

Horch: From the work that Burgess and I have done in the adult cat, it turns out that the amount of sprouting you see if you leave the skin undamaged and don't apply noxious stimuli to the denervated area skin is very small. Using a mapping method, where we know exactly where the receptors are and therefore can eliminate any question of stimulus spread, the reinnervation is limited to the very border of the denervated area. By and large, the central area of denervation remains denervated for at least a year if the severed axons are restricted from reappearing; even if you let them regrow, they don't fill in the field completely and there are patches of the field that are essentially denervated as described by Dr. Tupper. It's as if a neuron can only send a sprout out so far and then it gives up, similar to the situation in the central nervous system where these collateral sprouts will only move a few millimeters at the most, and then give up.

Jewett: What is it that controls sprouting at the cut end of a nerve?

Sunderland: I think this has a very simple answer: we don't know. We can only speculate on the axon as it leaves the endoneurial tube. The proximal stump is now in an entirely different medium or matrix where the predominant tissue is collagen. The manner in which the collagen is aligned, so to speak, will determine the initial direction taken by the axon. When it meets an obstacle, it will branch and move around, but that's sheer speculation. There's no doubt whatsoever that there is a prolific sprouting and branching of axons at the proximal stump of the severed nerve, but what is responsible for it, controls it, or terminates it I just don't know.

Editor: One wonders if we crush the nerve to a muscle, will further sprouting and innervation occur as might be desirable in polio? Or is it that motoneurons sprout maximally in such a disease?

Editor: Are the terminal endings of the axons in the salamander and/or the rat surrounded by endoneurial tubes, and, if so, how do collaterals and/or sprouts of the axons cross this barrier?

Diamond: Although we have not studied this in detail, in the salamander the non-neural supporting cells do not seem to accompany the final axon terminal as it penetrates the basal lamina to enter the epidermis. However, we do *not* know exactly where collateral sprouting begins, only where it ends. New branches might take off from the parent axon in the dermis or even below it. The point is an excellent one. I believe that sprouting axonal branches, be they collateral or those that Dr. Sunderland referred to at the proximal stump of a severed nerve, will not get far as *naked* extensions. They need their supporting cells. Perhaps it is these latter cells that regulate the extent of sprouting by "staying put" as it were. Conversely, when the non-neural cells divide and migrate readily, then the axon terminal can get further in its growth. Perhaps the initiation of *regeneration*, which as I said may promote innervation far beyond that achieved by the collateral sprouting of remaining undamaged axons, really affects the supporting cells. These are stimulated by damage and so "unleash" the axon whose extension they can follow into otherwise "foreign" territory. Who knows?

13

Reinnervation of skeletal muscle: restoration of the normal synaptic pattern

Joshua R. Sanes, Lawrence M. Marshall, and U. J. McMahan

Motor axons branch within the skeletal muscles that they innervate, supplying each muscle fiber with at least one, and usually exactly one, contact or neuromuscular junction (nmj). Damage to the axons leaves the muscle denervated, but the axons can regenerate from the point of injury to reinnervate the muscle and restore neuromuscular function. The success of reinnervation varies with a number of factors, including the way in which the axon is injured and the length of time that the muscle stays denervated. Under optimal conditions, however, reinnervation can be remarkably complete and precise—that is, nearly every fiber in the muscle is reinnervated, and the new nmj's that are formed look and perform very much like the original ones did. This chapter summarizes our studies on the extent to which the normal synaptic pattern is reestablished when skeletal muscles are reinnervated and on the factors that guide the regenerating axons as they grow into the muscle and form new nerve terminals. Our methods and results are detailed elsewhere,[8-12] and extensive references to other relevant articles can be found in reviews that have recently appeared.[1,4,5,14]

THE NORMAL NEUROMUSCULAR JUNCTION

The motor axon loses its myelin sheath as it approaches the muscle fiber and terminates in an array of branches on the fiber's surface (Fig. 13-1, A). The patterns formed by these branches vary from muscle to muscle and species to species, but most vertebrate nmj's (including those in human muscle) are similar in their ultrastructure (Figs. 13-1, B, and 13-2). The nerve terminal lies in a shallow groove or gutter on the muscle fiber's surface and is capped by the processes of a Schwann cell. A synaptic cleft, about 50 nm wide, separates the nerve from the muscle. A sheath of basal lamina (sometimes called basement membrane) surrounds each muscle fiber and runs through the synaptic cleft. The basal lamina is a collagenous, extracellular sheath, not a cellular membrane,[7] and as such it is permeable to neurotransmitter that is released from the nerve terminal. The Schwann cell also has a basal lamina, and the basal laminae of Schwann and muscle cells fuse at the edges of the nerve terminal.

Both nerve and muscle are specialized in their region of contact. The nerve terminal, for example, contains large numbers of membrane-bound, 50 nm-diameter vesicles and is, in this respect, distinguishable from preterminal portions of the axon, which contain few vesicles. Some of these synaptic vesicles, which probably contain the neurotransmitter, acetylcholine, are clustered near thickened patches of the presynaptic membrane called active zones. Active zones are the sites from which acetylcholine is thought to be released. There are no active zones in preterminal portions of the axon.

The muscle fiber is also differentiated in the region of the synapse. Its surface is

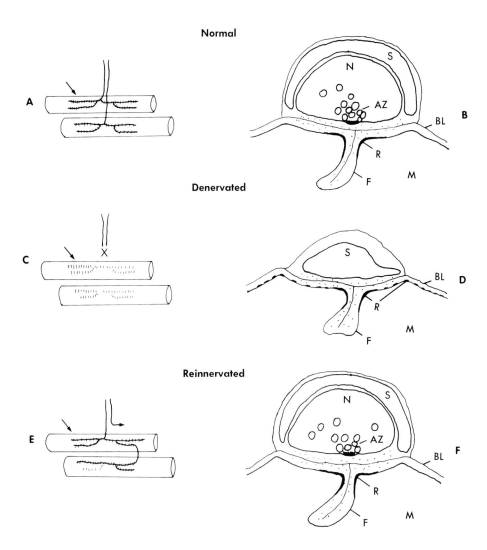

Fig. 13-1. Normal, denervated, and reinnervated end-plates. **B, D,** and **F** sketch electron microscopic cross sections taken at levels indicated by arrows in **A, C,** and **E. A** and **B,** In normal muscle, axons terminate in spray of fine branches at the neuromuscular junction. Nerve terminals, *N*, are capped by processes of Schwann cell, *S*, and are separated from muscle fiber, *M*, by 50 nm synaptic cleft. Vesicles and active zones, *AZ*, in terminal lie opposite mouths of junctional folds, *F*, that indent muscle fiber's surface. Sheet of basal lamina, *BL*, passes through synaptic cleft and extends into folds. Acetylcholine receptors, *R*, are concentrated at the crests of the folds. **C** and **D,** Nerve terminals degenerate in denervated muscle, folds widen, and some receptors appear extrasynaptically, but Schwann cell and specialized features of postsynaptic membranes persist. **E** and **F,** During reinnervation, axons regenerate to fill original synaptic sites and form new neuromuscular junctions. Extrasynaptic acetylcholine receptors disappear. Branching pattern of regenerating axons is sometimes aberrant, but ultrastructure of new nerve terminals is quite normal.

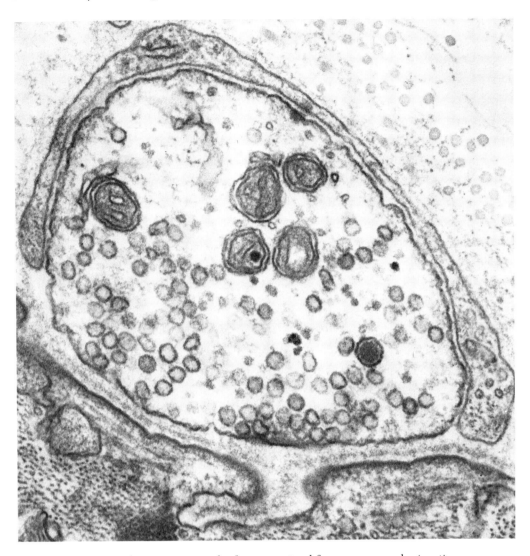

Fig. 13-2. Electron micrograph of cross-sectional frog neuromuscular junction.

thrown into folds beneath the nerve terminal, and the basal lamina of the synaptic cleft
extends into the folds. Active zones in the
nerve terminal almost invariably lie directly
opposite the mouths of these junctional folds.
Acetylcholine receptors, with which acetylcholine combines to activate the muscle, are
concentrated in the subsynaptic membrane
of the muscle fiber. Thickenings and specializations of this subsynaptic membrane, some
of which may correspond to acetylcholine receptors, can be seen by thin-section and
freeze-fracture electron microscopy. The en-

zyme acetylcholinesterase, which inactivates
acetylcholine after it has acted, is also concentrated at the nmj, and when muscles are
treated with a histochemical stain for this enzyme, reaction product fills the synaptic
cleft. At least some of the acetylcholinesterase of the nmj is associated with the basal
lamina of the cleft.[10]

DENERVATED MUSCLE

When the motor axons that supply a muscle are damaged, their distal portions degenerate, and the muscle is left denervated (Fig.

13-1, *C*). The nerve terminals are phago-cytized by Schwann cells. Neuromuscular transmission can fail within a few hours of nerve damage, and the terminal is generally removed within a few days. (These processes vary with the distance between the site of nerve injury and the nmj's. In mammals transmission fails roughly 2 hours later for every extra centimeter of nerve stump length.)

The muscle is profoundly affected by denervation—its mechanical, electrical, and metabolic properties are all altered, and ul-timately the muscle fiber atrophies. Despite these changes, however, the subsynaptic re-gion of the muscle fiber retains several of its specialized properties (Fig. 13-1, *D*). Junc-tional folds become wider and shallower after denervation but they, and the projections of basal lamina that extend into them, persist. Acetylcholinesterase levels decline, but his-tochemically demonstrable enzyme remains at the end-plate for many months after the muscle is denervated. Acetylcholine recep-tors appear throughout the plasma mem-brane of denervated myofibers, but they re-main at their highest concentration in the postsynaptic membrane. Finally, processes of Schwann cells remain behind after they have phagocytized the nerve terminal and come to abut the original postsynaptic mem-brane. If denervation is prolonged these processes eventually retract, but even then their sheaths of basal lamina persist.

PRECISE REINNERVATION OF ORIGINAL SYNAPTIC SITES

The new nmj's that form when denervated muscle is reinnervated are similar in their geometry (Fig. 13-1, *E*) and ultrastructure (Fig. 13-1, *F*) to the original nmj's. Further-more, new nmj's generally form precisely at those sites on the muscle fibers where the original nmj's had been. The early light mi-croscopic studies in which this pattern was first documented[6] have more recently been confirmed and extended by electron micros-copy. Either the histochemical stain for acetylcholinesterase or the presence of junc-tional folds can be used to identify original synaptic sites. In the electron microscope,

one finds that reinnervation is precise at a submicron level: new nerve terminals lie di-rectly above the junctional folds of the origi-nal synaptic sites.

The preference of regenerated nerve ter-minals for original synaptic sites varies from one experimental situation to another, and in some cases large numbers of completely new nmj's are formed far from the sites of the orig-inal nmj's.[1,5,14] Generally, however, most of the new nmj's are formed at original synaptic sites. In our study of frog muscle,[8,12] in which the nerve was crushed (rather than cut) and the injury was inflicted very near the nerve's entry into the muscle, over 98% of the axonal processes that approached muscle fibers made their contacts precisely at original synaptic sites (Fig. 13-3, *A*).

It is also worth noting that reinnervation can be quite complete: in our experiments, functional neuromuscular transmission was restored to over 95% of the muscle fibers within 3 weeks of nerve crush, and over 90% of the original synaptic surface was covered by regenerated nerve terminals (Fig. 13-3, *B*)

The precision and completeness of rein-nervation are especially striking in light of the fact that original synaptic sites occupy only about 0.1% of each muscle fiber's sur-face. How do growing axons find and recog-nize these sites? Some guidance is provided by the surviving perineurial and endoneurial sheaths of the nerves through which the re-generating axons generally grow. However, regenerating axons growing outside of their original pathways can pass over long stretches of extrasynaptic muscle membrane to form synapses at original sites. One sort of pattern sometimes encountered in reinner-vated muscle is diagrammed in Fig. 13-1, *E*. Regenerating axons, unlike normal axons, often continue to grow after they have formed a nmj. Their so-called "escaped fibers,"[6] which are clearly not confined to any preexisting pathways, almost invariably form additional synapses only when they again en-counter original synaptic sites. Thus there must be factors at the original site itself that account, at least in part, for its precise rein-nervation.

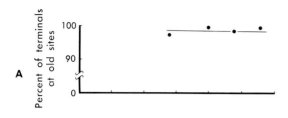

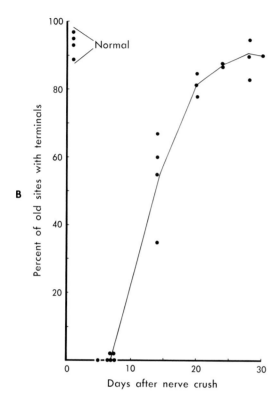

Fig. 13-3. Precision and completeness of reinnervation of frog muscle, at various times after nerve crush. **A,** Percentage of all nerve terminals seen in electron microscope that lie within 0.1 μm of original synaptic site (marked by histochemical stain for acetylcholinesterase) provides a measure of precision of reinnervation. **B,** Because virtually all nerve terminals are located at original synaptic sites, percentage of such sites that are opposed by terminals provides a measure of completeness of reinnervation.[8,12]

PRECISE REINNERVATION OF ORIGINAL SYNAPTIC SITES IN DAMAGED MUSCLE

The factors that guide the precise reinnervation of original synaptic sites might be in (or be) any of several structures. One obvious candidate is the muscle cell itself—for example, the nerve might be attracted by substances released by the muscle from its endplate, or it might recognize molecules in the postsynaptic membrane. In order to examine these possibilities, we studied the reinnervation of muscles in which the muscle cells had been killed.[9,12]

If skeletal muscle is damaged in any of a number of ways (for example by mechanical, ischemic, or pharmacological injury), the muscle cells in the region of damage degenerate and are phagocytized.[3] The sheaths of basal lamina, which are extracellular structures, remain behind, however, as do precursor cells within the sheaths, which can divide and differentiate to form new myofibers.[2,3] The basal lamina of the original myofibers thus serves as a scaffold to ensure the orderly regeneration of the damaged muscle (Fig. 13-4, *A*).

If muscles are denervated and damaged simultaneously, regeneration of nerve and muscle proceed concurrently. Myofibers regenerate within the sheaths of basal lamina, axons grow back to their surface, and functional new nmj's are established (Fig. 13-4, *B*). Because the basal lamina survives denervation and damage, it is possible to determine where the original nmj's had been: the acetylcholinesterase that is bound to the basal lamina of the synaptic cleft can be demonstrated histochemically after degeneration of nerve and muscle, and the projections of basal lamina that once extended into the junctional folds provide an independent marker of original synaptic sites. Using these markers, we found that new nmj's were formed preferentially at original synaptic sites, even though the original muscle cell has long since degenerated and been removed. In fact (at least in our experiments, in which the nature and extent of damage was carefully controlled), reinnervation of regenerated muscle was as precise as reinnervation of undamaged muscle: over 95% of the axonal processes that approached the basal lamina sheaths made their contacts at original synaptic sites. Thus, neither the integrity of the

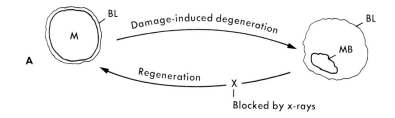

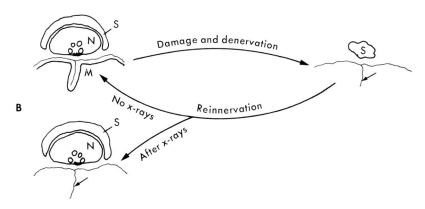

Fig. 13-4. A, Muscle cells, M, degenerate and are phagocytized after they are damaged, but their sheaths of basal lamina, BL, survive. Myoblasts, MB, within sheaths divide and differentiate to produce new muscle fibers, but this process of regeneration can be blocked by x-irradiation. **B,** Nerve terminals, N, and muscle cells, M, both degenerate after muscles are denervated and damaged. X-irradiation prevents regeneration of muscle but not that of nerve. Projections of basal lamina that once extended into junctional fields (arrows), as well as acetylcholinesterase in basal lamina and Schwann cell processes, mark sites where synapses had been even after nerve and muscle have been removed.

original muscle cell nor any appreciable portion of its contents is necessary for the precise reinnervation of original synaptic sites in denervated skeletal muscle. Quite possibly, factors in the basal lamina itself play some role in guiding the growth of the regenerating axon.

Although reinnervation of damaged muscle is precise, it is not complete. A sizable fraction of the original synaptic sites on the basal lamina remained denervated long after myofibers had regenerated and nearby sites had been reinnervated. Our guess is that access to some sites was blocked by connective tissue that built up after surgery. A similar explanation has been advanced to account for the incomplete reinnervation of atrophied mammalian muscle.[6,14]

DIFFERENTIATION OF THE REGENERATING AXON

The precision of reinnervation is manifested not only in the growth but also in the differentiation of the regenerating motor axon. Only those portions of the regenerating axons that approach within about $0.1\ \mu$ of the muscle's fiber's surface acquire active zones and concentrations of synaptic vesicles. Preterminal portions of the axons, or portions that have grown beyond a muscle (for example, Fig. 13-1, E), contain few vesicles and bear no active zones. The mechanisms for transmitter release appear and mature in the reinnervated muscle and, although no direct evidence is available, these mechanisms are presumably also confined to the terminal portions of the regenerated axons.

Within each terminal branch, differentiation proceeds in a precise and orderly fashion. The junctional folds that indent the muscle fiber's surface survive denervation and are eventually covered by the regenerating axons. As the new terminals mature, active zones form and synaptic vesicles accumulate precisely above the mouths of these surviving junctional folds, thus reconstituting the pattern seen in normal muscle. This correspondence between "new" active zones and "old" junctional folds provides strong evidence that factors in or near the muscle fiber's surface guide the transformation of a regenerating axon into a nerve terminal.

FORMATION OF MOTOR NERVE TERMINALS IN THE ABSENCE OF MUSCLE CELLS

Regeneration of nerve and muscle proceed by fundamentally different mechanisms: axons elongate by addition of cytoplasm and membrane to their growing tips, while myofibers form by the mitotic divisions and subsequent fusion of myogenic cells. It is therefore possible to inhibit muscle regeneration selectively by the use of agents such as x-rays, which block cell division.[13] We continued our studies of reinnervation by x-irradiating muscles after we had damaged and denervated them (Fig. 13-4, A). We could then ask whether regenerating axons formed differentiated nerve terminals in the absence of their normal postsynaptic targets, the muscle cells.[12]

Axons regenerated to the "empty" sheaths of basal lamina that persisted in damaged denervated, irradiated muscle (Fig. 13-4, B). The axons contacted the basal lamina precisely at original synaptic sites (marked by acetylcholinesterase or the basal lamina of junctional folds), confirming that the muscle cell need not be present for precise reinnervation to occur. Once returned to the basal lamina sheaths, the regenerating axons differentiated. They acquired active zones and concentrations of synaptic vesicles (Fig. 13-5, B) and in this way became distinguishable from other portions of the axons, which had few vesicles and no active zones (Fig. 13-5,

A). Thus, even though muscle cells had been completely removed from the basal lamina sheaths by the time reinnervation occurred, the axons were able, by morphological criteria (their physiological capabilities have not yet been tested), to differentiate into nerve terminals at an appropriate place and in an organized manner.

As noted above, synaptic vesicles and active zones in normal and reinnervated muscles are concentrated directly opposite the mouths of the junctional folds. In damaged muscle, these sites can be recognized as points where the projections of basal lamina that once lined the folds join the basal lamina of the synaptic cleft (Fig. 13-4, B). When regenerating axons differentiated at original synaptic sites in damaged muscle, their vesicles and active zones were preferentially associated with these points of intersection (Fig. 13-5, B). From this correspondence, one can conclude that there are molecules in the basal lamina of the original synaptic cleft that play a role in triggering or organizing the differentiation of a regenerating axon into a nerve terminal.

PRECISE REINNERVATION OF SKELETAL MUSCLE: THE ROLE OF THE MUSCLE CELL

One can define and study the precision of reinnervation in any of several ways. We have not considered the extent to which axons return to their appropriate muscles after nerve damage or the extent to which motor units within a muscle are correctly reconstituted. Evidence from experimental and clinical studies suggests that reinnervation is often quite imprecise in these regards, although axons can "choose" among various targets and preferentially reinnervate the "correct" muscles or muscle fibers in some situations.[4,5]

We have focused on the precision of reinnervation at the level of individual axons and muscle fibers—that is, without considering whether or not the "correct" axon and muscle fiber are being matched. Although nmj's in reinnervated muscle can be distinguished from normal nmj's (for example, by their "es-

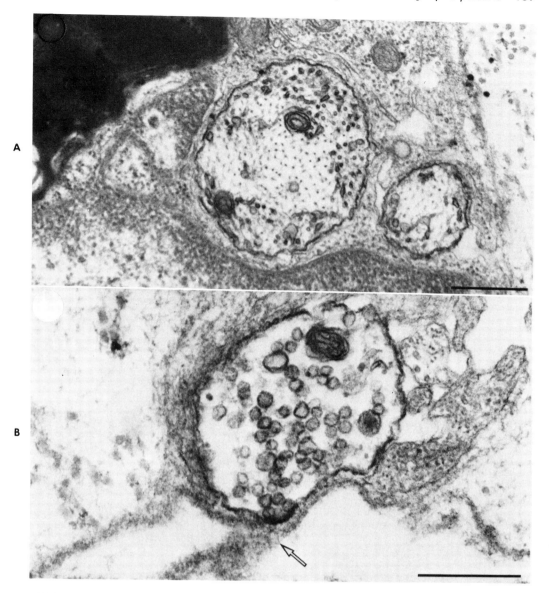

Fig. 13-5. Preterminal and terminal portions of axons reinnervating basal lamina sheaths in damaged, irradiated muscle. **A,** Axons in nerve trunk, wrapped by Schwann cell, contain many neurofilaments and microtubules but few synaptic vesicles. **B,** Nerve terminal, apposed to basal lamina of myofiber sheath, contains numerous synaptic vesicles, some of which are focused on active zone that lies opposite intersection (arrow) of synaptic cleft and junctional fold of basal laminae. Bar is 0.5 μm. (From Sanes, J. R., Marshall, L. M., and McMahan, U. J.: J. Cell Biol. **78:**176, 1978.)

caped fibers"; see Fig. 13-1, *E*), they are quite normal in their geometry, ultrastructure, and function. The restoration of the normal synaptic pattern occurs in large part because the regenerating axons are guided by factors near the muscle fiber's surface and at the original synaptic site. In ways that we do not yet understand, these factors orient the growth and the differentiation of the regenerating axons.

Our experiments on damaged muscle show that some of these factors are not contained within the muscle cell but are associated with the basal lamina that lies just beyond the myofiber's plasma membrane. This is not to minimize the importance of the muscle cell. The myofiber produces and secretes at least some portion of the basal lamina during embryogenesis and thus may be the source of the factors that guide the axons. (It is intriguing, however, to consider the possibility that the axon or Schwann cell may contribute to the basal lamina of the synaptic cleft.) Furthermore, it is our impression that axons do not mature completely or survive indefinitely in the absence of muscle cells—that is, on the basal lamina sheaths of damaged, irradiated muscle. Although alternative explanations have not yet been ruled out, it is possible that motor axons can return to their target areas and differentiate "on their own," but they require trophic support from the muscle cell for their maintenance. Nevertheless, the demonstration that regenerating motor axons can behave normally, in several respects, in the absence of muscle cells draws attention to structures whose importance in the formation of the nmj had previously received little attention—the connective tissue framework that ensheaths each myofiber and especially the basal lamina of the synaptic cleft.

REFERENCES

1. Bennett, M. R., and Pettigrew, A. G.: The formation of neuromuscular synapses, Cold Spring Harbor Symp. Quant. Biol. **40:**409, 1975.
2. Bischoff, R.: Regeneration of single skeletal muscle fibers in vitro, Anat. Rec. **182:**215, 1975.
3. Carlson, B. M.: The regeneration of skeletal muscle—a review, Am. J. Anat. **137:**119, 1972.
4. Fambrough, D. M.: Development of cholinergic innervation of skeletal, cardiac, and smooth muscle. In Goldberg, A. M., and Hanin, I., eds.: Biology of cholinergic function, New York, 1976, Raven Press, p. 101.
5. Fischbach, G. D.: Some aspects of neuromuscular junction formation. In Cox, R. P., ed.: Cell communication, New York, 1974, John Wiley & Sons, Inc., p. 43.
6. Gutmann, E., and Young, J. Z.: The reinnervation of muscle after various periods of atrophy, J. Anat. (Lond.) **78:**15, 1944.
7. Kefalides, N. A.: Structure and biosynthesis of basement membranes, Int. Rev. Connect. Tissue Res. **6:**63, 1973.
8. Letinsky, M. S., Fishbeck, K. H., and McMahan, U. J.: Precision of reinnervation of original postsynaptic sites in muscle after a nerve crush, J. Neurocytol. **5:**691, 1976.
9. Marshall, L. M., Sanes, J. R., and McMahan, U. J.: Reinnervation of original synaptic sites on muscle fiber basement membrane after disruption of the muscle cells, Proc. Natl. Acad. Sci. USA **74:**3073, 1977.
10. McMahan, U. J., Sanes, J. R., and Marshall, L. M.: Cholinesterase is associated with the basal lamina at the neuromuscular junction, Nature **271:**172, 1978.
11. Rotshenker, S., and McMahan, U. J.: Altered patterns of innervation in frog muscle after denervation, J. Neurocytol. **5:**719, 1976.
12. Sanes, J. R., Marshall, L. M., and McMahan, U. J.: Reinnervation of muscle fiber basal lamina after removal of myofibers. Differentiation of regenerating axons at original synaptic sites, J. Cell Biol. **78:**176, 1978.
13. Williams, R. T., and Pietsch, P.: Time-related inhibition of mammalian muscle regeneration by x-irradiation, Anat. Rec. **151:**434, 1965.
14. Zacks, S. I.: The motor endplate, New York, 1973, R. E. Krieger Publishing Co., Inc.

DISCUSSION

Wiley (Solana Beach): You have suggested that the basal lamina reappeared as the nerve grew to that region. Is it at all possible that the basal lamina is partially a secretion of a differentiated nerve terminal?

Sanes: We believe that the *old* basal lamina persists after the muscle degenerates and is contacted by the regenerating nerve. However, it is certainly possible that the basal lamina contains contributions from the nerve terminal. We are intrigued by the possibility that when the nerve develops embryonically, it contributes some substance to the basal lamina at the original synaptic site, and in that way the synaptic site becomes specialized and recognizable later during reinnervation. One of the first signs of the embryonic neuromuscular junction is the appearance of a little bit of cleft material that may be basal lamina in between the nerve and the muscle. Later, as the muscle differentiates, basal lamina appears extrasynaptically all the way around the muscle fiber. So, although there is some evidence that the basal lamina is predominantly secreted by the muscle cell, one possibility is that there is some special component contributed by either the nerve terminal and/or by its associated Schwann cell.

Stein: Considering the idea of a trophic substance in regeneration, is it possible that acetylcholinesterase, for example, was the thing that guided the nerve back to the basal lamina?

Sanes: Yes, that is possible. It is an interesting idea. In one experiment we blocked the active site of acetylcholinesterase at the time we damaged and denervated the muscle, using an irreversible inhibitor, DFP. Under those conditions the nerve still came back just as precisely to the old site, in fact reinnervating it just as completely. Therefore acetylcholinesterase *activity* was not necessary for reinnervation. However, the acetylcholinesterase molecule is a very large one, and we were blocking only a very small portion of it. So I do not think this experiment really rules out the possibility you raise.

Ochs: With regard to the localization of acetylcholinesterase in the basal lamina, we and others have seen a fast transport of acetylcholinesterase in the motor neurons and we have speculated in the past as to the possibility that it may leave the motor terminal and go into the muscle, but we did not quite envision it as staying in the basal lamina and possibly acting as a directing force. It is an interesting possibility, and I would encourage a little bit more of a study along that line.

Anonymous: In reinnervation of the neuromuscular junction what happens if you have the wrong motor axon reach the muscle? It has been shown in fishes, for example, that if you take the inferior oblique muscle and reunite it with the superior oblique nerve, you will have the wrong motor axon regrowing into the muscle and the eye will rotate in the wrong direction. However, after just a month or so, you will have the right nerve growing down and creating a second population of neuromuscular junctions that will take over, and the first population with the wrong axons will be silent. In this case there is functional restitution with two populations of neuromuscular junctions, whereas in mammals we know that if you have aberrant reinnervation in the eye muscles, you will never have that functional restoration. Can you tell us what the difference is between mammals and lower species?

Sanes: My understanding of that literature is that this issue is complex and somewhat controversial. I think it is not quite entirely clear yet to what extent repression can occur in salamanders, frogs, or fish nor whether it is completely absent in mammals. As far as foreign nerves go, in the situation that I was describing, we have transplanted foreign nerves. In particular we took the nerve from the arm and ran it to the cutaneous pectoris muscle of the chest. Those axons went as precisely to original synaptic sites as did the axons of the normal nerve. The reason we did that experiment was that we wanted to avoid limiting ourselves to what has been described as a type II injury. In this case clearly the foreign axons were not confined to any perineurial or endoneurial tubes. What we saw though is that they had a marked affinity for the remaining perineurial tubes of the old muscle. They often entered them intramuscularly, since they could enter them more or less at will, yet all the same they rejected extrasynaptic membrane, chose synaptic membrane, and differentiated only where they touched down.

Aguayo: Did irradiation affect the Schwann cells? Could these cells be part of the guidance mechanism?

Sanes: It is likely that the irradiation affected not only the muscle cells, but that we also inhibited the divisions of the Schwann cell that occur following transection of the nerve. Nevertheless, the Schwann cells that were originally at the neuromuscular junction remained there in many cases, following muscle damage and irradiation. Also, the Schwann cells eventually retracted from the neuromuscular junctions after prolonged denervation, as also occurs in undamaged muscle. We have no way of clearly distinguishing between the basal lamina and the Schwann cell in the guidance. The one argument we have to suggest it is the basal lamina is that we know that after long periods of denervation, Schwann cells retract from the original synaptic site. Yet Letinsky, Fishbeck, and McMahan have shown that even after long periods of denervation when the Schwann cells are gone, the reinnervation of old synaptic sites is complete and precise. We are on firmer ground when looking at the differentiation of the nerve terminals. Here, we are sure that the basal lamina is involved instead of the Schwann cells because we saw active zones directly above sites on the basal lamina that marked the junctional folds.

Editor: It would be of great interest to know if there were "domains" that limit the reinnervation of muscle, in a manner similar to that in skin as described in Chapter 12.

14

A critical review of histological methods used in the study of nerve regeneration

Michael G. Orgel

Much of our understanding about peripheral nerve regeneration after injury has been derived from research involving histological methods. Careful work describing regeneration of myelinated fibers occurred earlier in this century, and technological advances have now made it possible to quantitate regeneration of these fibers. More recently, the advent of the electron microscope has made it possible to quantitate regeneration of the unmyelinated C fibers.

The aim of this presentation is to familiarize the reconstructive surgeon with various histological techniques utilized in the study of nerve regeneration, identify possible sources of error associated with these techniques, and describe a method of combined electrophysiological and morphological study that may eliminate some of these problems. Thus armed, the surgeon can critically assess the results of animal experimentation and apply these results to nerve regeneration after injury in man.

HISTOLOGICAL TECHNIQUES

Silver impregnation techniques have been widely used for the morphological study of the peripheral nervous system since being described by Ramón y Cajal[22] and Bielshowsky[5] at the beginning of this century. Ranson[23] modified Cajal's technique utilizing a pyridine-silver method and was the first to demonstrate the distribution of unmyelinated fibers in somatic nerves. Later in this century Gutmann and Sanders[13] popularized Flem-

ming's solution (chromium trioxide-osmium tetroxide-glacial acetic acid-water) as a fixative for tissue that was then embedded in paraffin. Four- to five-micron sections were cut and stained with a modified Weigert hematoxylin method.[13] Resolution of the myelinated fibers is quite good with the latter technique, and it continues to be used for certain aspects of the study of such fibers (Fig. 14-1).

However, significant problems are associated with these methods when quantitation of nerve regeneration is desired. First, the thickness of the paraffin sections presents the problem that different parts of the nerve will be located in different planes on the section requiring refocusing of the microscope while viewing various parts of the slide. It therefore becomes difficult to accurately photograph all the fibers within a cross section of the nerve bundle for counting purposes. In addition, it is not possible to demonstrate the unmyelinated component well with these techniques, and since the smallest unmyelinated fibers are beyond the resolution of the light microscope, these fibers can only be quantitated by electron microscopy.[1]

An interesting technique for qualitative study of the peripheral nervous system involves the use of methylene blue as an intravital dye.[15,20,24] This substance selectively stains nervous tissue in the living animal by an interaction with the myelin sheath (Fig. 14-2, A) that is not well understood.[18] By utilizing a stereomicroscope, it is possible,

141

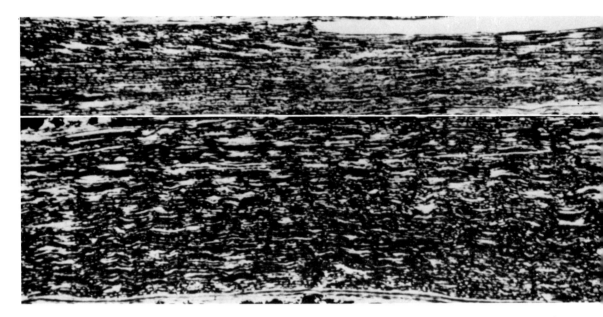

Fig. 14-1. Longitudinal paraffin-embedded section, 5 μ. Fixed in Flemmings solution and counterstained with modified (Weigert) hematoxylin. Note myelinated fibers (black) in this preparation of two fascicles. Rabbit sciatic nerve.

for example, to view all the ramifications of the cutaneous nerves from the subcutaneous tissue to the corpuscular nerve endings after an infusion of methylene blue (Fig. 14-2, *B*). In addition methylene blue preparations can be used to study the "geographic pattern" of recovery after nerve injury and repair.[20]

Longitudinal sections of nerve fibers crossing suture lines or other injuries are necessary adjuncts to quantitative transverse section study but cannot be taken alone as accurate "counts" of nerve fiber regeneration. Simpson and Young[27] have noted that it is "surprisingly easy to draw false conclusions by simple visual or qualitative judgment . . ." of the degree of myelination. Isolated qualitative or "semiquantitative" histological studies of nerve regeneration should be viewed with some skepticism.

Electron microscopic technology has revolutionized the study of myelinated and unmyelinated fibers in nerve regeneration work. Schwann cell axonal relationships remained obscure until defined by this entity, and it was not until quite recently that the formation of myelin[12] and the relationship of

the Schwann cell to the unmyelinated axon was demonstrated.[11] The technique involves now-standard methodology with buffered glutaraldehyde fixation, postfixation in osmium tetroxide, dehydration in graduated alcohols, and embedding in an epoxy resin.[20] For light microscopy, 1 μ sections are counterstained with phenylenediamine (for phase microscopy) (Fig. 14-3, *A*) or methylene or toluidine blue (Fig. 14-3, *B*). Improved resolution, with all myelinated axons being located in one plane, is standard with these preparations (Fig. 14-3, *B*). Another advantage of the plastic embedded material is the availability of an ultrathin contiguous section to be used for electron microscopy. In addition to its use for quantitative study, the 1 μ section is used to determine the most profitable area of the cross section of the nerve bundle to be studied by electron microscopy.

Concomitant with electron microscopic technology, methods have developed for more rapid quantitation of nerve regeneration. In 1961 Espir and Harding[9] introduced an apparatus for measuring and counting myelinated fibers. Dyck and co-workers[8] cal-

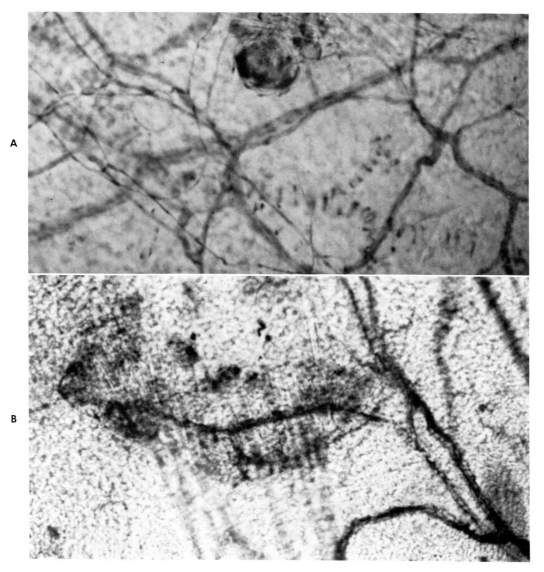

Fig. 14-2. Intravital methylene blue dye. **A,** Horizontal full-thickness preparation of rabbit ear skin. Note polygonal ramifications that become smaller as surface is approached. (×100) **B,** Detail of nerve bundle that is branching and entering corpuscular nerve ending.

culated the area covered by myelinated fibers in nerve bundles. Aguayo and co-workers,[1] using an improved fiber-sizing device,* described methods for the quantitative study of the total fiber population (myelinated and unmyelinated). Nerve fiber circumference as well as the parameters can now also be measured using computer technology.[7]

Our technique[19] for the quantitative histologic study of nerve regeneration after injury will be briefly described. Myelinated fiber sizes and counts are taken from light photomicrographs (1 μ sections) enlarged 1000 times (Fig. 14-3). Measurements are done with a Zeiss (TGZ-3) particle-size analyzer. From this data fiber caliber histograms can be constructed, and the area of each nerve bundle occupied by myelinated fibers

*Zeiss TGZ-3 particle-size analyzer.

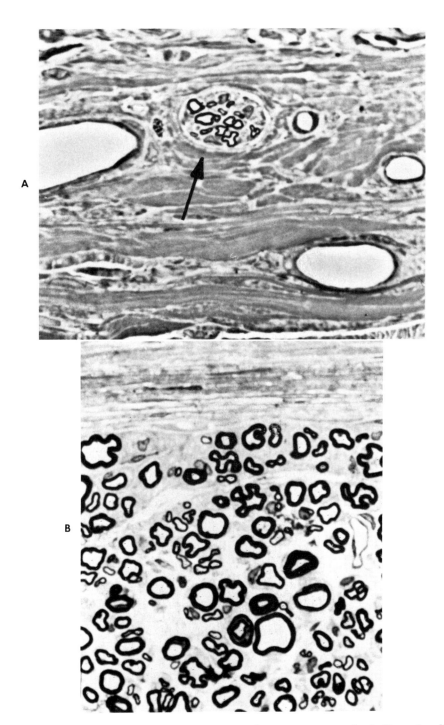

Fig. 14-3. Transverse epon-embedded 1 μ sections for quantitative study. **A,** Nerve bundle in dermis of rabbit ear (arrow). Phase photomicrograph counterstained with phenylenediamine. ($\times$300) **B,** Portion of central fascicle of rabbit sciatic nerve with perineurial sheath. Light photomicrograph counterstained with toluidine blue. ($\times$1000)

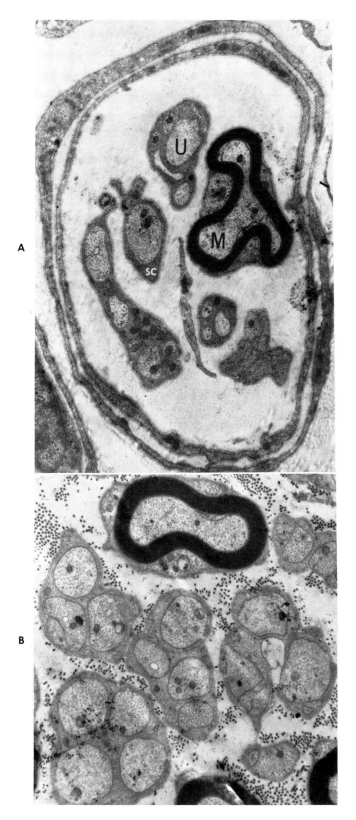

Fig. 14-4. Ultrathin transverse epon-embedded electron microscopic sections. **A,** Nerve bundle in dermis of rabbit ear. Note myelinated fiber, *M,* and unmyelinated fibers, *U,* (which can be quantitated by this technique); *SC,* Schwann cell process. (×8000) **B,** Small portion of central fascicle of rabbit sciatic nerve demonstrating groups of unmyelinated axons within Schwann cell process. (×10,000)

can be calculated. Be defining the total area of the nerve bundle with planimetry, the number of myelinated fibers per square millimeter can be calculated.

Unmyelinated fiber counts are taken from electron photomicrographs enlarged 10,000 times (Fig. 14-4). Similar data and calculations are then derived for this fiber population. In addition, the number of unmyelinated fibers per axon/Schwann cell complex* and the number of these complexes per square millimeter can be determined.

A relatively unexplored morphological technique in nerve regeneration studies concerns the use of the scanning electron microscope.[28] This tool will add another dimension to the qualitative surface study of nerve regeneration when the problem of the masking connective tissue sheaths can be solved.

SOURCES OF ERROR

It is not often possible to obtain detailed quantitative morphology in man; thus nerve regeneration studies present a somewhat unique research challenge. The reconstructive surgeon needs the ability to interpret these studies and relate applicable data to the treatment of the patient. Therefore the sources of error associated with quantitative nerve regeneration studies must be appreciated.

Unavoidable error

Sources of unavoidable error consist of problems with histological technique, magnification, and counting and fiber sizing technique. Each study should be scrutinized to determine if standard methods were used and if repeat checks of magnification were taken so that these errors are kept constant.[13,27] In addition, it is important that each animal serve as its own control, and that data be gathered from the same level of nerves to be compared.

---

*A cross-sectional electron micrograph entity defined as one or more axons, and the associated Schwann cell process, totally enclosed by basal lamina.[2]

Sampling techniques

To decrease the significant amount of effort required to harvest the data from such a project, various authors[7,13,25,27] have sampled a portion of the cross section of nerve for quantitative study. Certain biases may be introduced into the study if optimum sampling techniques have not been used. This kind of study must account for the nonrandom distribution of nerve fibers of different size, the tendency to overestimate small fibers when measurements are taken from electron photomicrographs, and the underestimation of small fibers if only light microscopy is used. These biases can be diminished by sampling enough fibers and surveying large areas of the nerve in question.[7] They can be avoided altogether by complete cross-sectional fiber counts, especially when the fiber density is uneven.

Unmyelinated fibers

Since unmyelinated fibers considerably outnumber myelinated fibers in the mammalian peripheral nervous system,[17] modern morphological studies of nerve regeneration should include counts of these fibers. However, study of the total unmyelinated fiber population presents a monumental undertaking, so sampling methods must be used.[6,7,21] Other problems in the study of these fibers include rare occurrences of unmyelinated axonal bands being invaded by a regenerating axon that may later become myelinated and Schwann cell process that may be mistaken for unmyelinated axons.[16] Again, care must be taken to ensure that these errors remain constant throughout the study. An interesting but unaccountable aspect of unmyelinated nerve fiber regeneration is the phenomenon of preferential but misdirected growth along the more abundant Schwann cell sheaths of degenerated myelinated fibers.[10,14]

Myelin sheath thickness/axonal diameter

Regenerating fibers do not have a constant ratio of myelin sheath thickness to axonal diameter as is found in normal mammalian myelinated nerve fibers.[26] Myelin sheath thickness remains diminished after nerve transection and repair although axonal diameters may approach normal values. A decrease in myelin sheath thickness would theoretically decrease conduction velocity more than a decrease in axonal diameter, and the known deficit in conduction velocity of a regenerating nerve may be due to this fact. However, few studies[7,26] have acknowledged this information.

Fiber maturation

Failure of the regenerating fiber to meet its correct end-organ will retard an increase to normal size in that fiber.[2,4,30] After nerve repair many fibers never reach their terminus and remain immature. A valid longitudinal study of nerve regeneration must therefore encompass a long enough period to take this fact into account. It may be apropos to study end-organ morphology as a more accurate arbiter of nerve regeneration.

COMBINED ELECTROPHYSIOLOGY AND MORPHOLOGY

Because of inherent errors in the study of nerve regeneration by isolated morphological or electrophysiological methods, it is desirable to combine these techniques. Recent investigative tools have made it possible to study both structural and functional nerve regeneration by quantitative techniques. These methods can be applied to the comparison of various kinds of treatment after nerve injury.[19,21] A brief description of the methodology involved will demonstrate a means of combined study that may eliminate some of the problems that have been noted.

Once a question to be answered by the method has been chosen, enough animals are selected to satisfy statistical needs. The animals are divided into groups and treated in exact fashion except for the repairs to be compared. All surgical procedures are done by one investigator under microscopical control. The animals are boarded for their designated period of study and then randomized.

The study nerves are then reexposed and submitted to electrophysiological recordings.[19,29] Platinum stimulating electrodes are placed on individual fascicles distal to the repair, and recordings are taken from corresponding fascicles in the proximal nerve segment. The thresholds for stimulation and response are determined, and the shape, amplitude, and latency of the evolved signals are analyzed. Distance between electrodes is measured to determine conduction velocities of the compound action potentials.

All animals are then subjected to aortic perfusion with 3% cacodylate-buffered glutaraldehyde. The nerve, including neuroma and proximal and distal stumps, is excised. Transverse biopsies, 1 mm, are taken from a representative fascicle at the site or sites to be studied. This tissue is then processed by accepted electron microscopical technique as noted above.

The type of repair in each animal is coded and is unknown to the electrophysiological or morphological investigator. All of the data are analyzed and tabulated prior to breaking the code. This model has been used to study several problems in nerve regeneration of interest to the clinician[19,21] and could be utilized for the study of other traumatic peripheral neuropathies.

SUMMARY

Various histological techniques utilized in nerve regeneration studies have been reviewed, and the possible sources of associated error have been outlined. In addition, a method for combined quantitative electrophysiological and morphological study has been described. It is hoped that the reconstructive surgeon will utilize this information to critically assess experimental work. Only in this manner will it be possible to relate nerve regeneration after injury in animals to the clinical situation.

REFERENCES

1. Aguayo, A. J., and Bray, G. M.: Pathology and pathophysiology of unmyelinated nerve fibers. In Dyck, P. J., Lambert, E. H., and Thomas, P. K., eds.: Peripheral neuropathy, Philadelphia, 1975, W. B. Saunders Co., p. 363.
2. Aguayo, A. J., Peyronnard, J. M., and Bray, G. M.: A quantitative ultrastructural study of regeneration from isolated proximal stumps of transected un-

myelinated nerves, J. Neuropathol. Exp. Neurol. **32:**256, 1973.

3. Aitken, J. T.: The effect of peripheral connexions on the maturation of regenerating nerve fibers, J. Anat. **83:**32, 1949.

4. Aitken, J. T., and Thomas, P. K.: Retrograde changes in fiber size following nerve section, J. Anat. **96:**121, 1962.

5. Bielschowsky, M.: Die Silberimprägnation der Neurofibrillen, J. Psychol. Neurol. (Leipz.) **3:**169, 1904.

6. Bray, G. M., and Aguayo, A. J.: Regeneration of peripheral unmyelinated nerves. Fate of the axonal sprouts which develop after injury, J. Anat. **117:**517, 1974.

7. Bronson, T. B., Bishop, Y., and Hedley-Whyte, E. T.: Contribution to the electron microscopic morphometric analysis of peripheral nerve, J. Comp. Neurol. **178:**177, 1978.

8. Dyck, P. J., et al.: Histologic and teased-fiber measurements of sural nerve in disorders of lower motor and primary sensory neurons, Mayo Clin. Proc. **43:**81, 1968.

9. Espir, M. L. E., and Harding, D. T. C.: Apparatus for measuring and counting myelinated nerve fibers, J. Neurol. Neurosurg. Psychiatry **24:**287, 1961.

10. Evans, D. H. L., and Murray, J. G.: Orientation of regenerating non-medullated nerves, J. Physiol. (Lond.) **120:**52, 1953.

11. Gasser, H. S.: Properties of dorsal root unmedullated fibers on the two sides of the ganglion, J. Gen. Physiol. **38:**709, 1955.

12. Geren, B. B.: The formation from the Schwann cell surface of myelin in the peripheral nerves of chick embryos, Exp. Cell. Res. **7:**558, 1954.

13. Gutmann, E., and Sanders, F. K.: Recovery of fiber numbers and diameters in the regeneration of peripheral nerves, J. Physiol. (Lond.) **101:**489, 1943.

14. King, R. H. M., and Thomas, P. K.: Electron microscope observations on aberrant regeneration of unmyelinated axons in the vagus nerve of the rabbit, Acta Neuropathol. (Berl.) **18:**150, 1971.

15. Miller, M. R., Ralston, H. J., and Kasahara, M.: The pattern of cutaneous innervation of the human hand, Am. J. Anat. **102:**183, 1958.

16. Ochoa, J.: Microscopic anatomy of unmyelinated nerve fibers. In Dyck, P. J., Lambert, E. H., and Thomas, P. K., eds.: Peripheral neuropathies, Philadelphia, 1975, W. B. Saunders Co., p. 131.

17. Ochoa, J., and Mair, W. G. P.: The normal sural nerve in man. I. Ultrastructure and number of fibers and cells, Acta. Neuropathol. (Berl.) **13:**197, 1969.

18. Orgel, M. G.: Nerve regeneration in free skin transplants, Masters thesis, McGill University, 1971.

19. Orgel, M. G., and Terzis, J. K.: Epineurial vs. perineurial repair: an ultrastructural and electrophysiological study of nerve regeneration, Plast. Reconstr. Surg. **60:**80, 1977.

20. Orgel, M. G., Aguayo, A., and Williams, H. B.: Sensory nerve regeneration: an experimental study of skin grafts in the rabbit, J. Anat. **111:**121, 1972.

21. Orgel, M. G., Robillard, D. M., and Terzis, J. K.: Nerve regeneration across nerve graft vs. end-to-end suture: an ultrastructural and electrophysiological study. In press.

22. Ramón y Cajal, S.: Un sencillo método de coloración selectiva del retículo proto plasmico, Trab. Lab. Recherch. Biol. Univ. **2:**129, 1903.

23. Ranson, S. W.: Non-medullated nerve fibers in the spinal nerves, Am. J. Anat. **12:**67, 1911.

24. Richardson, K. C.: The fine staining of autonomic nerves after vital staining with methylene blue, Anat. Rec. **164:**359, 1969.

25. Sanders, F. K., and Young, J. Z.: The influence of peripheral connexion on the diameter of regenerating nerve fibers, J. Exp. Biol. **22:**203, 1946.

26. Schröder, J. M.: Altered ratio between axon diameter and myelin sheath thickness in regenerated nerve fibers, Brain Res. **45:**49, 1972.

27. Simpson, S. A., and Young, J. Z.: Regeneration of fiber diameter after cross-unions of visceral and somatic nerves, J. Anat. **79:**48, 1945.

28. Spencer, P. S., and Lieberman, A. R.: Scanning electron microscopy of isolated peripheral nerve fibers, Z. Zellforsch. **119:**534, 1971.

29. Terzis, J. K., Dykes, R. W., and Hakstian, R. W.: Electrophysiological recordings in peripheral nerve surgery: a review, J. Hand Surg. **1:**52, 1976.

30. Weiss, P., Edds, M. V., and Cavanaugh, M.: The effect of terminal connections on the caliber of nerve fibers, Anat. Rec. **92:**215, 1945.

DISCUSSION

Editor: Does the particle analyzer measure axonal diameter or the outside diameter of the stained myelin? Which diameter do you feel is more useful for nerve studies?

Orgel: The particle size analyzer can measure either axonal diameter or outside diameter of the fiber. Since there is a discrepancy between myelin sheath thickness and axonal diameter in regenerating nerves, both should probably be measured. This has only been done by a few authors as I noted in the text.

Editor: How good is count/recount agreement of the same slide in standard counts?

Orgel: An estimate of between 5% to 10% is probably close to the error in recounting fibers.

Editor: How should the diameter of fibers be dealt with when the axon has been cut at an angle and it appears oval? How good are area measurements under these circumstances?

Orgel: It is important to be consistent in one's decision about oval fibers. Dr. Aguayo and myself always use the smallest diameter in these fibers. Others have taken the average between the largest and smallest diameters. I do not know which is "right," but if treated consistently, it can then be disregarded as a problem. Area measurements are undoubtedly more accurate but require a computer or individual fiber planimetry. My area determinations are made mathematically from diameter measurements.

Editor: Has anyone studied the errors in automatic techniques compared with an exhaustive hand count?

Orgel: I do not know of a comparative study between "automatic" techniques and hand counts. However, one looks at each fiber with the particle size analyzer. It is merely a device for sizing and counting fibers at a more rapid pace.

Editor: How can proximal/distal comparisons ever tell the number of fibers connected centrally if branching occurs? Many studies show higher counts distally than proximally.

Orgel: Branching is a phenomenon of the early regeneration of nerve fibers. As distal connections are made, the higher counts regress and the fibers assume greater diameters. In fact, a greater number of small fibers in the distal segment is a sign of immaturity and lack of distal connections. This is another reason that end-organ morphology needs to be a part of a complete nerve regeneration study.

15

Physiological methods of evaluating experimental nerve repairs

Joseph M. Rosen and Don L. Jewett

New nerve repair techniques should only be introduced and accepted into general practice if they can be conclusively demonstrated to improve the results obtained by previous techniques. To reach this goal, evaluation methods are required that will provide an objective measure of the level of recovery.

Useful recovery of nerve function is defined with respect to man and his capabilities; therefore it is best evaluated in clinical studies. However, there are several significant difficulties with clinical evaluation of the end result of nerve repair techniques. Clinical studies of nerve repair are complicated by the existence of many variables, such as the type of nerve injured, extent of the injury, age of the patient, and level of nerve injury and any associated injuries. Since no two patients provide the same nerve injury and potential for recovery, it is very difficult in clinical studies to isolate the effects of the different types of repair being compared from the other concurrent variables. Another significant obstacle is the difficulty of defining and objectively measuring useful recovery in clinical studies. Although numerous methods of determining clinical end-result function exist, there is little agreement as to what is the best method of evaluation.

Compared with clinical studies, animal experimentation permits greater control of many of the variables influencing recovery; hence each variable can be subjected to separate study and evaluation. Animal experiments also provide objective methods to evaluate the early phases of recovery in a manner not presently obtainable in clinical studies. Some of the available physiological methods of evaluation will be discussed in this chapter.

PHASES OF RECOVERY

An understanding of the phases of functional recovery is a prerequisite to understanding the value and limitations of experimental evaluation methods for nerve repair. Recovery may be divided into three phases (Table 15-1): axonal regeneration, simple function, and complex function (see Chapter 37).

The phases of regeneration are not independent steps. They form a continuum in which each new phase builds on the preceding phase of recovery. The first phase comprises two steps, axonal regeneration across the repair site and the reconnection of axons to the peripheral end-organs. In the first phase axons may succeed in crossing the repair site, or they may regenerate blindly into the connective tissue outside of the endoneurial tubes. The axons that succeed in finding distal endoneurial tubes will only be useful if they establish functionally appropriate connections. Thus the first phase determines the available population of neurons for the subsequent phases of recovery.

AXONAL REGENERATION

A number of fiber types may be generated by nerve repair. We may categorize these types as either connected or unconnected

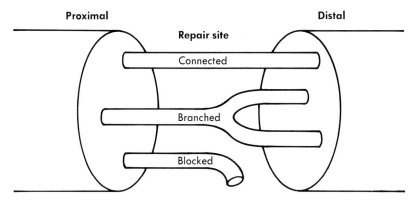

Fig. 15-1. Schematic representation of axon types at repair site: proximal nerve on left and distal nerve on right with connected and unconnected axons illustrated at repair site. "Connected" proximal axon (top) represents axon with single distal connection. Connected proximal "branched" axon (middle) has multiple distal connections. Unconnected "blocked" axon (bottom) has *no* distal connections.

Table 15-1. Phase of recovery (based on Sunderland, Chapter 37).

Phase	Definition	Time course
Axonal regeneration	Reconnection of axon across anastomosis with subsequent reestablishment of connection with peripheral end-organ	Within 3 years
Simple function	Motor: Reappearance of contractions in individual muscles in response to voluntary effort Sensory: Return of protective sensation to denervated skin	Within 3 years
Complex function	Motor: Return of complex movements requiring the coordinated activity of groups of muscles Sensory: Return of discriminative aspects of sensation	Greater than 3 years

axons (Fig. 15-1). The connected axons include proximal axons with one distal connection (Fig. 15-1, top) and proximal axons with multiple distal connections—branched axons (Fig. 15-1, middle). The unconnected axons are proximal axons with no distal connection—blocked axons (Fig. 15-1, bottom). Many other fiber types are possible, but connected and unconnected axon types are sufficient to illustrate the difficulties that must be dealt with by any evaluation method for axonal regeneration.

The functional capacity of regenerated axons is probably altered in multiple ways by the changes in structural geometry that occur during regeneration[15] (see Chapter 19). For example, axon branching acts to compensate for the unconnected proximal axons by allowing the remaining connected axons to innervate multiple distal endoneurial tubes. However, as a consequence of branching after nerve injury, the functional capability of both sensory and motor systems may be reduced.

Branched fibers in the sensory system will result in a decreased specificity of the signals from the skin. If a number of sensory organs in different locations are reinnervated by the same proximal axon, then the information from these sensory receptors is transmitted along the same axons proximal to the repair site. This in turn may prevent discrimination between stimuli originating from different locations on the skin.

Branched fibers in the motor system may also result in a decreased specificity of muscle function. In the normal motor system multiple branchings of axons exist at the level of the muscle. In the repaired nerve a motor proximal axon may branch into multiple endoneurial tubes at the repair site, and the motor signal traveling down this proximal axon may result in stimulation of muscles in different locations. This may lead to a loss in independent control of motor activity or loss in coordinated activity.

In addition, fibers that decrease in diameter distal to the repair site may not function normally when they have reinnervated the distal structure, since smaller diameter axons are limited in their speed of conduction and capacity to fire at higher frequencies.[22]

Fibers with an abrupt decrease in diameter at the repair site may have a decreased functional capacity. At the extreme, if the change in diameter is great enough, the axon may conduct centrifugally but not centripetally.[15] In such a case the functional effect would be greatest in sensory fibers in contrast to motor fibers, and the fiber would act like a blocked (unconnected) axon.

The overall effect on clinical function of these changes is unknown at present, but it is clear that regenerated axons with changed structure both with respect to branching, internodal length, axon diameter to myelin ratio, nodal area, and so on, undoubtedly alter the functional capacity of the regenerated nerve (see Chapter 19).

Experimental evaluation methods are of value in predicting certain of these structural changes and connections. However, detection and quantification of most of the characteristics of newly regenerated axons remain beyond the capacities of presently available evaluation methods.

Objective evaluation methods for axonal regeneration may be based on histology, biochemistry, or physiology. Representative

methods are listed in Table 15-2. Each of these methods will be discussed with respect to its values and limitations for evaluation of axonal regeneration.

Histology

Histological evaluation methods can determine the number and diameter of the axons proximal and distal to the repair site (for a review of these methods, see BeMent and Olson[3] and Chapter 14). These have classically been important in exploring the mechanisms of degeneration and regeneration.[23] Histology continues to contribute to our knowledge of nerve regeneration, but it is limited in its ability to compare various nerve repair techniques because of the difficulty in determining the number of proximal axons with distal connections. Examination of Fig. 15-1 will show why histological counts of the number of fibers proximal and distal to the repair zone cannot indicate how many of the *proximal* fibers are capable of approaching normal function. The presence of branched fibers (connected) and fibers that end in the scar (unconnected) makes the straight comparison of the number of myelinated axons proximal and distal to the repair site an uncertain approximation; the axons that end in the scar are blocked and are thus nonfunctioning, but the distal axon count may not reveal such fibers because the branched axons fill the empty endoneurial tubes and elevate the distal count. It is not uncommon for the distal count to be 150% or more of the proximal count.[17,19,23,26,28] Since individual axons can branch into as many as 20 distal fibers,[17] such histological analysis gives no indication as to how many proximal axons are functionally connected with the periphery

If there are a significant number of blocked axons that are not detected by the counting procedure, then this method of study will give a poor reflection of the possible functioning of the nerve, since blocked axons offer no useful information to the animal and cannot be physiologically compensated for by the branched axons despite their number.

Proximal diameter histograms may provide

Table 15-2. Evaluation methods for axonal regeneration (myelinated axon population)

Method	Value	Limitation
Histology		
Axon counts	Measure of number of axons present	Cannot differentiate between connected and unconnected proximal axons
Axon diameter distribution (histogram)	Measure of number and diameter of axons present	Cannot differentiate between connected and unconnected proximal axons for entire population
	Can differentiate between connected and unconnected proximal axons in largest diameter group	
	Can provide a measure of branching by determining mean axon size distal to repair site	
Biochemistry		
Myelin assay	Quantifies myelin as measure of maturation of axons	Cannot quantify number of axons or differentiate between connected and unconnected proximal axons
Physiology		
CAP		
Conduction velocity	Determines maturation of largest diameter axons and connections across repair site	Cannot determine number of axons connected across repair site
Peak height	Measure of subpopulation of number of axons that cross repair site	Cannot differentiate change in height owing to number from change in height owing to conduction velocity; measure only of subpopulation of proximal axons
Area	Measure of total number of axons that cross repair site	Cannot differentiate contribution of various subpopulations to CAP
Single unit studies	Determines more information about conduction characteristics of individual axon and end-organ connections	Samples axonal population with bias for large diameter axons

information with respect to fibers that fail to cross the repair site, since large diameter proximal axons that fail to cross the repair site may change in diameter sufficiently to shift to smaller axon diameter groups.[1,16] If one can accurately establish the given population histogram of the large diameter group before injury, then the shift to smaller fibers after injury provides a measure of the number of fibers in the largest groups that fail to cross the anastomosis.

Distal axon diameter histograms provide a measure of the number and maturation of distal axons. This might provide a measure of

branching: as branching increases, the demand on any proximal axon increases, and the resulting distal diameters may be smaller (see Chapter 14).

Biochemistry

Biochemical analysis is an important method for investigating the role and quantity of specific nerve substances during nerve regeneration. Recent advances in biochemistry have resulted in techniques that can differentiate sensory and motor fibers (see Chapter 3). Biochemical analysis of the quantity of myelin in repaired nerves has been used as a quantitative measure of regeneration.[6] This biochemical technique, like the histological techniques just described, is also limited in its value for comparing nerve repair techniques with respect to the number of proximal axons with distal connections.

Physiology

Electrophysiological methods provide a measure of nerve activity in the normal and repaired state. Electrical stimulation of a nerve results in the propagation of action potentials in the component axons. Each axon that is stimulated above its activation threshold produces an SFAP (single fiber action potential). This SFAP has a characteristic waveform (duration and height) and conduction velocity dependent on the anatomical and physiological state of the stimulated axon. The relationship of the axon to its electrical response (SFAP) has been investigated.[3,5] The conduction velocity is a function of the structure of the axon (diameter, myelin-to-axon ratio, nodal area, internodal distance) and the physiological state (temperature and metabolism) (see Chapter 19). In normal nerves the conduction velocity is related to axon diameter, but this relationship is altered in regenerated nerves. The wave form of the SFAP is also correlated with axonal diameter in normal nerves.[22] This relationship may also be altered as the geometry and physiological state of the nerve are changed in the injured and repaired nerve.

A nerve may be studied by stimulating or recording from single axons, or both, or by recording from the entire nerve. Although the techniques of single fiber study provide more information about individual axons than can be obtained with CAP recordings, the limitations of single unit techniques restrict their usefulness for studying the entire population (see "Single Fiber Action Potentials" at the end of this chapter).

Compound action potential

The CAP (compound action potential) is the algebraic sum of the SFAP's of the axonal population being stimulated (Fig. 15-2). The size and shape of the CAP is determined by the amplitude and duration of the SFAP's, the number of axons in the nerve, the range and distribution of axon CV's (conduction velocities), and the distance the impulse must travel along the nerve. The CAP may be reconstructed from the axon diameter distribution (histogram) if the relationships of

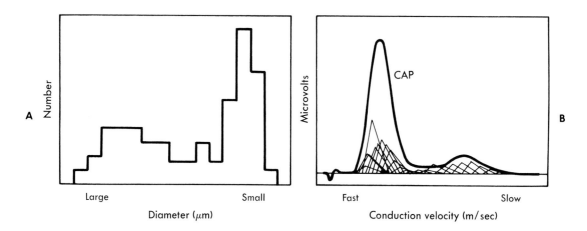

Fig. 15-2. Compound action potential, *CAP*, comparison of CAP, constituent single fiber action potentials (SFAP's), and axon diameter histogram (based on Gasser and Grundfest,[13] cat saphenous nerve). **A,** Axon diameter histogram—number of axons within each diameter class that comprise CAP. **B,** CAP—SFAP's that algebraicly sum to form waveform of CAP.

axonal diameter to SFAP waveform and conduction velocity are known.[3,14]

The CAP is the most commonly used physiological measure to determine information about peripheral nerve function.[27] The CAP latency, peak height, area, and waveform may be measured. Each of these methods will be described in the following sections.

The experimental method for physiological evaluation of the CAP requires a set of stimulating and recording electrodes (Fig. 15-3). The nerve may be studied in a recording chamber or within the animal. The recording electrode is located at the proximal portion of the nerve, and the stimulating electrodes are located proximal and distal to the repair site. The CAP may be recorded biphasically or monophasically by crushing the proximal end. Both connected and unconnected axons are stimulated at the proximal electrode, but stimulation at the distal electrode activates only those proximal axons that are functionally connected across the repair site. Therefore by comparing CAP's recorded from stimulation at the proximal electrode (connected and unconnected axons) with that CAP from stimulation at the distal electrodes (connected axons only) a measure of axonal regeneration may be obtained. Note that in this technique the position of the recording electrodes does not vary.

Conduction velocity (latency). The distance the CAP travels divided by the latency to the onset of the CAP determines the CV (conduction velocity) of the fastest fibers in the axon population (Fig. 15-4). This technically simple measure allows evaluation of axonal regeneration with respect to maturation of the fastest fibers,[27] but it gives little indication of the number of fastest fibers in the population or any indication of the CV and number of axons in the rest of the population.[20]

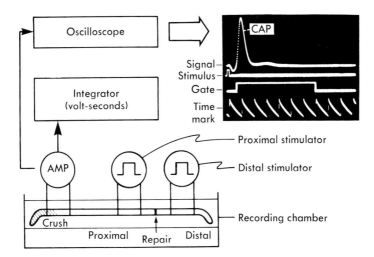

Fig. 15-3. Experimental method for physiological evaluation of CAP (in vitro). Nerve is schematically represented in recording chamber with repair site and distal and proximal regions labeled. Nerve may be stimulated either distal or proximal to repair site and CAP from these stimulations recorded from proximal end of nerve, which has been crushed to provide monophasic CAP's. Impulses may be amplified and then analyzed by integrator or computer (not shown here) or may be displayed on oscilloscope to determine CAP parameters (latency, height, and area). Diagram in upper right represents oscilloscope display with signal (CAP), stimulus, time window (section of signal being integrated), and reference time marks.

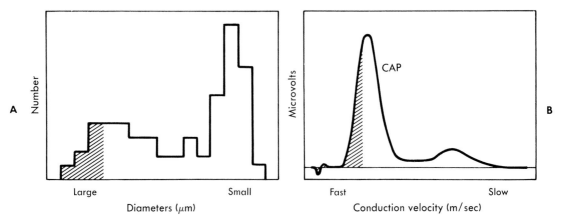

Fig. 15-4. Conduction velocity of CAP—measure of fastest axons. **A,** Axon diameter histogram with representation of fastest axons (diagonal lines) measured by conduction velocity of CAP. **B,** CAP with representation of SFAP's (diagonal lines) contributing to conduction velocity measurement.

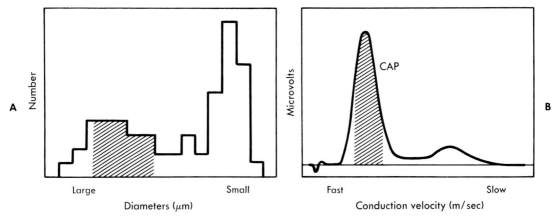

Fig. 15-5. Amplitude of CAP: a measure of a subpopulation. **A,** Axon diameter histogram with representation of axons (diagonal lines) measured by peak height of CAP. **B,** CAP with representation of SFAP's (diagonal lines) contributing to amplitude measurement.

In regenerating nerves the CV is altered by changes in structure (see Chapter 19). The alteration in structural parameters cannot be predicted accurately for a given diameter at a given time. Conduction velocity may remain normal in spite of functional decrements, or function may improve without consequent improvement in CV.[12] For example, in crush injuries where the normal distribution of axons is regained[16] the CV remains reduced by 25%.[9] Clinical studies comparing sensory return measured by two-point discrimination with conduction velocity of the fastest fibers have shown no positive correlation between the two evaluation methods.[2]

Amplitude (peak height). The amplitude of the CAP is a quantitative measure of the number of axons within a subpopulation of the total population (Fig. 15-5). This quantitative measure can be easily calculated and gives an indication of axonal regeneration with respect to the number of axons conduct-

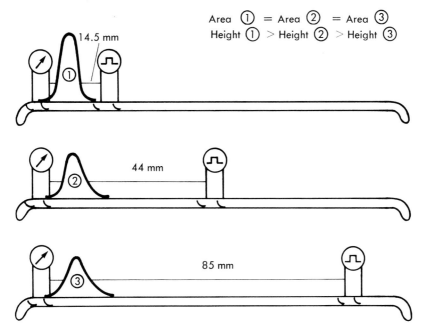

Area ① = Area ② = Area ③
Height ① > Height ② > Height ③

Fig. 15-6. Change of CAP waveform with increasing conduction distances (based on Erlanger, Bishop, and Gasser[12]). At increasing conduction distances (CAP[*1*] 14.5 mm, CAP[*2*] 44 mm, CAP[*3*] 86 mm) the amplitude of the CAP decreases, with amplitude *1* greater than *2* greater than *3*. The area remains the same in each case: area *1* equals area *2* equals area *3*. Stimulating electrodes on right, recording electrodes on left, with schematic representation of normal nerve.

ing across the repair site (see Fig. 15-3). Amplitude measurements are limited in their ability to predict the number of proximal axons with distal connections. These potential limitations are a consequence of several factors: (1) changes in CV in the regenerating nerve, (2) changes in the diameter of proximal axons that do not connect, and (3) possible selectivity of repair techniques for either large or small diameter axons with respect to regeneration across the repair site.

Amplitude is not only a function of the number of axons firing, but it is also a function of conduction velocity and conduction distance. It is well known that any changes in either conduction distance or conduction velocities can influence the waveshape and hence the amplitude.[5,13] In normal nerves the waveshape of the CAP broadens, and amplitude declines as conduction distance increases (Fig. 15-6). To compare the proximal and distal stimulations, a correction must

be made for the increased distance from the distal stimulation to the recording electrode. However, in the regenerating nerve the changes in the structure of the axons (that is, diameter, axon-to-myelin ratio, internodal length) may alter the conduction velocity and thus influence the amplitude. There is no known way in which amplitude measurements may be accurately corrected for such changes. Thus at present it is not possible to separate conduction velocity changes from changes in the number of functioning axons by means of amplitude measurements alone; however, measurements of the area of the CAP do not have this limitation. Both the amplitude of the CAP and the area under the curve may also be influenced by changes in the diameter of the proximal population (which alter amplitude both directly and also indirectly by altering CV) or by a selective bias of a repair technique for a given axon diameter size (see next section—"Area").

Despite these limitations, the height of the CAP is used both experimentally and clinically because it does give some indication of the function of the population of axons in the nerve.[27] However, there are large variations in the normal amplitude of human sensory nerves, which makes clinical interpretation of functional impairment difficult unless there are severe neuronal losses.[7]

Area. The area under the *monophasic* compound action potential does not significantly change when its height and waveshape are clearly altered by increasing conduction distance (see Fig. 15-6). This indicates that as long as the recording electrode position is not altered, the area measure gives the same value when the same population of normal axons is activated, despite changes in waveshape (caused by conduction distance or changes in conduction velocity).[13] By direct extension, the area will not change if axons distal to the repair site have a slower conduction velocity or are delayed at the repair site as long as they functionally connect to the proximal axons being recorded and thus contribute to the proximally recorded CAP. The area under the monophasic CAP may be computed from the recorded signal on the oscilloscope. An alternative method[25] is to electronically integrate the CAP (see Fig. 15-3).

Thus the area of the CAP can provide a measure both of the total population of proximal (connected and unconnected) axons (Fig. 15-7) and of the proximal myelinated axons with distal connections (connected) without being influenced by differences in conduction or conduction velocity. This method has recently been applied to experimental nerve evaluation[25] (also see Chapters 16 and 36).

Description of method. For purposes of simplicity, let us assume that we have a nerve that contains only branched and blocked axons (see Fig. 15-1) and we wish to determine what proportion of the proximal axons are connected. We can record proximally and compare the area obtained from stimulation just proximal to the nerve repair site with that obtained by stimulation just distal to the repair site (see Fig. 15-3). Stimulation at the proximal stimulator (if it is supramaximal) will activate all proximal axons (branched and blocked), whereas stimulation at the distal stimulator can only activate axons that connect across the repair site (branched axons, with one or more branches). A measure of the proportion of proximal connected axons to the total number of proximal axons (both connected [branched] and unconnected [blocked]) may be obtained by determining the ratio of the distal area to the proximal area.

For the area ratio to be directly proportional to the number of axons, the area (or mean area) contribution to the CAP of the

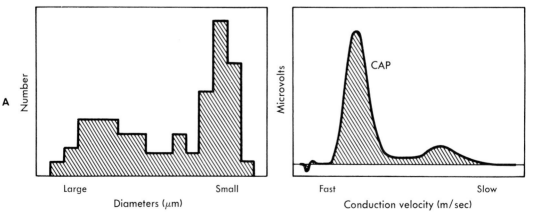

Fig. 15-7. Area of CAP: measure of total population. **A,** Axon diameter histogram, with representation of axons (diagonal lines) measured by area of CAP. **B,** CAP with representation of SFAP's (diagonal lines) contributing to area measurement.

SFAP's from the connected and unconnected axons must be the same. Any factor during injury and repair that changes the mean area of a subpopulation of axons that contribute to the proximally recorded CAP will yield inaccurate estimates of the populations, unless specifically accounted for. The location or position of the axons could affect the mean area. For example, axons at the periphery of the nerve contribute a greater mean area than axons at the center of the nerve. The axon population activated at the stimulating electrodes should be randomly intermixed at the proximal end of the nerve (see Chapter 3) where the CAP is recorded (see Fig. 15-3), and this factor should not interfere with the area evaluation.

The predictive value of the area method may be affected by changes in the structure of the subpopulation of the proximal axons that do not reconnect across the repair site if this alters the mean SFAP area. The proximal axons that fail to reestablish distal connections (unconnected) will decrease in diameter[8,16,18] (also see Chapter 16). This "shrinkage" may result in a decreased mean SFAP area for the unconnected population compared with the connected population. The area ratio compares the SFAP area of connected axons (numerator) to the summed SFAP areas of the connected and unconnected axons (denominator). A decrease in the SFAP area of the unconnected axons (denominator) will effectively increase the ratio without changing the actual numerator or number of connected axons. The area ratio will predict a greater proportion of connected axons than that which actually exists.

The magnitude of the discrepancy between area ratio and actual proportion of axons may be calculated for a given percentage of shrinkage of the unconnected axons.[11] Shrinkage will act to reduce the observed differences between two repair methods. The differences in SFAP area ratio between two methods will therefore be as predicted (if we assume no shrinkage) or greater than what is predicted (if shrinkage has occurred). The discrepancy from shrinkage will only produce false negatives and will not provide false positives.

The predictive value of the area ratio method may be affected if the repair techniques being compared select populations of axons according to size, that is, if one repair technique selects large diameter axons and the other selects small diameter axons. The magnitude of this potential error may be calculated.[11] The area ratio method may predict a false positive if a repair technique that selects large diameter axons results in a greater area ratio than a repair technique that selects small diameter axons, when in fact the repair technique that selects small diameter axons actually results in a greater number of connected axons than the repair technique that selects large axons.

A discrepancy between the predicted area ratio and the actual proportion of connected axons may result from changes in the mean area of the SFAP's of a subpopulation of axons. This problem may be overcome by analyzing the contribution of the subpopulation of SFAP's that contribute to the CAP Methods are now available to estimate the axon conduction velocity distribution of normal and nontraumatic peripheral neuropathies.[10,20,21] These methods have not yet been applied to traumatic peripheral neuropathies.

Clinical application. The preceding evaluation method (recording of the area under the CAP) requires a *monophasic* CAP and a *nonconductive* external medium for the nerve. This technique is directly applicable to intraoperative evaluation of incontinuity nerve lesions. The nerve may be lifted on electrodes into air and the monophasic signal obtained by applying a local anesthetic agent (lidocaine) to the most proximal electrode of the pair of recording electrodes.[24]

Single fiber action potentials

Another method of analyzing nerve regeneration involves recording from single fiber action potentials by nerve splitting or microelectrode techniques. In such experiments it is possible to determine the physiological properties of each fiber in a manner that is not possible with CAP studies (as described in foregoing sections). Such studies following nerve repair have indicated reinnervation patterns for sensory nerves and central connection changes (see Chapter 11).

There is a "selectivity" in SFAP techniques toward the larger fibers of the population.[4] The single unit method might well be utilized for "sampling" the population of fibers diagrammed in Fig. 15-1. However, if we wish to consider the full fiber spectrum, single unit studies cannot determine the spectrum of fibers that comprise the regenerated population unless correction is somehow made for the inherent "selectivity."

SUMMARY

Experimental evaluation methods are of significant value in comparing nerve repair techniques if their specific limitations are understood and respected.

The measurement of the proximal population of myelinated axons that connect across the repair site provides a comparison of different nerve repair techniques with respect to axonal regeneration.

In the animal model the many variables present in clinical nerve injury may be controlled. This enables a comparison of the effect of a new repair technique with a conventional technique under standard conditions for the age of the animal, level of repair, associated injury, and nerve injured. This is not readily possible in clinical studies.

The physiological measurements of axonal regeneration that we have described do not differentiate axonal connections that are appropriate (that is, sensory to sensory and motor to motor) from axonal connections that are inappropriate (that is, sensory to motor and motor to sensory). If inappropriate connections are made and are not corrected, physiological conduction may occur across the repair site, but no useful function will result.

The measurement of axonal regeneration across the site of repair provides a measure of the surgeon's ability to anatomically reconnect the severed ends of the nerve. It does not test his ability to match functionally appropriate fascicles and axons.

Axonal regeneration is the first phase of a complex maturation process. The results of animal experimentation serve a definite role as a testing ground for new techniques in nerve repair. However, the final acceptance of any new technique still rests on conclusive evidence that it results in superior functional recovery in humans.

REFERENCES

1. Aitken, J. T., and Thomas, P. K.: Retrograde changes in fibre size following nerve section, J. Anat. **96:**121, 1962.
2. Almquist, E., and Eeg-Olofsson, O.: Sensory-nerve-conduction velocity and two-point discrimination in sutured nerves, J. Bone Joint Surg. **52A:**791, 1970.
3. BeMent, S. L., and Olson, W. H.: Quantitative studies of sequential peripheral nerve fiber diameter histograms and biophysical implications, Exp. Neurol. **57:**827, 1977.
4. Biedenbach, M. A., Beuerman, R. W., and Brown, A. C.: Graphic-digitizer analysis of axon spectra in ethmoidal and lingual branches of the trigeminal nerve, Cell Tissue Res. **157:**341, 1975.
5. Blair, E. A., and Erlanger, J.: A comparison of the characteristics of axons through their individual electrical pulses, Am. J. Physiol. **106:**524, 1933.
6. Bora, F. W., Pleasure, D. E., and Didzian, N. A.: A study of nerve regeneration and neuroma formation after nerve suture by various techniques, J. Hand Surg. **1:**138, 1976.
7. Buchthal, F., and Rosenfalck, A.: Evoked action potentials and conduction velocity in human sensory nerves, Brain Res. **3:**1, 1966.
8. Cragg, B. G., and Thomas, P. K.: Changes in conduction velocity and fibre size proximal to peripheral nerve lesions, J. Physiol. (Lond) **157:**315, 1961.
9. Cragg, B. G., and Thomas, P. K.: The conduction velocity of regenerated peripheral nerve fibers, J. Physiol. (Lond) **171:**164, 1964.
10. Cummins, K. L.: Estimation of nerve-bundle conduction velocity distribution: methods based on a linear model of the compound action potential, Ph.D. thesis, Stanford University, 1978.
11. Cummins, K. L., and Rosen, J. M.: Unpublished data, 1978.
12. Dyck, P. J., Thomas, P. K.: and Lambert, E. H., eds: Peripheral neuropathy, Philadelphia, 1975, W. B. Saunders Co.
13. Erlanger, J., Bishop, G. H., and Gasser, H. S.: Experimental analysis of the simple action potential wave in nerve by the cathode ray oscillograph, Am. J. Physiol. **78:**537, 1926.
14. Gasser, H. S., and Grundfest, H.: Axon diameters in relation to the spike dimensions and the conduction velocity in mammalian A fibers, Am. J. Physiol. **127:**393, 1939.
15. Goldstein, S. S., and Rall, W.: Changes of action potential shape and velocity for changing core conductor geometry, Biophys. J. **14:**731, 1974.

16. Gutman, E., and Sanders, F. K.: Recovery of fibre numbers and diameters in the regeneration of peripheral nerves, J. Physiol. (Lond) **101:**489, 1943.

17. Holmes, W., and Young, J. Z.: Nerve regeneration after immediate and delayed suture, J. Anat. **77:**63, 1942.

18. Kiraly, J. K., and Krnjevic, K.: Some retrograde changes in function of nerves after peripheral section, Q. J. Exp. Physiol. **44:**244, 1959.

19. Lavarack, J. O., Sunderland, S., and Ray, L. J.: The branching of nerve fibers in human cutaneous nerves, J. Comp. Neurol. **94:**293, 1951.

20. Lee, R. G., et al.: Analysis of motor conduction velocity in the human median nerve by computer simulation of compound muscle action potentials, Electroencephalogr. Clin. Neurophysiol. **39:**225, 1975.

21. Liefer, L. J., et al.: Nerve-bundle conduction velocity distribution measurement and transfer function analysis, Proc. IEEE **65:**747, 1977.

22. Paintal, A. A.: Conduction in mammalian nerve fibers. In Desmedt, J. E., ed.: New developments in electromyography and clinical neurophysiology, vol. 2, Basel, 1973, Karger, p. 19.

23. Ramón y Cajal, S.: Degeneration and regeneration of the nervous system, London, 1928, Milford.

24. Rosen, J. M.: Unpublished data, 1978.

25. Rosen, J. M., et al.: Fascicular sutureless and suture repair of peripheral nerves: a comparison study in laboratory animals, Orthop. Rev. **8:**85, 1979.

26. Shawe, G. D. H.: On the number of branches formed by regenerating nerve fibers, Br. J. Surg. **42:**474, 1955.

27. Terzis, J. K., Dykes, R. W., and Hakstian, R. W.: Electrophysiological recordings in peripheral nerve surgery: a review, J. Hand Surg. **1:**52, 1976.

28. Watrous, W. G.: Axon branching after nerve regeneration, Proc. Soc. Exp. Biol. Med. **44:**541, 1940.

DISCUSSION

Horch: The idea of estimating how many fibers cross a transection neuroma by the use of compound action potential recordings is an attractive one. I have spent considerable time working with the method in which stimulating electrodes are placed on the nerve on both sides of the neuroma, the compound action potential is recorded proximal to the proximal stimulating electrode, and its area measured for stimulation from each of the two stimulating sites. However, I have abandoned this technique for a number of reasons, the most compelling of which follows.

The contribution a fiber makes to the area of the compound action potential depends on its size—small fibers contributing less than large fibers. Therefore an uncorrected areal measurement is more sensitive to the population of large fibers than it is to small fibers. Transected axons that have not reestablished functional connection with the skin are atrophied throughout their length[*] and will make a smaller contribution to the total compound action potential area than their numbers would suggest. This also means that fibers that have not crossed the neuroma are not likely to be uniformly distributed within the compound action potential elicited from the proximal stimulation site.

In principle one could compensate for this by weighing the different components of the compound action potential, but in practice it is not easy to determine what the correct weighing function should be. Even if it could be accurately determined, such a weighing function would be of no use for stimulation distal to the neuroma. The fibers in the distal stump are permanently decreased in size and slowed in conduction velocity,[*] and the reduction in conduction velocity is not the same for all the fibers. As a result, the relative position in which individual fibers are represented in the proximally recorded compound action potential changes. Moreover, even with signal averaging, it is difficult to get a good measure of the number of small fibers because the potentials are small and they tend to be spread out in time, especially when stimulating distal to the neuroma.

However, information is currently available that allows us to estimate how many neurons regenerate across an unrepaired transection lesion of a cutaneous nerve in cats. From data of the type shown in my contribution to this volume, I have found that, on the average, about 60% of the cutaneous type I sensory fibers reestablish functional connections with type I receptors after *unrepaired* nerve transection. These axons regenerate less well then those innervating other cutaneous receptors,[†] which means that at least 84% of the myelinated sensory fibers in an unrepaired, transected, feline cutaneous nerve regenerate back to the skin. This agrees well with a preliminary study I have done on transected sural nerves in cats using single unit analysis, which indicated that 87% of the axons recorded had crossed the transection site. The data from this study also suggest that, in spite of the limitations described above, measurements of compound action potential areas can give a reasonable *relative* measure of regeneration success when comparing different types of nerve repair, provided that the same nerve is used in all the subjects.

---

[*]Gutmann, E., and Sanders, F. K.: J. Physiol. **101**:489, 1943. Horch, K. W.: Unpublished observations.
[†]Burgess, P. R., and Horch, K. W.: J. Neurophysiol. **36**:101, 1973.

---

[*]Horch, K. W.: Brain Res. **117**:19, 1976.

16

Differential atrophy of sensory and motor fibers following ligation or resuture of cat hindlimb nerves

J. A. Hoffer, T. Gordon, and R. B. Stein

In our study of the degenerative and regenerative events that follow nerve section (see Chapter 17) we mentioned that the severity of the injury appeared to be greater in sensory fibers than in motor fibers of the same peripheral nerve. This suggestion arose from the more incomplete recovery of total sensory fiber discharge levels during locomotion in peripheral nerves that had been sectioned and resutured. Evoked compound action potentials from whole nerves could not render the sensory fiber contribution separately from the motor fiber contribution. We therefore developed a method based on measurements of compound action potentials recorded at dorsal and ventral roots, which allowed us to measure the response to axotomy and regeneration separately in myelinated motor and sensory fibers.

METHODS

In six cats with implanted peripheral nerve electrodes, in which one or two nerves had been sectioned and either ligated, resutured, or grafted into muscles, we performed final acute experiments several months after nerve section. Under deep anesthesia the spinal cord was exposed, an oil pool was formed, and the dorsal and ventral roots L6, L7, and S1 were prepared bilaterally for recording on platinum hooks. Nerves in the unoperated hindlimb were prepared for stimulation to serve as controls, while the experimental nerves were stimulated through their implanted electrodes.

As each nerve was stimulated we recorded monophasic compound action potentials from the corresponding roots. Typical potentials are shown schematically in Fig. 16-1. Notice that in the experimental side root potentials occurred later than in the control side because of the lower conduction velocity in fibers that had atrophied following nerve section. The peak amplitude was usually smaller in experimental nerves for similar reasons.

Comparison of potential amplitudes recorded from different roots is not meaningful unless the electrical impedance of each root filament is taken into account. In Fig. 16-1 notice in the diagrams at the far left that the S1 roots are considerably thinner than the L7 roots, while the L6 roots are shorter. Therefore the electrical resistance of the tissue over which the potentials develop is markedly different, as shown in the second column. We measured impedances using a 10 kHz test signal, and scaled the potential amplitudes appropriately. The corrected values, in units of *current* now, are shown in the middle diagrams.

Finally, as was shown by Erlanger and Gasser[1] and also observed by Rosen and Jewett in Chapter 15, the peak amplitude of a compound potential, which will vary with conduction distance and conduction velocity dispersion, is not as good an indicator of fiber

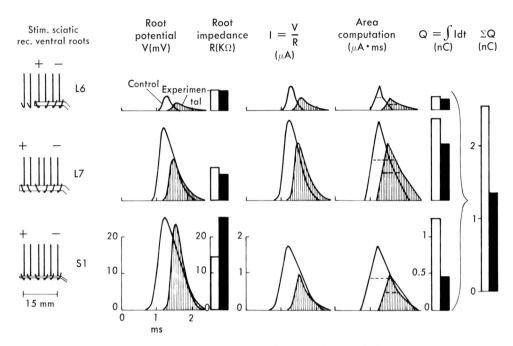

Fig. 16-1. Schematic representation of compound potentials recorded from roots in experimental side (filled areas) and control side (open areas) when each sciatic nerve was stimulated. Recording configurations are shown at left. Sequence of measurements and calculations that provided a measure of total charge delivered at each root is further described in text.

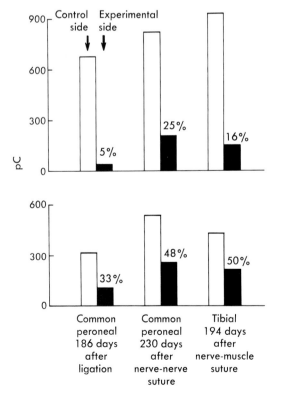

Fig. 16-2. Total charge delivered at dorsal roots L6, L7, and S1 (top) and ventral roots L6, L7, and S1 (bottom) following stimulation of experimental nerves (filled bars) and contralateral controls (open bars) is compared for cases of nerve section followed by ligation, resuture, and graft into muscle. Percents are expressed in terms of control values obtained in same preparation.

population response as is the *area* under the potential. Computing the area under each curve was equivalent to integrating current over time, giving units of *charge*—we thus obtained a measure in nanocoulomb (nC) of the discharge of myelinated fibers projecting from each nerve onto each root.

Values of charge are proportional to the number of fibers present in a nerve and to the average fiber diameter. In contrast to peak voltages, these values of charge are truly additive, and the contributions of each nerve onto all dorsal roots and all ventral roots could be added separately.

RESULTS

Our findings are shown in Fig. 16-2, where the effects of nerve section followed by ligation, resuture, and suture into muscle are compared. Ligation predictably posed the most serious test, for after 186 days the total charge delivered by all sensory fibers in a ligated common peroneal nerve was reduced to 5% of control, while the motor fiber contribution was down to 33%. Sensory fibers were six times more severely affected than motor fibers.

Results from resutured nerves reflected the classic findings of the 1940's[2,3]: fiber shrinkage that follows nerve section is a reversible process if fibers are given a chance to reinnervate peripheral structures. Sensory fibers in these nerves were still more affected than motor fibers, but the process of recovery was apparent after both nerve resuture and nerve graft into muscle. The latter procedure may have accounted for sensory fibers having fared less well when the tibial nerve, a mixed nerve with a large cutaneous fiber compo-

nent, was sutured into the long plantar flexor muscles, leaving many sensory fibers in want for suitable end-organs to resupply. Motor fibers seemed to recover equally well after either nerve suture procedure.

We have thus demonstrated that myelinated sensory fibers are more severely affected by injury to peripheral nerves than are motor fibers. The possible reasons for such a difference are intriguing. Sensory fibers may be more dependent on trophic factors from the periphery transported along the axon. Alternatively, the electrical silencing that nerve division imposes on sensory fibers, but not on motor fibers, suggests a role for electrical activity in the regulation and maintenance of nerve cells.

The implications of this finding in the clinical situation are not yet clear. Our data from nerves resutured immediately after section showed substantial recovery in sensory fibers several months later. However, the reestablishment of sensory function may be more adversely affected by long delays than the return of motor function if fibers are allowed to atrophy markedly before having a chance to reinnervate. This point awaits further experimental evidence.

REFERENCES

1. Erlanger, J., and Gasser, H. S.: Electrical signs of nervous activity; Philadelphia, 1937, University of Pennsylvania Press.
2. Gutmann, E., and Sanders, F. K.: The recovery of fibre size and numbers during nerve regeneration, J. Physiol. **101**:489, 1943.
3. Weiss, P., Edds, M. V., and Cavanaugh, M.: The effect of terminal connections on the caliber of nerve fibers, Anat. Rec. **92**:215, 1945.

17

Long-term recordings from cat peripheral nerves during degeneration and regeneration: implications for human nerve repair and prosthetics

R. B. Stein, T. Gordon, J. A. Hoffer, L. A. Davis, and D. Charles

Our group has been interested for a number of years in methods for recording chronically from nerve fibers.[6,7,14] This interest arose naturally from our work on motor control and in the function of various types of sensory and motor fibers in normal motor behavior.[12] Once we had succeeded in being able to record for months and even years from mammalian nerves, we realized that these techniques provided a valuable and unique tool for studying long-term trophic interactions between nerve and muscle and for providing the possibility of neuroelectrical control and sensory feedback to amputees in the control of powered prostheses. This chapter will outline the recent progress we have made toward these two goals.

The goals are closely related, for if an amputee is to use neural signals from cut nerves, either for motor control or sensory feedback, three basic questions must be answered about the response of nerve cells disconnected from target organs: (1) Do nerve cells survive more or less indefinitely when they have no chance of reinnervating a suitable end-organ? (2) If they survive, do nerve fibers retain the ability to conduct action potentials for periods of years? (3) If they can still conduct action potentials, do motor fibers continue the apparently useless task of generating impulses to a neuroma during

phases of movements where they have been active prior to amputation?

Some of these questions have been studied since the end of the last century, although we know of only one other attempt to do this with chronic recordings.[2] Reviewing an already sizable literature in 1906, Ranson[10] suggested that some nerve fibers survive axotomy for many years. What percentage survives has been difficult to determine. Sunderland,[15] in his major work on nerve and nerve injuries, quotes studies in which between 6% and 83% of nerve fibers survived. Although various factors that are known to affect the survival of fibers have been outlined, it remains unclear to what extent they can account for the wide variation observed. In addition to the quantitative variation, the question of long-term survival is still an open one, since a scientist such as Ernst Gutmann, who has been concerned with these questions since the second world war, assumes that, "If no regeneration is possible after section of the nerve, the stimuli for proteosynthesis cease, the nerve cell atrophies and is replaced by neuroglial cells surrounding the neuron."[4]

There is more agreement on the second question. When nerve fibers survive, at least some of them retain the ability to conduct impulses, although at a lower velocity. In cut

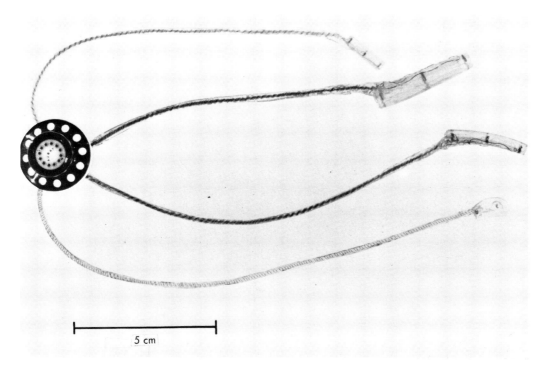

Fig. 17-1. Device for implantation in cats containing three neural recording cuffs and one EMG probe connected to a twelve-pin socket in a vitreous carbon button that serves as a skin interface. (From Stein, R. B., et al.: Brain Res. **128**:21, 1977.)

nerves that end in neuromas, the conduction velocities proximal to the point of section are reduced to between 50% and 80% of control values 300 or more days after axotomy.[1] The scatter in the data from different animals suggests that methods allowing single animals to be followed chronically might be helpful in dealing with this question.

The third question, whether amputated nerves continue to fire during movements in which they previously participated, is an interesting and important one. In addition to well-known changes in the diameter of nerve axons and cell bodies associated with the chromatolytic reaction, changes in the presynaptic connections onto motoneurons following axotomy have recently been described. The connectivity between individual muscle spindle primary afferent fibers and individual motoneurons dropped from 94% to 70% within 1 to 2 months after axotomy.[8] In the sympathetic system, Purves[9] found a 70% loss of synaptic connections after cutting the postganglionic fibers, so that over a quarter of the ganglion cells could not be activated even with supramaximal electrical stimuli to the preganglionic nerve. Thus there remains a real question whether neurons do in fact retain the ability to generate nerve impulses synaptically during behavior, even if they survive and can conduct action potentials following axotomy.

METHODS

Fig. 17-1 illustrates a chronic recording device that we developed to study these questions. In this example, there are three nerve cuffs of different sizes to fit around different peripheral nerves and an EMG probe. The nerve cuffs each contain three-standard Teflon-coated platinum-iridium electrode wires that are spiralled around Dacron threads to form a cable. The neural cuffs, the EMG probes, and the sleeves surrounding the cables are all constructed from medical grade Silastic. The cables end in a socket that is epoxied into a hard smooth carbon button, which serves as a skin interface.[11] Further details on the design and construction of these devices have been published elsewhere.[14]

Once these cuffs were implanted in the hindlimb of a cat, we could monitor various aspects of nerve function. Under halothane (Fluothane) anesthesia we could stimulate each nerve, such as the lateral gastrocnemius–soleus nerve (LGS) as shown in Fig. 17-2, and record the latency and amplitude of the compound action potential on the sciatic nerve. Furthermore, we could record the EMG produced in the ankle extensors, and by enclosing the foot in a metal boot, we could measure the contractile prop-

erties of the muscles stimulated. Finally, we could record from the same nerves while the cats were performing a stereotyped behavioral task on a treadmill. This activity consisted of sensory and motor impulses from all the fibers in the nerve.

We could sort out the proportion of impulses arising in the large sensory and motor fibers during this voluntary activity using the technique of cross-correlation shown in Fig. 17-3.[5] To do this we recorded from two sets of three electrodes in a single cuff, as shown in Fig. 17-3, or if there was insufficient length, we recorded from two cuffs, one on the sciatic nerve and the other on one of its branches. The reasons for having three electrodes in each set, and for connecting them to separate preamplifiers as shown, involve the necessity to isolate the neural signals from

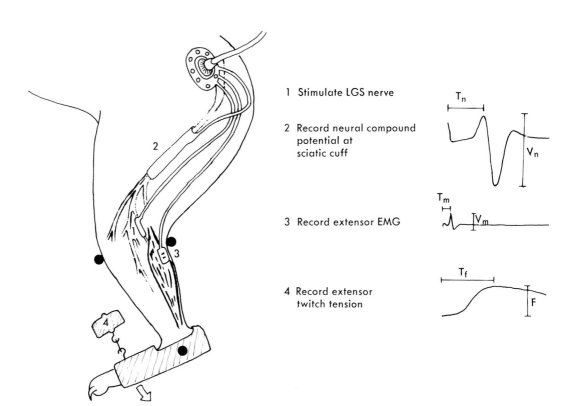

1 Stimulate LGS nerve

2 Record neural compound potential at sciatic cuff

3 Record extensor EMG

4 Record extensor twitch tension

Fig. 17-2. Methods for measuring nerve and muscle activity in chronic animal experiments. In example shown, nerve cuffs were implanted on sciatic and lateral gastrocnemius–soleus nerves and EMG probe was implanted on ankle extensors. Tension could be measured when required with a specially designed boot.

the much larger EMG signals in surrounding muscles, as has been described previously.[13] The idea of the cross-correlation is that if sensory impulses conduct from left to right with velocity, v, they will arrive at one set of electrodes a short time, $\Delta t = l/v$, before they arrive at the second set of electrodes, where l is the distance between the central electrodes in each set. On the other hand, motor impulses will conduct from right to left and will arrive at the first set of electrodes a short time after they arrive at the second set of electrodes. Thus, in the cross-correlation function, we see two positive peaks—one a short time to the left (sensory) and one a short time to the right (motor) of the origin. The cross-correlation function was calculated by the spectral analysis method, as described in French and Holden.[3] We therefore had a variety of methods available to test nerve function before and after nerve section and repair.

COMPOUND ACTION POTENTIALS

Following implantation, the condition of the nerves was monitored periodically, both with measurement of evoked compound action potentials under anesthesia and during locomotion on a treadmill. In some animals the values remained steady for many months after implantation. In others there was a transient nerve block caused by trauma during surgery or slight movement after implantation such that pressure block occurred during subsequent activity. Even when a complete block occurred in the sense that tension could no longer be elicited, as in Fig. 17-4, we could follow the full-time course of the changes in the neural activity during the recovery from nerve block, which happened either spontaneously or as a result of further surgical intervention to repair the damage. The onset of nerve block was variable, but the recovery followed a simple exponential curve with a time constant of about 2 months. Surgical intervention did not affect the time course of recovery but increased the final value to which the nerve recovered. This is shown in Table 17-1 based on 14 nerves studied. A few months after operation, the repaired nerves had recovered to 62% of control values, whereas the nerves that were not repaired had only recovered to 38% of control values. Since the recovery curves were

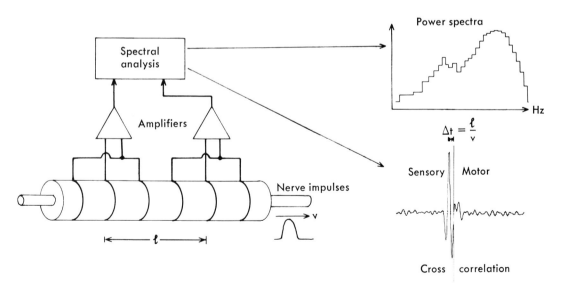

Fig. 17-3. Using two sets of recording electrodes and methods of spectral analysis, sensory nerve impulses conducting from left to right can be distinguished from motor nerve impulses conducting from right to left. Amount of each type of activity during a behavioral task can be measured from peaks in cross-correlation function on right.

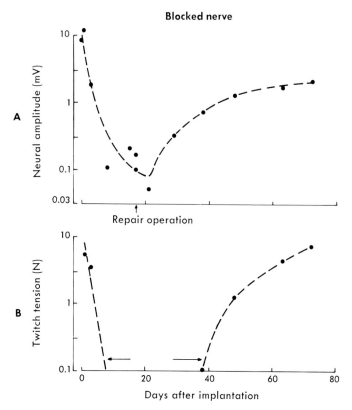

Fig. 17-4. Compound neural potential, **A,** and twitch tension, **B,** recorded after nerve block on common peroneal nerve. Full-time course of changes in nerve could be studied even during period when neuromuscular transmission was blocked (horizontal arrows). Nerve began to recover shortly after repair operation, but eventual recovery of tension was more complete. Ordinates are logarithmic.

Table 17-1. Recovery from nerve block of nerves that were not surgically repaired in subsequent operation

	Repaired nerves	Unrepaired nerves
No.	7	7
Initial mV	1.88	2.27
Minimum mV (%)	0.08 (4)*	0.09 (4)*
Last mV (%)	1.17 (62)	0.87 (38)*
Projected mV(%)	1.90 (101)	1.15 (51)*

NOTE: Initial, minimum, last measured and projected values (using a computed exponential fit) are given as geometric means in millivolts (mV) and in brackets in percent (%) of initial values before block. Values that were significantly different from the initial values before block are indicated by * with P < 0.001.

exponential, we could project the final values that would eventually be attained. For the repaired nerves, the mean projected value was to control levels, whereas for unrepaired nerves, the projected values were still significantly reduced at 51% of control levels. However, even when the amplitude of the compound action potential did not recovery fully, as in Fig. 17-4, the tension often recovered to control values. This result could be due to those motoneurons, which were successful in regenerating back to the muscle, sprouting to reinnervate all available muscle fibers.

When the neural amplitude reached a steady value, further surgical procedures were performed. Some nerves were cut and ligated and a segment of the nerve distal to the tie was removed to further hinder regen-

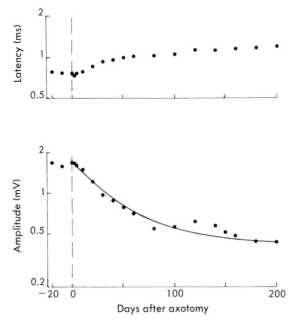

Fig. 17-5. Mean latency to first peak and amplitude of compound action potentials for three ligated nerves that were followed for over 200 days after axotomy. Decline in amplitude is fitted with single exponential with time constant of 45 days and final value one fourth of control value before axotomy.

eration. The average results for nerves treated in this way are shown in Fig. 17-5. The latency increased about 30% and the amplitude of the compound action potentials decreased to about a quarter of control values. Again, the changes in amplitude could be fitted with a simple exponential curve with a time constant of 45 days. Individual nerves were followed for periods of more than a year and showed no further change. This result shows clearly that nerve fibers do survive and retain the ability to conduct action potentials for long periods of time, even if there is no opportunity for regeneration to suitable end-organs.

Other nerves were cut cleanly and resutured to their distal stumps, as is done in surgical nerve repair. Still other nerves were cut and sutured into the fascia of nearby muscles that were denervated in the same operation.

Following nerve-nerve sutures and nerve-muscle sutures, some motoneurons and sensory fibers grew out and reinnervated appropriate end-organs. As shown in Fig. 17-6, two exponentials were now required to fit the average results. The exponential decay process had the same time constant as for tied nerves, but in addition there was an exponential recovery with a time constant of 3 to 4 months. This was somewhat longer than that for the recovery from nerve block and the recovery was not usually as complete. No significant differences were observed between the results of the nerve-nerve and nerve-muscle sutures. Thus, as long as some nerve fibers were able to reinnervate appropriate end-organs, a recovery was observed in the compound action potentials and a decrease in the latency of conduction (that is, an increase in conduction velocity).

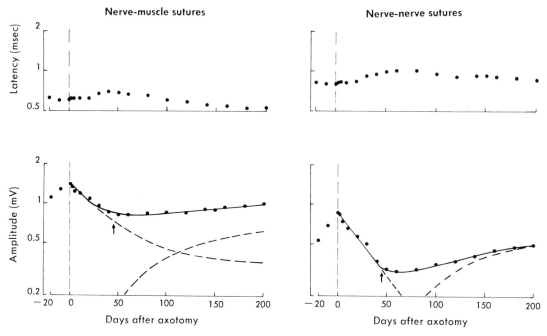

Fig. 17-6. Changes in latency and amplitude, as in Fig. 17-5, when nerves were cut and either sutured into muscle (left) or resutured to distal nerve stumps (right). Arrows indicate mean time at which reinnervation occurred. Note recovery in amplitude and decline in latency that began within a week or so of innervation. Dashed lines in each part represent decaying exponential with same time constant as in Fig. 17-5 and exponential recovery curve with longer time constant (3 to 4 months). Solid lines represent sums of these two exponential curves.

NEURAL ACTIVITY DURING LOCOMOTION

Compound action potentials evoked by electrical stimuli do not tell us how a nerve is used during behavior. To study this, we recorded the asynchronous nerve impulses occuring during locomotion under constant conditions on a treadmill. Fig. 17-7 shows data for three individual nerves in which the activity on the treadmill was compared with the compound action potentials measured for the same nerves under anesthesia. The asynchronous activity during locomotion was much smaller in amplitude (measured in μV rather than mV). Also, when the motor component is determined through the cross-correlation technique, it depends on the product of the amplitudes at the two sets of electrodes (that is, μV^2 are the units in Fig. 17-7

for the peaks of the cross-correlation functions). For comparison, we multiplied the values of the compound action potentials recorded on the same set of electrodes to get a value in mV^2 in Fig. 17-7. The compound action potentials in the top half of each part of the figure declined for the ligated nerves, as described previously, and recovered for the nerve that was resutured. The activity during locomotion followed the same general pattern but with two exceptions. First, the motor signals tended to decline more rapidly during the first month or so than did the evoked potentials, but then they either declined less rapidly beyond the first couple of months or recovered more rapidly. This is seen most clearly in the case of the peroneal nerve on the bottom, which had been ligated. The evoked potentials declined as ex-

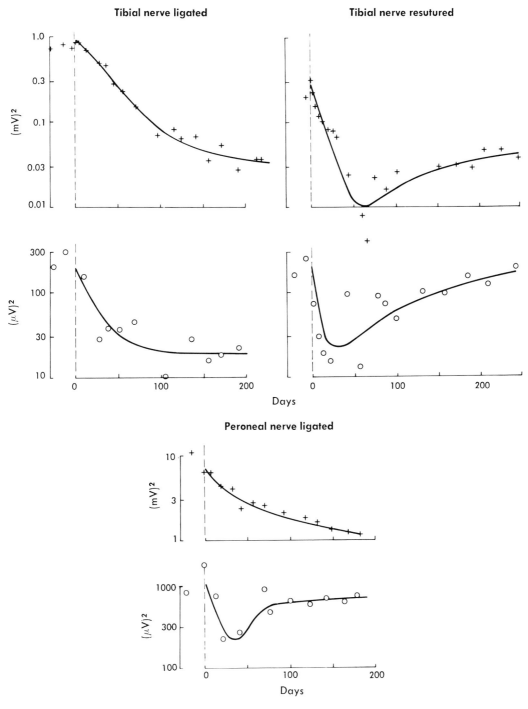

Fig. 17-7. Comparison of compound action potentials (upper traces in mV²) and asynchronous motor activity (lower traces in μV²) from cats walking on treadmill. Motor activity was measured using cross-correlation technique between two sets of electrodes (see "Methods") and compound action potentials measured at same two sets of electrodes were multiplied for comparison. Note that motor activity declines more than compound action potentials in first month but declines less (or recovers more) at later times (100 to 200 days). Transformer with approximate voltage gain of 20 was used during walking for reasons described previously.[13] Values in lower traces have not been corrected for this factor.

pected, whereas the motor activity first declined more rapidly and then actually recovered somewhat, while the evoked signals continued to decline.

The same trends have been observed in other animals, but the number of animals studied to date is not great enough for the differences to be statistically significant. Nonetheless, the rapid decline in motor signals over the first months is consistent with the idea that was mentioned earlier of synaptic contacts being lost from motoneurons as part of the chromatolytic reactions. The improved performance of the motor signals at 150 days suggests that these synaptic contacts return, perhaps even where regeneration to a suitable end-organ is prevented by ligating a nerve. However, other explanations can be suggested. The evoked potentials depend on contributions from both the impulses of sensory and motor fibers. At 30 days there was no sensory activity during locomotion because reinnervation of sense organs had not yet occurred. However, even at 150 days, sensory activity during locomotion was much lower than would be expected from the evoked potentials. Thus, nerve section may have more severe effects on sensory fibers than motor fibers. Evidence for this observation was obtained in terminal experiments (see Chapter 16). Dorsal root fibers were found to have atrophied more severely than ventral root fibers following distal section and ligation or section and resuture of peripheral nerves.

Whatever the explanation of these detailed results, it seems clear that we can answer all three questions that were raised previously in the affirmative. Nerve fibers do appear to survive nerve section, even if they have no opportunity to grow back to suitable end-organs. They do retain the ability to conduct nerve impulses, and motoneurons do continue to generate nerve impulses during motor behavior.

IMPLANTATION IN A HUMAN AMPUTEE

The positive answers obtained above and the good survival of the devices in experi-

mental animals for up to 2 years to date suggested that a clinical trial of these methods to help amputees control powered artificial limbs was warranted. On October 19, 1977, the first such device was implanted in a 62-year-old man whose left arm was amputated just below the elbow during World War II. The device contained four EMG probes that were sutured to remaining portions of wrist extensor, wrist flexor, supinator and pronator muscles close to their motor points. The amputee had previously used surface EMG electrodes over the flexor and extensor muscles to control an Otto Bock electric hand with fair reliability, but because of the shortness of the stump, he had no way to control a powered wrist, which he wished to be able to do. In addition to the EMG probes, a nerve cuff was placed on the ulnar nerve to offer the possibility of sensory feedback.

Fig. 17-8, *A*, shows the left arm of this patient in February, 1978. The stump has healed well, including the skin interface where electrical connections can be made to the internal electrodes. Fig. 17-8, *B*, shows the patient wearing his prosthesis. A cable connects the socket within the skin interface to four preamplifiers built into the prosthesis. The EMG preamplifier gains are adjusted so that the patient can control the motors that open and close the hand and turn the wrist in two directions. Rechargeable batteries provide power for the motors.

The long-term success of this operation cannot yet be assessed, but the results to date are very encouraging. The amputee can generate clearly separated EMG signals on each of the four EMG probes of sufficient amplitude to control each function reliably and independently. Finally, the patient can sense brief electrical stimuli applied to the ulnar nerve. These stimuli are reported as arising from the fourth and fifth fingers of the hand that was amputated over 30 years ago. A detailed mapping has not yet been done, but the general area is the usual sensory innervation of the ulnar nerve. This indicates that at least some sensory fibers have survived amputation for this period of time, despite the

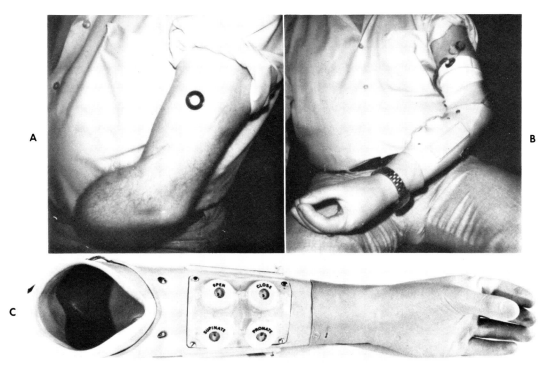

Fig. 17-8. Short below-elbow amputee in whom EMG probes and neural recording cuff were implanted in October 1977. Condition of stump is shown in Feburary 1978, **A.** Note healing around skin interface. Patient is shown wearing his prosthesis, **B,** and prosthesis is seen in more detail in **C.** It contains preamplifiers and signal processing circuits for controlling an electric hand and wrist, together with a cable and plug for connecting to implanted electrodes.

fact that the nerve ended in a large neuroma. Since an important shortcoming of current electrical prostheses is the inability of the amputee to sense the action of his prosthesis without visual attention and concentration, a technique that can provide a sense of "feeling" is an important advance. The prospect of reliable and simple feedback using neural cuffs is most encouraging. The results to date thus offer a good prospect for being able to help amputees regain more function than was previously thought possible.

SUMMARY

Methods have been developed for recording chronically from mammalian nerves and muscles. These methods have been applied to study long-term "trophic" interactions between nerve and muscle and to improve the methods available for amputees to control powered artificial limbs.

Following pressure block of cat hindlimb nerves, the amplitudes of compound action potentials elicited by supramaximal electrical stimuli recover with an exponential time constant of about 2 months. If the block is repaired surgically, the extent of the recovery is increased without affecting its time course.

Following ligation of a nerve, the compound action potentials proximal to the ligation decline exponentially to about a fourth of control values with a time constant of 45 days. If regeneration is permitted by resuturing a cut nerve to its distal end or directly to muscle, a second exponential recovery process is observed with a time constant of 3 to 4 months following the exponential decline.

Using a cross-correlation technique, asynchronous motor activity was also measured in these nerves during a stereotyped motor task in which cats walked on a treadmill at constant speed. Motor signals in the freely moving animal tend to decline more rapidly that the evoked compound action potentials over the first month but are less reduced at later times (5 months). Possible explanations in terms of synaptic changes or differential effects of denervation on sensory and motor fibers are discussed.

The success of these long-term recording methods suggests that neural signals can be used in addition to EMG for control of powered artificial limbs. Nerves can also be used to provide sensory feedback. Successful results with implanted neural and EMG probes in one amputee to date are presented.

REFERENCES

1. Cragg, B., and Thomas, P. K.: Changes in conduction velocity and fibre size proximal to peripheral nerve lesions, J. Physiol. **157:**315, 1961.
2. DeLuca, C. J., and Gilmore, L. D.: Voluntary nerve signals from severed mammalian nerves: long-term recordings, Science (N.Y.) **191:**193, 1976.
3. French, A. S., and Holden, A. V.: Frequency domain analysis of neurophysiological data, Comp. Prog. Bio.-Med. **1:**219, 1971.
4. Gutmann, E.: Histology of degeneration and regeneration. In Licht, S. H., ed.: Electrodiagnosis and electromyography, ed. 3, New Haven, 1971, E. Licht, p. 113.
5. Heetderks, W. J., and Williams, W. J.: Partition of gross peripheral nerve activity into single unit responses by correlation techniques, Science (N.Y.) **188:**373, 1975.
6. Hoffer, J. A.: Long-term peripheral nerve activity during behaviour in the rabbit: the control of locomotion, Ph.D. Thesis, Johns Hopkins University, Baltimore, 1975.
7. Mannard, A., Stein, R. B., and Charles, D.: Regeneration electrode units: implants for recording from single peripheral nerve fibres in freely moving animals, Science (N.Y.) **183:**547, 1974.
8. Mendell, L. M., Munson, J. B., and Scott, J. B.: Alterations of synapses on axotomized motoneurones, J. Physiol. **255:**67, 1976.
9. Purves, D.: Long-term regulation in the vertebrate peripheral nervous system, Int. Rev. Physiol. **10:**125, 1976.
10. Ranson, S. W.: Retrograde degeneration in the spinal nerves, J. Comp. Neurol. **16:**265, 1906.
11. Stanitski, C. L., and Mooney, V.: Osseus attachment to vitreous carbons, J. Biomed. Mater. Res. **4:**97, 1973.
12. Stein, R. B.: The peripheral control of movement, Physiol. Rev. **54:**215, 1974.
13. Stein, R. B.: Principles underlying new methods for chronic neural recording, Can. J. Neurol. Sci. **2:**235, 1975.
14. Stein, R. B., et al.: Stable long-term recordings from cat peripheral nerves, Brain Res. **128:**21, 1977.
15. Sunderland, S.: Nerve and nerve injuries, London, 1972, Churchill Livingstone.

DISCUSSION

Carlo DeLuca (Boston): I just want to add some additional information that we have available. We have been working with a similar problem in Boston for several years and we performed an experiment somewhat parallel to Dr. Stein's. That is, we actually transected a nerve, performed an axotomy, and then placed an electrode cuff similar to Dr. Stein's, and we can keep recording voluntary nerve signals for up to 142 days thus far. However, in the first 3 or 4 weeks there is a severe decrease in the amplitude of the action potentials of the voluntary signals, which then tends to flatten out. We suspect that this loss is not due to local effects in the electrode cuff.

18

Ectopic generation of impulses in pathological nerve fibers

Michael Rasminsky

Symptoms of peripheral nerve injuries fall into two broad categories: (1) *negative symptoms*, that is, sensory loss, muscle weakness, and localized loss of autonomic regulation; (2) *positive symptoms*, that is, pain, paresthesias, muscle fasciculations, and localized signs of autonomic hyperactivity.

Negative symptoms are readily understood in terms of complete or partial interruption of impulse traffic through the site of injury. Positive symptoms are in general less readily understood in these terms. In order to explain positive symptoms of peripheral nerve pathology solely as a consequence of *decreased* nerve impulse traffic, it is essential to invoke mechanisms involving the central nervous system.

The purpose of this chapter is to review some of the recent evidence that *increased* nerve impulse traffic is generated in the peripheral nervous system by various types of pathological nerves; the obvious clinical implication is that such increased impulse traffic may be reflected in positive symptoms of peripheral nerve disease.

ACUTELY AND CHRONICALLY INJURED NERVE
Acute effects of nerve transection

Almost half a century ago, Adrian[1] reported that acute sectioning of mammalian nerve provoked persistent discharges of impulses in some nerve fibers. The patterns of discharge observed were: (1) continuous high-frequency discharge at greater than 150 Hz, (2) continuous lower frequency discharge, and (3) bursting activity. Although there is no question that acute nerve transection frequently provokes a short burst or a few seconds discharge of impulses, subsequent workers have not in general observed persistent activity following nerve section.[30] However, Wall and Devor[26] report that a stump of a severed nerve may begin to generate spontaneous activity as early as 3.5 hours following nerve section.

Acute effects of nerve ischemia and compression

Kugelberg[15] found that ischemic nerve compression with a pneumatic tourniquet led to repetitive EMG activity distal to the tourniquet that was caused by repetitive firing of nerve fibers at the compression site. Reduction of serum calcium by hyperventilation enhanced the repetitive firing. The paresthesias associated with the onset and interruption of compression ischemia have been attributed to generation of impulses at the compression site.[15,17]

Chronic effects of nerve transection

Following transection of a peripheral nerve the cut axons ultimately sprout and either regenerate along the course of the original nerve or form a neuroma at the site of transection. Such neuromas may give rise to pain at rest and are exquisitely sensitive to mechanical stimulation. The physiological properties of neuromas have been exten-

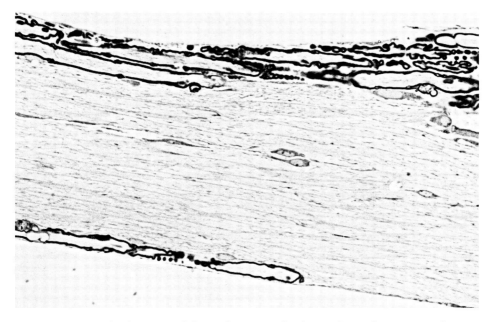

Fig. 18-1. Longitudinal section of dystrophic mouse lumbosacral spinal root. Magnification ×480.

sively studied by Wall and co-workers[5,28,29] and recently summarized by Wall and Devor.[27]

Regenerating nerve terminals within a neuroma can be excited by both mechanical and electrical stimulation and some terminals generate spontaneous activity.[28,29] Fibers excited by stimulation of a neuroma are those with conduction velocity in the A delta or C fiber range.[5] This may reflect a predilection for small diameter fibers to form a neuroma. However, it is also possible that sprouts of large diameter fibers would be dysfunctional because of their inability to excite the parent axons; the current generated by excitation of a relatively small diameter unmyelinated sprout may be sufficient to excite a small diameter parent myelinated fiber but insufficient to excite a larger diameter fiber[5] (see also Chapter 19).

The spontaneous nerve impulse activity generated within neuromas is suppressed by application of local anesthetics and after invasion of the neuroma by a brief antidromic tetanus. Ongoing activity is highly dependent on maintenance of adequate blood flow. Activity is enhanced by systemic administration of the α-active sympathetic amine noradrenalin but is not by the β-active sympathetic amine isoprenaline.[28,29]

SPINAL NERVE ROOTS OF DYSTROPHIC MICE

In genetically dystrophic mice, the cervical and lumbosacral spinal nerve roots contain many axons that are bare, closely apposed to one another, and devoid of any Schwann cell investment[3,4,24] (Fig. 18-1). The pathology is most striking in midroot; near the spinal cord and the exit from the spinal canal most axons are myelinated, albeit with myelin inappropriately thin for the axon diameter.[4] The spectrum of axon diameters in the dystrophic roots is similar to that of normal animals.[3] Conduction velocity of nervous impulses is greatly reduced in these fibers[13,22]; both saltatory and continuous conduction occur in the same single fiber, presumably in the myelinated and bare portions, respectively.[22]

Generation of ectopic activity

When spontaneous nerve impulse activity is recorded biphasically from spinal roots, the direction of spontaneous impulse traffic can be inferred from the polarity of the biphasic action potentials that are recorded, initial negativity being recorded at the electrode first traversed by the impulse. In normal mice all spontaneous impulse traffic in lumbosacral dorsal roots is toward the spinal cord (centripetal), and all spontaneous impulse traffic in lumbosacral ventral roots is away from the spinal cord (centrifugal). In lumbosacral ventral roots of dystrophic mice, spontaneous impulse activity is largely centrifugal near the exit from the spinal cord; in some ventral roots near the spinal cord a substantial proportion of the spontaneous activity is centripetal (Fig. 18-2). Since few if any centripetal impulses traverse the more distal portion of ventral roots, this centripetal activity must originate in midroot, in the region of the major pathology in the roots. The activity originating ectopically in midventral root is reduced but usually not abolished if the normal centrifugal activity is eliminated by plac-

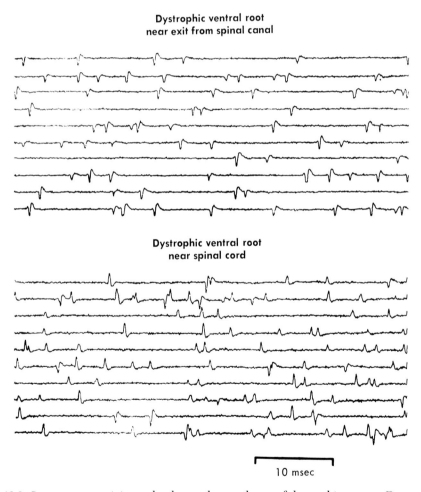

**Dystrophic ventral root
near exit from spinal canal**

**Dystrophic ventral root
near spinal cord**

10 msec

Fig. 18-2. Spontaneous activity on lumbosacral ventral root of dystrophic mouse. Downward deflections are impulses traveling away from spinal cord (centrifugal); upward deflections are impulses traveling toward spinal cord (centripetal). Centripetal activity is seen near spinal cord but not near exit from spinal canal. (Reproduced with permission from Rasminsky, M.: Ann. Neurol. **3:**351, 1978.)

ing local anesthetic on the root at its emergence from the spinal cord or by cutting the root near its origin.[19] The midroot site of origin of spontaneous activity in either ventral or dorsal roots of dystrophic mice can be more explicitly demonstrated by simultaneous recording from two pairs of bipolar electrodes placed on either side of the ectopic site of origin of spontaneous activity (Fig. 18-3, *A*). Ectopic activity in single fibers arises as single impulses, in bursts, or as continuous firing.[19] These patterns are similar to those originally observed by Adrian[1] in acutely injured peripheral nerve and by Kugelberg[15] in acute ischemic compression lesions.

Cross talk

Ephaptic interactions between artificially apposed invertebrate axons were first described 40 years ago[2,14] and were subsequently reported to occur in acutely injured mammalian nerve by Granit and co-workers.[9,10] Although the concept of cross talk between pathological nerve fibers has gained wide currency in the clinical neurological and neurosurgical literature,[6,8,31] physiologists have in general taken a more skeptical view of the experiments of Granit and co-workers,[9,10] both because of difficulties in reproducing these experiments[30] and because of the questionable relevance of a

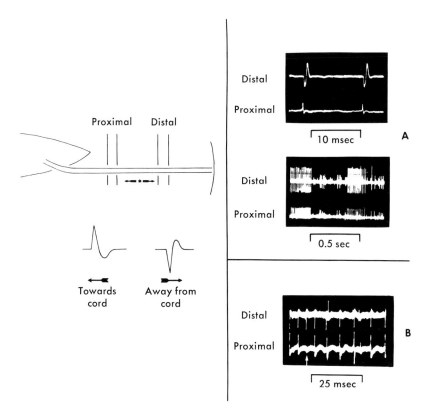

Fig. 18-3. Spontaneous activity originating between proximal and distal electrode pairs applied to same root is recorded as upward deflection at proximal electrodes and downward deflection at distal electrodes. **A,** Spontaneous activity on dystrophic mouse ventral root. Slower sweep speed (below) illustrates bursting activity of fiber for which only two impulses are shown at faster sweep speed (above). **B,** Spontaneous activity of fiber from rat ventral root demyelinated with diphtheria toxin. Note failure of third impulse in burst to traverse proximal electrodes (arrow). This reflects failure of demyelinated fiber to transmit all impulses in train.[21]

short-lived effect in an acute preparation to chronic pathological states.[19,25]

The concept of cross talk in pathological nerves has recently been revived by Huizar and co-workers,[13] who showed that stimulation of one of the tibial and common peroneal nerve branches of the sciatic nerve in dystrophic mice invariably produced discharges in the other nerve branch even after section of the appropriate dorsal roots. Abolition of the response when the appropriate ventral roots were sectioned far enough distal to the spinal cord suggested that side-to-side communication occurred within spinal roots or just outside the spinal column. I subsequently showed that cross talk could in fact occur between single fibers in the spinal roots of dystrophic mice[19] (Figs. 18-4 and 18-5). It remains to be established whether such cross talk occurs between adjacent and closely apposed bare axons, between bare axons and adjacent myelinated axons, or between adjacent (abnormally) myelinated axons.

DEMYELINATED NERVE

The extensive literature on the physiology of demyelinated nerve fibers has been almost exclusively concerned with the impaired ability of such fibers to transmit nerve impulses. The extreme consequence of demyelination is blockage of conduction; other well-characterized properties of less severely affected demyelinated nerve fibers include de-

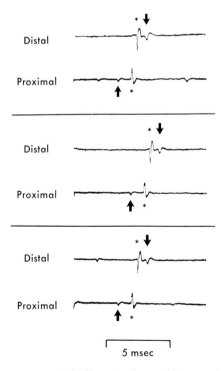

Fig. 18-4. Cross talk between two single fibers in dystrophic ventral root. Three separate occurrences of same complex simultaneously recorded from proximal and distal electrode pairs are illustrated. Impulse originating in midroot* is associated with impulse traveling away from spinal cord (arrows) (see Fig. 18-5). (Reproduced with permission from Rasminsky, M.: Ann. Neurol. **3:**351, 1978.)

creased condution velocity, increased refractory period of transmission, decreased ability to transmit trains of impulses, posttetanic depression, and reversible conduction block with increased temperature in the physiological range.[20] It has recently became apparent that demyelinated nerve fibers are also capable of ectopic generation of nerve impulses.

Howe and co-workers[11] have shown that if a mammalian peripheral nerve is chronically injured (presumably demyelinated) with a gut ligature,[16] the site of injury can become a point of reversal in direction or reflection of nervous impulses entering the lesion. The postulated mechanism of this reflection is that slowing of the impulse at the site of pathology is so marked as to permit reexcitation of the portion of the fiber from which the impulse has just entered the lesion, this normal adjacent portion having passed through its postexcitation refractoriness before the impulse in the injured zone has made significant forward progress.[11] Although axons chronically injured with this technique are only rarely spontaneously active, they are much more readily excited by mechanical stimulation than normal axons.[12]

In preliminary experiments on rat spinal root fibers demyelinated with intrathecal injection of diphtheria toxin,[21] I have found that ectopically generated activity can frequently be observed (Fig. 18-3, *B*). Just as in the dystrophic mouse spinal root fibers, such ectopic activity occurs as single isolated impulses, in bursts at frequencies that may approach 400 Hz, or as continuous firing.

DISCUSSION

The examples presented indicate that generation of nerve impulses is not an exclusive property of nerve cell bodies or normal sensory terminals. Nerve impulses can also be generated in several types of pathological nerve—both by the unmyelinated sprouts of regenerated nerve in a neuroma and at the site of pathological abnormality in congenitally abnormally myelinated nerves or demyelinated nerves.

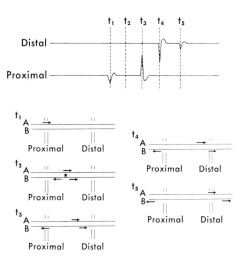

Fig. 18-5. Diagrammatic reconstruction of cross talk illustrated in Fig. 18-4. At time t_1 centrifugal impulse in fiber *A* traverses proximal electrode pair, causing downward deflection. At time t_2 fiber *B* is excited in midroot* initiating impulse that travels in both directions. At time t_3 impulse in fiber *B* traverses proximal electrode pair, causing upward deflection. At time t_4 impulse in fiber *B* traverses distal electrode pair, causing downward deflection. At time t_5 impulse in fiber *A* traverses distal electrode pair, causing second downward deflection. (Reproduced with permission from Rasminsky, M.: Ann. Neurol. 3:351, 1978.)

The ability of pathological peripheral nerve to generate ectopic activity is of obvious relevance to some clinical manifestations of nerve injuries that are the subject of this volume. Nerve injury eventuating in axonal transection may result in neuroma formation—the work of Wall and his collaborators[5,27,28] has now made it clear that much of the troublesome symptomatology of neuromas is due to the high level of spontaneous activity emanating from the neuroma and the enhancement of this activity by minimal stimuli.

Ochoa and co-workers[18] have shown that if axonal transection does not ensue, the ultimate consequence of nerve compression is demyelination. The sudden dysesthesias experienced by patients with compression neuropathies on percussion of the compression site (Tinel's sign) presumably reflect the increased sensitivity of demyelinated nerve to stimulation by pressure.[12] Patients with the carpal tunnel syndrome characteristically complain of being awakened from sleep with dysesthesias in the affected hand. It is possible that the additional edema that accumulates during sleep increases pressure on the nerve sufficiently to provoke or increase spontaneous impulse traffic originating at the compression site.

Positive symptoms of central nervous system demyelinating disease may also reflect ectopic impulse generation in pathological central nerve fibers.[20] The exacerbation of such symptoms by hyperventilation[26] may reflect increased ectopic impulse generation caused by membrane hyperexcitability, which is provoked by the hyperventilation-induced fall in ionized serum calcium. In principle positive symptomatology in peripheral nerve disorders could be treated by therapeutic use of pharmacological agents that reduce membrane excitability. Tic douloureux and the painful components of some peripheral neuropathies can be successfully treated with drugs such as carbamazepine.[7] It is possible that the therapeutic effectiveness of these drugs on peripheral nerve symptomatology is related to their depressant effects on membrane excitability of peripheral nerve[23] rather than to other effects that they may have in the central nervous system.

This chapter has emphasized ectopic generation of nerve impulses as a cause of positive symptoms, particularly sensory symptoms, in peripheral nerve injuries. Other peripheral mechanisms for generation of such symptomatology may also be of importance; these include alterations in properties and innervation of receptors, changes in the spectrum of fiber sizes within pathological nerves, altered patterns of connectivity of spinal cord projections of sensory fibers, and altered reactivity of the postsynaptic mechanisms in the spinal cord.[27] It is also possible, and perhaps at times necessary, to account for positive symptomatology in terms of as yet rather vaguely defined changes within the central nervous system.

The attractiveness of the ectopic generator as a possible (but not necessarily exclusive) source of symptomatology is two-fold: (1) such generators are amenable to detailed experimental examination and (2) the activity of at least some ectopic generators is subject to physiological and pharmacological manipulation.[28,29,30]

SUMMARY

Impulses are generated ectopically in chronically injured nerve fibers, congenitally dysmyelinated nerve fibers, and demyelinated nerve fibers. In some cases ectopic activity in single nerve fibers is provoked by impulses traversing neighboring fibers; in most cases activity arises *de novo* in single pathological fibers but may be modified by metabolic conditions and drugs. Ectopic impulse activity arising in pathological nerve may be an important mechanism in the production of the positive symptomatology of peripheral nerve disease.

ACKNOWLEDGMENT

The research for this chapter was supported by the Medical Research Council of Canada.

REFERENCES

1. Adrian, E. D.: The effects of injury on mammalian nerve fibers, Proc. R. Soc. B. **106:**596, 1930.
2. Arvanitaki, A.: Réactions déclenchées sur un axone

au repos par l'activité d'un autre axone au niveau d'une zone de contact; conditions de la transmission de l'excitation, C. R. Soc. Biol. (Paris) **133**:39, 1940.

3. Bradley, W. G., and Jenkison, M.: Abnormalities of peripheral nerve in murine muscular dystrophy, J. Neurol. Sci. **17**:227, 1973.

4. Bray, G. M., and Aguayo, A. J.: Quantitative ultra-structural studies of the axon–Schwann cell abnor-mality in spinal nerve roots from dystrophic mice, J. Neuropathol. Exp. Neurol. **34**:517, 1975.

5. Devor, M., and Wall, P. D.: Type of sensory nerve fibre sprouting to form a neuroma, Nature (Lond) **262**:705, 1976.

6. Doupe, J., Cullen, C. H., and Chance, G. Q.: Post traumatic pain and the causalgic syndrome, J. Neurol. Neurosurg. Psychiatry **7**:33, 1944.

7. Espir, M. L. E., and Millac, P.: Treatment of paroxysmal disorders in multiple sclerosis with car-bamazepine, J. Neurol. Neurosurg. Psychiatry **33**:528, 1970.

8. Gardner, W. J.: Cross talk—the paradoxical trans-mission of a nerve impulse, Arch. Neurol. **14**:149, 1966.

9. Granit, R., and Skoglund, C. R.: Facilitation inhibi-tion and depression at the artificial synapse formed by the cut end of a mammalian nerve, J. Physiol. (Lond) **103**:435, 1945.

10. Granit, R., Leksell, I., and Skoglund, C. R.: Fibre interaction in injured or compressed regions of nerve, Brain **67**:125, 1944.

11. Howe, J. F., Calvin, W. H., and Loeser, J. D.: Im-pulses reflected from dorsal root ganglia and from focal nerve injuries, Brain Res. **116**:139, 1976.

12. Howe, J. F., Loeser, J. D., and Calvin, W. H.: Mechanosensitivity of dorsal root ganglia and chron-ically injured axons: a physiological basis for the radicular pain of nerve root compression, Pain **3**:25, 1977.

13. Huizar, P., Kuno, M., and Miyata, Y.: Elec-trophysiological properties of spinal motoneurones of normal and dystrophic mice, J. Physiol. (Lond) **248**:231, 1975.

14. Jasper, H. H., and Monnier, A. M.: Transmission of excitation between excised non-myelinated nerves: an artificial synapse, J. Cell Comp. Physiol. **11**:259, 1938.

15. Kugelberg, E.: "Injury activity" and "trigger zones" in human nerves, Brain **69**:410, 1946.

16. Lehmann, H. J., and Ule, G.: Electrophysiological findings and structural changes in circumspect inflammation of peripheral nerves, Prog. Brain Res. **6**:169, 1964.

17. Lewis, T., Pickering, W., and Rothschild, P.: Cen-tripetal paralysis arising out of arrested blood flow to the limb, including notes on a form of tingling, Heart **16**:1, 1931.

18. Ochoa, J., Fowler, J. T., and Gilliatt, R. W.: Anatomical changes in peripheral nerve compressed by a pneumatic tourniquet, J. Anat. **113**:433, 1972.

19. Rasminsky, M.: Ectopic generation of impulses and cross-talk in spinal nerve roots of "dystrophic" mice, Ann. Neurol. **3**:351, 1978.

20. Rasminsky, M.: Physiology of conduction in de-myelinated axons. In Waxman S. G., ed.: Physiol-ogy and pathobiology of axons, New York, 1978, Raven Press, p. 361.

21. Rasminsky, M., and Sears, T. A.: Internodal con-duction in undissected demyelinated nerve fibres, J. Physiol. (Lond) **227**:323, 1972.

22. Rasminsky, M., et al.: Conduction of nervous im-pulses in spinal roots and peripheral nerves of dys-trophic mice, Brain Res. **143**:71, 1978.

23. Schauf, C. L., Davis, F. A., and Marder, J.: Effects of carbamazepine on the ionic conductances of Myxicola giant axons, J. Pharmacol. Exp. Ther. **189**:538, 1974.

24. Stirling, C. A.: Abnormalities in Schwann cell sheaths in spinal nerve roots of dystrophic mice, J. Anat. **119**:169, 1975.

25. Thomas, P. K., and Cavanagh, J. B.: Neuropathy due to physical agents. In Dyck, P. J., Thomas. P. K., and Lambert, E. H., eds.: Peripheral neuro-pathy, vol. II, Philadelphia, 1975, W. B. Saunders Co., p. 734.

26. Toyokura, Y., Sakuta, M., and Nakanishi, T.: Pain-ful tonic seizures in multiple sclerosis, Neurology (Minneap.) **26** (no. 6, part 2): 18, 1976.

27. Wall, P. D., and Devor, M.: Physiology of sensation after peripheral nerve injury, regeneration and neuroma formation. In Waxman, S. G., ed.: Physiology and pathobiology of axons, New York, 1978, Raven Press, p. 377.

28. Wall, P. D., and Gutnick, M.: Properties of afferent nerve impulses originating from a neuroma, Nature (Lond), **248**:740, 1974.

29. Wall, P. D., and Gutnick, M.: Ongoing activity in peripheral nerves: the physiology and pharmacology of impulses originating from a neuroma, Exp. Neurol. **43**:580, 1974.

30. Wall, P. D., Waxman, S., and Basbaum, A. I.: On-going activity in peripheral nerve: injury discharge, Exp. Neurol. **45**:576, 1974.

31. White, J. C., and Sweet, W. H.: Pain and the neurosurgeon, Springfield, Ill., 1969, Charles C Thomas, Publisher.

19

Structure-function relations in nerves and nerve injuries

Stephen G. Waxman

This chapter will deal with structure-function relations along normal and injured nerve fibers. In particular, it will deal with the structural determinants of conduction properties in normal and pathological axons. In doing so, we will concentrate on the relation of morphology in the traditional sense (that is, with respect to those aspects of axonal structure that are discernible at the light and electron microscopical levels) to axonal physiology. It should be noted at the outset that altered function does not necessarily imply morphologically detectable abnormality of a nerve fiber. Metabolic abnormalities unaccompanied by morphological changes may alter nerve function. For example, nerve conduction velocities may be transiently and reversibly produced in patients receiving diphenylhydantoin therapy.[3] The time course of the changes is so rapid as to make a metabolic change much more likely as the factor responsible for alterations in conduction properties than a structural change. Rapidly reversible changes in nerve conduction can be demonstrated in patients with chronic renal failure before and after hemodialysis and are related to plasma electrolyte concentrations.[11] Similarly, in experimental diabetic neuropathy, decreases in conduction velocity may be seen in the absence of demonstrable structural abnormality when the fibers are examined by conventional light and electron microscopical techniques.[36] Conversely, it should be emphasized that altered structure does not

necessarily lead to pathological function in a given nerve fiber. Computer simulations[22] have shown that axonal conduction velocity its relatively insensitive to small changes in the area of the node of Ranvier or in the description of the excitable membrane processes at the node. This is consistent with the experimental observation that the slight widening of the nodes of Ranvier observed early in diphtheritic neuropathy is not necessarily accompanied by a decrease in motor axon conduction velocity.[23] Finally, we must note that abnormal function at the cellular level is not reflected by a clinical deficit in all cases. Thus it is not unusual to observe decreased nerve conduction velocities in asymptomatic patients with metabolic or familial neuropathies.

The preceding comments notwithstanding, it is clear that the structure of a given nerve will impose a set of boundary conditions that determine, within a range of variability, its conduction properties. Assuming that the compositions of the extracellular milieu and axoplasm are fixed and that specific membrane properties are invariant, it should be possible to define a set of relationships between structural parameters (for example, diameter, myelin thickness, internode length) and functional parameters (for example, conduction velocity, refractory period, ability to conduct trains of impulses) for each fiber. At present, conduction velocity is better understood, in terms of its relationship to structural substrates, than other aspects of conduction. Especially in view of the large and detailed body of data available concerning the structure of both normal and injured nerves, as exemplified by the meticulous observations of Sunderland,[39] it is appropriate to inquire as to what predictions concerning the physiology of conduction in a given axon can be made on the basis of observations of its morphology. This chapter will deal with this question, first for uniform fibers, that is, those in which properties do not change markedly along the course of the fiber, and then for nonuniform fibers, that is, those in which there are sudden changes in fiber properties. In the case of nonmyelinated fibers, uniformity implies that the fiber exhibits no changes in either diameter or shape, or in specific membrane properties, along its length. We will consider myelinated fibers to be uniform if all nodes and all internodes are identical.

Fig. 19-1 shows, in transverse section, the sequence that occurs during myelinogenesis in the mammalian peripheral nervous system. In peripheral nerve, as demonstrated by Geren[12] and Robertson,[32] the myelin-forming Schwann cell initially approaches the axon, then wraps around it in a spiral manner so as to surround the axon with many layers of Schwann cell plasma membrane, and finally exudes the cytoplasm and most of the extracellular space from this membrane spiral so as to form the compact myelin sheath. The myelin sheath is punctuated periodically by nonmyelinated gaps (the nodes of Ranvier) extending less than 2μm along the axis of the fiber. For a detailed description of the node, the reader is referred to Berthold.[2]

In normal myelinated fibers the myelin, as a result of its high resistance and low capacitance, shunts the majority of the action current through the nodes of Ranvier, and spike electrogenesis is confined to the nodes so that conduction is saltatory, that is, progresses in a discontinuous fashion from node to node.[19] The myelin is of functional significance in several respects: In peripheral nerve myelinated fibers conduct more rapidly than nonmyelinated fibers of similar diameter. In addition, the energetic requirements for trans-

mission are less in myelinated fibers.[16] Finally, as noted below, in normal myelinated fibers, the Na^+ channels are concentrated at the nodes, and the density of Na^+ channels in the internodal axon membrane beneath the myelin is so low that this portion of the axon membrane may, in the absence of myelin, not support conduction unless there is a redistribution, or production, of additional channels.

CONDUCTION IN UNIFORM AXONS

In general for uniform myelinated fibers in which specific membrane properties are constant, and in which (1) the nodal length is nearly constant, (2) internodal distance (the distance between nodes of Ranvier) is proportional to fiber diameter, and (3) the myelin thickness varies linearly with axon caliber, the conduction velocity will be approximately proportional to fiber diameter[33,45] (Fig. 19-2). Myelinated fibers in most normal mammalian peripheral nerves conform to these criteria for "structural similarity." There are, however, some differences in the ratio of conduction velocity to diameter in large as compared to small diameter fibers. For example, Boyd and Davey[6] found a ratio of 4.5 between conduction velocity (in m/sec) and diameter (in μm) in small diameter axons, compared to a value of 5.7 in large diameter fibers. This may reflect a variation from structural similarity, or it may be due to differences in membrane properties among fibers of different size.

A number of studies have addressed the relation between myelin thickness and conduction velocity. For any given axon, conduction velocity will increase monotonically with myelin thickness.[37] However, for a fiber with *fixed* total diameter (that is, diameter of axon plus myelin sheath), there is an optimum ratio of myelin thickness to axon diameter. If the myelin is too thin, there will be excessive internodal current loss as a result of the transverse conductance and capacitance. Increased myelin capacitance is more important than increased conductance in decreasing the conduction velocity.[22] If the myelin is too thick, on the other hand, the axial lon-

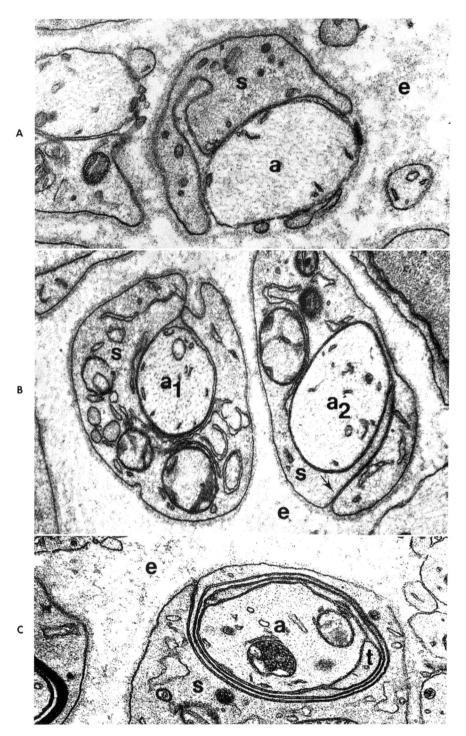

Fig. 19-1. Electron micrographs in this and following figures show cross sections of axons from baby mouse sciatic nerve at various stages of myelination. **A,** Schwann cell, *s*, has established one-to-one relationship with axon, *a*. *e*, Extracellular space. $KMnO_4$. (×36,000.) **B,** Two neighboring axons, a_1 and a_2, at early stages of myelination. Schwann cell, *s*, surrounds axon a_1 but has not yet formed spiral wrapping in this plane of section. Schwann cell surrounding axon a_2 has begun to form spiral mesaxon (arrow). $KMnO_2$. (×36,000.) **C,** Myelinating Schwann cell, *s*, that has formed approximately two loops around axon. Tongue of Schwann cell cytoplasm, *t*, extends longitudinally within noncompact sheath. $KMnO_4$. (×36,000.) **D,** Thin myelin sheath, *m*, that is nearly compact. Note that myelin remains connected to Schwann cell surface by mesaxon (arrow). *c*, Collagen. Glutaraldehyde. (×53,700.)

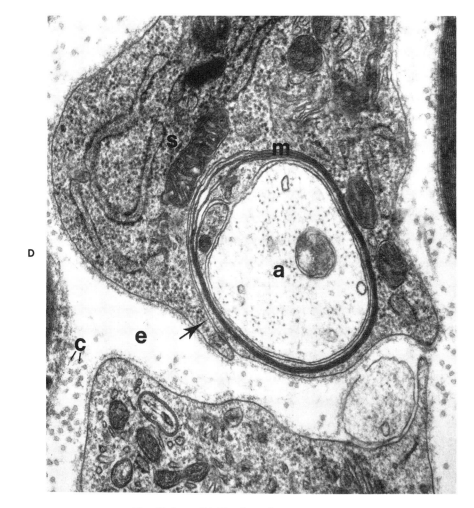

Fig. 19-1, cont'd. For legend see opposite page.

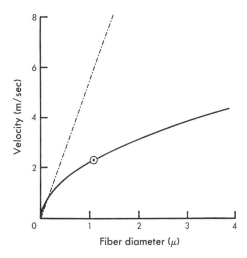

Fig. 19-2. Relationship between conduction velocity (on ordinate) and fiber diameter (on abscissa) for myelinated (broken line) and nonmyelinated (solid line) fibers. Above critical diameter of approximately 0.2 μm, myelinated fibers conduct more rapidly than nonmyelinated fibers of same diameter. Note that ratio between conduction velocities of myelinated and nonmyelinated fibers of a given diameter is not constant but increases with increasing fiber size. (Modified from Waxman, S. G., and Bennet, M. V. L.: Nature [New Biol.] **238**:217, 1972.)

gitudinal resistance of the axon will make conduction velocity less than maximal. Rushton[33] concluded from analytical arguments that the optimal value (in terms of maximizing conduction velocity) of the ratio g (axon diameter:total fiber diameter) should be 0.6 and that there should be only a 5% decrease in conduction velocity for variation in the value of g between 0.47 and 0.74. Our own studies[22] are in agreement, indicating a maximal conduction velocity when g = 0.62. Computations by Smith and Koles[37] also suggest that conduction velocity should be maximal at a value of g between 0.6 and 0.7, with a variation in velocity of less than 20% for values of g between 0.5 and 0.9 if total fiber diameter is held constant. Therefore, if total fiber diameter is constant, some variability in myelin thickness may occur without large reductions in conduction velocity. However, for very thinly or very thickly myelinated fibers, the conduction velocity will fall below the maximal value for that diameter. It should be pointed out, nevertheless, that despite a lowered conduction velocity, remyelination with even very thin myelin sheaths in previously demyelinated areas may permit saltatory conduction. Computer simulations by Koles and Ras-

minsky[21] suggest that remyelination with myelin as thin as 2.7% of normal thickness may restore conduction without block.

The relationship between conduction velocity and internode length[7] is shown in Fig. 19-3. Conduction velocity is maximized for any given diameter when the ratio L/d (internode distance/axon diameter) falls between the values of approximately 100 and 200, assuming that the nodes continue to exhibit normal specific membrane properties. For most normal peripheral axons the value of L/d does, in fact, fall within this range. Modest variations in L/d, as are observed in peripheral regenerated and remyelinated fibers, are accompanied by only small reductions in conduction velocity.[34] It should be noted in this context that for some specialized fibers within the normal CNS, values of L/d may be less than 10; these central axons are not designed so as to achieve maximal conduction velocity at their particular diameter but rather act as delay lines[42,43] and possibly modulate the invadability of presynaptic terminals.[46]

In contrast to myelinated fibers, for which conduction velocity is proportional to diameter, in nonmyelinated fibers the conduction velocity is proportional to the square root of

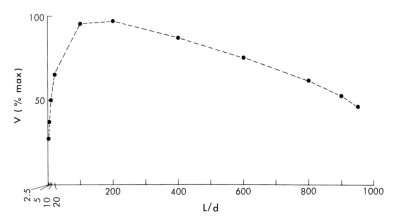

Fig. 19-3. Computed relation between conduction velocity (expressed as a percent of maximal conduction velocity) and the ratio *L/d* (internode distance/axon diameter). Internode distances of normal peripheral myelinated fibers are, in fact, such as to maximize conduction velocity. (Modified from Brill, M. H., et al.: J. Neurol. Neurosurg. Psychiatry **40:**769, 1977.)

the diameter (see references 33 and 45 and Fig. 19-2). Since the linear relation between conduction velocity and diameter for myelinated fibers must intersect the parabolic relation for nonmyelinated fibers at some point, there should be a minimal diameter, below which myelinated fibers do not conduct more rapidly than nonmyelinated fibers. Several arguments suggest that this initial diameter has a value close to 0.2 μm.[45] The value of 0.2 μm corresponds closely with the diameter of the smallest myelinated fibers present in the central nervous system.[4,45] However, in peripheral nerve, fibers are not myelinated until they achieve a diameter of approximately 1 μm (it should be noted, however, that diameter itself does not provide the signal for myelination; see Chapter 6). The difference in diameter of the smallest myelinated fibers in peripheral, as compared to central, tracts remains unexplained. It may reflect differences in the intrinsic membrane properties, in the nature of the extracellular milieu, in the geometry of the nodes of Ranvier, or still other factors.

A further consideration in terms of structure-function relations in uniform axons concerns the ability to conduct trains of impulses. In this context, it should be recalled that the recovery cycle of the axon in question will determine its ability to transmit trains of impulses. For most nerve fibers, the recovery cycle can be thought of as essentially triphasic: refractory period $\rightarrow$ supernormal period (increased excitability and conduction velocity) $\rightarrow$ subnormal period (decreased excitability and conduction velocity).[29,40,47] The characteristics of the recovery cycle are different for fibers of different diameters. Duration of the refractory period, for example, varies inversely with fiber size.[24,41] Similarly, duration of the supernormal period and the magnitude of the conduction latency decreases that occur during supernormality are inversely related to fiber size.[41] Raymond and Lettvin[29] observed that smaller fibers are more easily depressed; that is, subnormality is more easily produced in smaller axons. To the degree that axon diameter is altered distal to a site of injury, it

would therefore be reasonable to expect changes in the characteristics of the recovery cycle. Whether or not these changes would be functionally significant for any given fiber will depend on several factors, including the patterning of impulses during normal activity and the sensitivity of postsynaptic elements to the fine temporal patterning of impulses. It should further be noted that the recovery cycle is dependent, in part, on metabolic processes that can be blocked by agents such as ouabain.[29] In view of this, it is possible that abnormalities in the pattern of vascularization at or distal to a site of nerve injury might also be reflected by changes in impulse train transmission characteristics.

CONDUCTION IN NONUNIFORM AXONS

It is an all too common clinical observation that regeneration of a severed nerve may not be accompanied by functional recovery. Here one is struck by the disparity between outcome following nerve crush, in which the prognosis is not necessarily poor, and the outcome following nerve severance, in which the prognosis is much less optimistic. As noted elsewhere in this volume, clinical abnormalities persisting after nerve repair may reflect failure to reestablish appropriate peripheral connections. In addition, however, regeneration of an axon beyond a point of severance is not necessarily accompanied by the reliable transmission of neural information along the regenerated axon. A crucial site in the transmission of impulses along such regenerated axons would seem to be the site of anastomosis. This region presents a potential site for distortion or block of neural messages.

Let us consider, for example, the characteristics of impulse propagation past a region in which axonal diameter changes. As noted above, the conduction properties of two axonal regions of different diameter may not be equivalent, so that even if one were not to consider the transition zone itself, impulse trains might be expected to be handled differently (as a result of differences in refractory, supernormal, and subnormal periods) in large and small diameter regions of the axon. However, the transition region itself may also act in such a manner as to transform impulse trains by changing the fine temporal patterning of impulses, acting as a low-pass filter, or blocking transmission completely. In the case of normal central axons[8] and in some specialized peripheral axons,[48] it has been suggested that transformations in impulse patterning at sites of axonal nonuniformity may play a role in information transmission and coding. Chung, Raymond, and Lettvin,[8] for example, provide evidence that filtering impulse trains at axonal branch points may provide a mechanism for the transformation of temporal patterns of activity into spatial ones by the routing of impulses into appropriate parts of the axonal arborization. On the other hand, in regions of pathological nonuniformity at sites of nerve injury, changes in transmission properties may act so as to distort or block neural messages. There is both experimental[38,49] and computer simulation[14,20,25] evidence for conduction block or low-pass filtering at sites of abrupt increase in axon diameter. Lability of conduction at these sites probably reflects the electrical loading imposed by the region of increased diameter. In regions of nonuniformity where the increase in diameter is gradual rather than abrupt, conduction characteristics may be highly dependent on the geometry of the fiber. Parnas and coworkers[25] for example, showed that a change in diameter of 0.1 μm in a region of axonal tapering could significantly alter the safety factor for spike transmission through that region. In this regard, it should be emphasized that conduction properties through a region of nonuniformity are not necessarily symmetrical. Thus conduction from a small diameter region to a large diameter region may exhibit different properties than conduction in the other direction. This directionality may have important clinical implications. Regenerated axons are often of small diameter than their parent fibers. The question therefore arises as to whether differences in the pattern of recovery of sensory, as compared to motor, nerves reflect differences (conduction from

small to large diameter regions in regenerated sensory axons, conduction from large to small diameter regions in regenerated motor axons) related to the direction (distal-to-proximal vs. proximal-to-distal) of impulse conduction.

Two other points that have been demonstrated experimentally but not clinically in the case of nerve injury may be of some relevance to the issue of nerve repair. There is evidence in some experimental systems that the "critical ratio" of pre- and posttransitional diameters at which conduction will fail is dependent on temperature, with conduction becoming less secure as temperature increases.[49] This is similar to the reversible conduction block seen in some demyelinated fibers with increased temperature, which is probably due to decreased axonal current generation, and a consequent decrease in conduction safety factor, at higher temperature.[27] Finally, there is evidence that "reflected" impulses may arise at sites of axial inhomogeneity,[14,26] and these have also been observed at sites of experimental nerve injury[18] (see also Chapter 18).

A similar situation may occur in the absence of changes in diameter if there are changes in specific membrane properties or in the geometry of the myelin sheath. Thus, for example, conduction block may occur at sites of focal demyelination, even if the denuded axon membrane exhibits normal excitability (that is, has specific membrane properties like those of normal nodal membrane) as a result of inadequate current density in the demyelinated zone.[44] The effect is similar to what electrical engineers call "impedance mismatch." At these sites of conduction failure, computer simulations indicate that conduction may be facilitated by the interposition of internodes reduced in length proximal to the demyelinated zone.[46]

The degree of clinical deficit resulting from axonal nonuniformity will depend on several factors. The first is the severity and type of axonal nonuniformity. As noted above, even small changes in the geometry of the transition zone may affect the transmission properties of the axon. A major goal in nerve repair should be, then, the minimization of non-uniformity along the affected axons. As noted above, sensory and motor fibers may reflect structural pathology in different ways. Methods of nerve repair may therefore have to be matched to fiber type, as well as to the characteristics of the injury. The second factor is the nature of information coding in the axon under consideration. Given a simple frequency code (in which a parameter is coded by the average frequency of impulses), small changes in interspike interval may not distort the neural message. If information is, on the other hand, coded by the temporal patterning of impulses, even small temporal transformations may seriously interfere with reliable transmission of information. Finally, transmission characteristics through a region of low safety factor may be quite sensitive to metabolic factors and temperature.[35] It would be of interest, therefore, to determine whether the functional deficits encountered in peripheral nerve disease vary with body temperature or metabolic status.

MOLECULAR ARCHITECTURE OF THE AXON MEMBRANE

Although outside the scope of structure-function relations in the traditional sense, the organization of the axon membrane is an important determinant of conduction properties and will be briefly discussed. A more detailed account of the organization of the axon membrane can be found in Waxman.[44] Hodgkin[17] predicted that conduction velocity in non-myelinated fibers is dependent on the density of ionic channels in the axon membrane. In nonmyelinated mammalian fibers, the sodium channel density is approximately $110/\mu m^2$. In normal myelinated fibers, on the other hand, the sodium channels appear to be concentrated at the nodes, where channel density is approximately $10,000/\mu m^2$, in contrast to a channel density of less than $25/\mu m^2$ in the axon membrane beneath the myelin sheath in the internodes.[30] This heterogeneity of the axon membrane in myelinated fibers is important following demyelination, as may occur in a number of disorders in-

cluding pressure-induced nerve injury. In these cases, following loss of myelin, current may be shunted through the denuded internodal membrane, where electrical excitability may be so low that conduction failure will occur. There are, however, several lines of evidence that suggest that the axon membrane may be capable of reorganization following demyelination. In the case of *re*myelinated fibers, internode lengths are often reduced[9] and nodes are therefore located at the sites of former internodes. However, since remyelinated fibers often exhibit conduction velocities that are only mildly reduced and are consistent with their decreased internode distances,[7] some of the nodes formed during remyelination (which are located at previous internodal sites) must exhibit spike electrogenesis similar to that at normal nodes. This suggests a reorganization of the axon membrane at the new nodes formed during remyelination. There is also evidence suggesting that, under some conditions, conduction may occur in a continuous manner along *de*myelinated fibers. This suggestion arises in part from clinicopathological studies in multiple sclerosis[50] where demyelinated plaques may be clinically asymptomatic. There have also been recent electrophysiological demonstrations of possible continuous conduction along ventral root fibers demyelinated by exposure to diphtheria toxin[5] and in the amyelinated axons of dystrophic mice.[28] In the case of focally demyelinated axons, computer simulation studies suggest that it is not necessary to have as high a density of sodium channels as at normal nodes in the demyelinated region, but that channel density must be greater than at normal internodes.[46] It is not yet clear whether reorganization of the axon membrane following demyelination involves the production of new ionic channels or the redistribution of existing ones. Nor is it clear how often the prerequisites for conduction along demyelinated axons are met. This area is obviously an important one with respect to nerve injuries since specific membrane characteristics, which will depend on the number and distribution of channels, play an important role in the determination of conduction properties.

CONCLUSIONS

The clinical implications of decreases in conduction velocity will vary depending on the system involved and the mechanisms by which neural information is coded. In some systems, slowing of conduction velocity will clearly be accompanied by a clinical deficit. A striking example is provided by the electromotor system of the electric eel *Electrophorus*. In this system myogenic electrocytes located at varying distances from a command nucleus in the medulla all fire synchronously in response to a signal generated in the command nucleus. Despite the varying conduction distances involved, the conduction times to the various electrocytes are identical. This is accomplished via precise modulation of conduction times along the electromotor axons.[1,43] In a system such as this it would be expected that even small changes in conduction velocity would lead to desynchronization of the discharge and therefore to abnormal function. A common example encountered in the clinical domain is the loss of deep tendon reflexes in patients suffering from polyneuropathies or from nerve injuries. As noted by Gilliatt and Willison,[13] the deep tendon reflexes can be lost in patients with metabolic neuropathies in which conduction velocities are only minimally reduced; in this case even small changes in conduction velocity are sufficient to cause temporal dispersion of impulses in an ensemble of fibers and to interfere with the temporal summation mechanisms underlying normal reflex activity. On the other side of the coin, it should be recalled that in some cases in both the peripheral nervous system[10] and the central nervous system,[15] decreases in conduction velocity may be tolerated without the appearance of clinically manifest abnormalities.

Inability of a fiber to reliably conduct trains of impulses may also, of course, be a cause of significant clinical deficit. Complete conduction block represents the physiological equivalent of absence of connectivity. Intermittent conduction or low-pass filtering would be expected to lead to clinical deficit in systems that are designed to transmit high-frequency impulse trains in a one-to-one manner. Finally, even subtle changes in the patterning of impulses might have functional significance in systems that are finely tuned to the timing of impulses.[40]

The preceding discussion has focused on those aspects of axonal pathophysiology where morphophysiological correlations have been established. As noted in the first paragraph of this chapter, in some cases a clear correlation between structure and function cannot be made. In these instances we may hope that, as the structural analysis of nerve fibers becomes increasingly sophisticated, we may approach a higher degree of correlation between structure and function. In this regard, it seems likely that further advances in ultrastructure and freeze-fracture, membrane biophysics, computer simulations of nerve activity, and clinical electrophysiology will all lead to a better understanding of the structural bases of abnormal function in peripheral nerve injury.

ACKNOWLEDGMENTS

Work in the author's laboratory has been supported in part by grants from the U.S. Veterans Administration, the National Institutes of Health, and the National Multiple Sclerosis Society.

REFERENCES

1. Bennett, M. V. L.: Neural control of electric organs. In Ingle, D, ed.: The central nervous system and fish behavior, Chicago, 1968, University of Chicago Press, p. 147.
2. Berthold, C-H.: Morphology of normal peripheral axons. In Waxman, S. G., ed.: Physiology and pathobiology of axons, New York, 1978, Raven Press, p. 3.
3. Birket-Smith, E., and Krogh, E.: Motor nerve conduction velocity during diphenylhydantoin intoxication, Acta Neurol. Scand. 47:265, 1971.
4. Bishop, G. H., and Smith, J. M.: The sizes of nerve fibers supplying cerebral cortex, Exp. Neurol. 9:483, 1964.
5. Bostock, H., and Sears, T. A.: Continuous conduction in demyelinated mammalian nerve fibres, Nature 263:786, 1976.
6. Boyd, I. A., and Davey, M. R.: Composition of peripheral nerves, Edinburgh, 1968, E. & S. Livingstone.

7. Brill, M. H., et al.: Conduction velocity and spike configuration in myelinated fibres: computed dependence on internode distance, J. Neurol. Neurosurg. Psychiatry **40**:769, 1977.

8. Chung, S. H., Raymond, S. A., and Lettvin, J. Y.: Multiple meaning in single visual units, Brain Behav. Evol. **3**:72, 1970.

9. Dyck, P. J.: Pathological alterations of the peripheral nervous system of man. In Dyck, P. J., Thomas, P. K., and Lambert, E. M., eds.: Peripheral neuropathy, Philadelphia, 1975, W. B. Saunders, Co.

10. Eisen, A. A., Woods, J. F., and Sherwin, A. L.: Peripheral nerve function in long-term therapy with diphenylhydantoin, Neurology **24**:411, 1974.

11. Fleming, L. W., Lenman, J. A. R., and Stewart, W. K.: Effect of magnesium on nerve conduction velocity during regular dialysis treatment, J. Neurol. Neurosurg. Psychiatry **35**:342, 1972.

12. Geren, B. B.: The formation from the Schwann cell surface of myelin in the peripheral nerves of chick embryos, Exp. Cell Res. **7**:558, 1954.

13. Gilliatt, R. W., and Willison, R. G.: Peripheral nerve conduction in diabetic neuropathy, J. Neurol. Neurosurg. Psychiatry **25**:11, 1962.

14. Goldstein, S. S., and Rall, W.: Changes of action potential shape and velocity for changing core conductor geometry, Biophys. J. **14**:731, 1974.

15. Halliday, A. M., McDonald, W. I., and Mushin, J.: Visual evoked response in diagnosis of multiple sclerosis, Br. Med. J. **4**:661, 1973.

16. Hodgkin, A. L.: The conduction of the nerve impulse, Springfield, Ill., 1964, Charles C Thomas, Publisher.

17. Hodgkin, A. L.: The optimum density of sodium channels in an unmyelinated nerve, Philos. Trans. R. Soc. Lond. **270**:297, 1975.

18. Howe, J. F., Calvin, W. H., and Loeser, J. D.: Impulses reflected from dorsal root ganglia and from focal nerve injuries, Brain Res. **116**:139, 1976.

19. Huxley, A. F., and Stämpfli, R.: Evidence for saltatory conduction in peripheral myelinated nerve fibres, J. Physiol. **108**:315, 1949.

20. Joyner, R. W.: Temperature affects on neuronal elements, Fed. Proc. In press.

21. Koles, Z. J., and Rasminsky, M.: A computer simulation of conduction in demyelinated nerve fibres, J. Physiol. **227**:351, 1972.

22. Moore, J. W., et al.: Simulations of conduction in uniform myelinated fibers. Relative sensitivity to changes in nodal and internodal parameters, Biophys. J. **21**:147, 1978.

23. Morgan-Hughes, J. A.: Experimental diphtheritic neuropathy: a pathological and electrophysiological study, J. Neurol. Sci. **7**:157, 1968.

24. Paintal, A. S.: A comparison of the nerve impulses of mammalian non-medullated nerve fibres with those of the smallest diameter medullated fibres, J. Physiol. Lond. **193**:623, 1967.

25. Parnas, I., Hochstein, S., and Parnas, H.: Theoretical analysis of parameters leading to frequency modulation along an inhomogeneous axon, J. Neurophysiol. **39**:909, 1976.

26. Ramón, F., Joyner, R. W., and Moore, J. W.: Propagation of action potentials in inhomogeneous axon regions, Fed. Proc. **34**:1357, 1975.

27. Rasminsky, M.: The effects of temperature on conduction in demyelinated single nerve fibers, Arch. Neurol. **28**:287, 1973.

28. Rasminsky, M., et al.: Conduction of nervous impulses in spinal roots and peripheral nerves of dystrophic mice, Brain Res. **143**:71, 1978.

29. Raymond, S. A., and Lettvin, J. Y.: Aftereffects of activity in peripheral axons as a clue to nervous coding. In Waxman, S. G., ed.: Physiology and pathobiology of axons, New York, 1978, Raven Press, p. 203.

30. Ritchie, J. M., and Rogart, R. B.: The density of sodium channels in mammalian myelinated fibers and the nature of the axonal membrane under the myelin sheath, Proc. Natl. Acad. Sci. U.S.A. **74**:211, 1977.

31. Ritchie, J. M., Rogart, R. B., and Strichartz, G.: A new method for labelling saxitoxin and its binding to non-myelinated fibres of the rabbit vagus, lobster walking leg and garfish olfactory nerves, J. Physiol. **261**:477, 1976.

32. Robertson, J. C.: The molecular structure and contact relationships of cell membranes, Prog. Biophys. **10**:343, 1960.

33. Rushton, W. A. H.: A theory of the effects of fibre size in medullated nerve, J. Physiol. **115**:101, 1951.

34. Sanders, F. K., and Whitteridge, D.: Conduction velocity and myelin thickness in regenerating nerve fibres, J. Physiol. **105**:152, 1946.

35. Schauf, C. L., and Davis, F. A.: Impulse conduction in multiple sclerosis: a theoretical basis for modification by temperature and pharmacological agents, J. Neurol. Neurosurg. Psychiatry **37**:152, 1974.

36. Sharma, A. K., and Thomas, P. K.: Peripheral nerve structure and function in experimental diabetes, J. Neurol. Sci. **25**:1, 1974.

37. Smith, R. S., and Koles, Z. J.: Myelinated nerve fibers—computed effect of myelin thickness on conduction velocity, Am. J. Physiol. **219**:1256, 1970.

38. Spira, M. E., Yarom, Y., and Parnas, I.: Modulation of spike frequency by regions of special axonal geometry and by synaptic inputs, J. Neurophysiol. **39**:882, 1976.

39. Sunderland, S.: Nerves and nerve injuries, Edinburgh, 1968, E. & S. Livingstone, Ltd.

40. Swadlow, H. A., and Waxman, S. G.: Observations on impulse conduction along central axons, Proc. Natl. Acad. Sci. U.S.A. **72**:5156, 1975.

41. Swadlow, H. A., and Waxman, S. G.: Variations in conduction velocity and excitability following single and multiple impulses of visual callosal axons in the rabbit, Exp. Neurol. **53**:128, 1976.

42. Waxman, S. G.: Closely spaced nodes of Ranvier in the teleost brain, Nature **227**:283, 1970.

43. Waxman, S. G.: Integrative properties and design principles of axons, Int. Rev. Neurobiol. **18:**1, 1975.

44. Waxman, S. G.: Conduction in myelinated, un-myelinated, and demyelinated fibers, Arch. Neurol. **34:**585, 1977.

45. Waxman, S. G., and Bennett, M. V. L.: Relative conduction velocities of small myelinated and non-myelinated fibres in the central nervous system, Nature [New Biol.] **238:**217, 1972.

46. Waxman, S. G., and Brill, M. H.: Conduction through demyelinated plaques in multiple sclerosis: computer simulations of facilitation by short inter-nodes, J. Neurol. Neurosurg. Psychiatry **41:**408, 1978.

47. Waxman, S. G., and Swadlow, H. A.: The conduc-tion properties of axons in central white matter, Prog. Neurobiol. **8:**297, 1977.

48. Waxman, S. G., Pappas, G. D., and Bennett, M. V. L.: Morphological correlates of functional dif-ferentiation of nodes of Ranvier along single fibers in the neurogenic electric organ of the knife fish Sternarchus, J. Cell Biol. **53:**210, 1972.

49. Westerfield, M., Joyner, R. W., and Moore, J. W.: Temperature-sensitive conduction failure at axon branch points, J. Neurophysiol. **41:**1, 1978.

50. Wisniewski, H., Oppenheimer, D., and McDonald, W. I.: Relation between myelination and function in MS and EAE, J. Neuropathol. Exp. Neurol. **35:**327, 1976.

DISCUSSION

McCarroll: Distal regrown axons do not re-myelinate completely after nerve suture. What does this do to alter function in relation to that structure?

Waxman: That is a difficult question. I think all we can do is speculate a bit. Certainly, fibers that are nonmyelinated can conduct, so these sprouts may conduct. But I expect that they may show a distortion in terms of temporal patterning of the impulses of the sort that Dr. Jewett (in this volume) and others have described. The conduction properties of an axon are not fixed in time. They vary with the history of previous activities in that axon, and they vary in the following way. One sees the spike. That is followed by the refractory period. The refractory period is followed by a phase that is called the supernormal period, which in turn is followed by a subnormal period. The supernormal period is a period of increased conduction velocity and increased excitability. The subnormal period is a period of decreased excitability and decreased conduction velocity. The important point is this: if you plot the duration of the refractory period vs. axon diameter, there is a sharp inverse relationship. There is a similar inverse relationship between supernormal period duration and diameter and probably a similar relationship in the subnormal phase. If so, you would see much more depression after a spike in a small axon than in a large axon. I would expect that many of these small sprouts might therefore block at physiological frequencies, whereas the parent axon might not.

McCarroll: Is the fact that the sensory fiber is going to be a small myelinated one trying to fire its big component in the proximal stump going to make it a different situation from the motor fiber where a large nor-mally myelinated proximal stump is trying to fire a small myelinated distal fiber?

Waxman: This brings us into the area of variations in axonal caliber and their significance. Axons undulate, so that as one moves longitudinally along the course of a fiber there can be variations in caliber. Many of these variations are of little physiological significance; others are of significance. The most drastic type of variation you could get is that of a step function going from a small region to a big region. You probably have to have a three to six-fold difference in diameter before you get conduction failure for a single spike. What diameter changes will cause filtering and drop out every other spike or block trains of impulses I do not know. We also must remember that while some neural systems may code information by the fine temporal patterning of impulses, often systems may use a simple frequency code. These two types of systems will respond differently to pathological changes in impulse patterning.

Editor: It is conceivable that a regenerated axon may have a smaller diameter distal to a nerve repair. Since in this case an action potential in a sensory neuron would be traveling from a smaller diameter to a larger diameter, there could be full conduction block or at least trains block. This might be one of the reasons that sensory return in the forearm and hand is a greater problem than motor function. Other reasons include: proximal muscle groups that have shorter reinnervation paths, branching at muscle to substitute for loss of nerve fibers, and lesser standards of performance on the motor side compared with the sensory side from the clinical point of view.

Editor: The functional consequences of multiple branches* need to be considered in the light of branching following nerve repair. There may well be collisions of action potentials and altered branch-point excitability that could change the patterns of sensory inputs as well as restrict motor fiber maximum frequencies.

*Waxman, S. G.: Brain Res. **47:**269, 1972.

20

Functional blockade of impulse trains caused by acute nerve compression

Don L. Jewett

Function in an injured nerve is completely lost if axonal conduction cannot occur. Such is the case in nerve injuries of the second degree or higher in Sunderland's classification (see also Chapter 2).[13] With a first degree injury axonal conduction can occur despite local demyelination (see also Chapters 4 and 18). The purpose of this chapter is to indicate the possibility of even milder forms of injury that can affect nerve function without a histological change—possibly the basis for a "zero degree" form of injury. The effects on axonal function to be described here could occur as the result of relatively mild injury, or they could be the consequence of inadequate healing (see "Discussion" at the end of this chapter).

It is important to realize that rapid, repetitive action potentials place greater physiological demands on axons than does the conduction of a single action potential. The corollary of this principle is that mildly impaired axonal function is reflected in the inability of the axon to transmit action potentials closely spaced in time: the greater the impairment, the less the ability to conduct impulses at high frequencies. In experimental animals it is easiest to apply repetitive trains of impulses (with differing intratrain frequencies) as a test of an impairment of axonal conduction.

The inability of impaired axons to transmit trains of impulses has been clearly documented in the case of impairment caused by localized cooling.[5,10] These experiments can form a model of the impaired axon

under carefully controlled conditions. The analogy to nerve injury is reasonable since at sufficiently low temperatures complete blockage of axonal conduction occurs in both myelinated[10] and unmyelinated[5] fibers. Fig. 20-1 shows the type of data that can be obtained when a localized area of nerve is gradually cooled. This figure, taken from Franz and Iggo,[5] shows action potentials recorded from a single unmyelinated fiber. As a localized area between the stimulating and recording electrodes is cooled, the ability of the axon to conduct trains of impulses is impaired. The figure has been rearranged to show the single unit responses with increasing intratrain frequency from left to right and with decreasing temperature from top to bottom. As can be seen in Fig. 20-1, at normal temperature the axon is able to conduct all impulses in the trains at all frequencies up to the highest shown, 180 Hz. As the nerve is cooled, the axon loses its ability to transmit at higher frequencies first, while lower frequency trains are unaffected. However, as axonal conduction is further impaired by the cold, even the lower train frequencies are affected.

These results, as so far described, are readily intuited. What is surprising is the manner in which the trains of impulses are affected. It is to be noted that at the extreme, before complete axonal block, only the first impulse of the train traverses the cold region, while the rest of the impulses in the train are blocked. At lesser degrees of impairment the first action potential is always conducted;

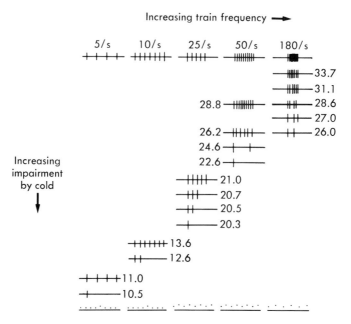

Fig. 20-1. Blocking pattern within trains of impulses in nonmyelinated axon (conduction velocity 0.9 m/sec) stimulated at different frequencies, which are indicated above each column. Control records with nerve at 37° C are shown in top row; nerve temperatures for other records are indicated at start of each trace. Repetitious traces have been omitted. Major time marks: 100 ms. (Adapted from Franz, D. N., and Iggo, A.: J. Physiol. (Lond.) **99**:319, 1968.)

then there can be varying amounts of block of the remaining portion of the train (Fig. 20-1). Paintal[10] has offered an explanation for this interesting behavior. Blockade of high frequencies usually would be thought to be due to an increased refractory period. However, since this can only block every other impulse or every third impulse (the so-called alternating block), it could not explain how only the first action potential in a train traverses a region (which will be called "trains block"). The most probable explanation[10] is that the most impaired node in the cool region fires an action potential with a significantly lower height when the action potentials are sufficiently close together. At this decreased height there is insufficient current to activate the next node, yet the impaired node continues to follow the high frequency with similar, small, abortive spikes. Thus, according to this explanation, it is paradoxical that there must be a firing, impaired node in order to block conduction of the latter part of the train of impulses.

Whatever the explanation, it is certainly clear that a blockage of nerve impulse trains (that is, "trains" block) can occur. Such behavior would have an extreme effect on the functioning of either sensory or motor axons and can account for some of the phenomena seen with first degree injuries.

The purpose of this chapter is to show that a blockade of nerve impulse trains can also occur as a result of impaired conduction from acute compression of the nerve. The clinical implications of this result will be described.

METHODS

Cats were anesthetized with intraperitoneal pentobarbital. A multilevel lumbar laminectomy provided intradural access to the lumbar dorsal rootlets. In the leg on either the posterior tibial or peroneal nerve, two sets of stimulating electrodes and a compression device were placed with the spacings shown in Fig. 20-2. All were kept under the surface of a mineral oil pool held by skin flaps.

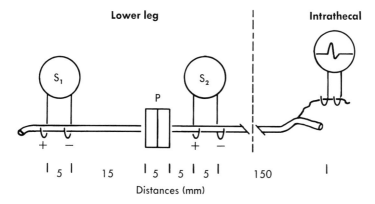

Fig. 20-2. Diagram of experimental arrangement, showing relationship of stimulating and recording electrodes. *P*, Balloon compression device, 5 mm long. S_1, Distal stimulating electrodes. Action potentials from here must conduct through compressed region. S_2, Proximal (control) stimulating electrodes.

Single units in the region of the lumbar laminectomy were hand-dissected under a binocular microscope beneath a mineral oil pool. All electrodes were Ag-AgCl. All single units were identified by their sharp threshold to stimulation (usually less than 0.1 volt) and their uniform spike height (not varying more than the baseline noise). The compression device was a plastic adapter fitted over the balloon of a urinary catheter. The amount of pressure was not measured but could be inferred physiologically (see "Results").

The arrangement of electrodes (Fig. 20-2) permitted stimulation of the axon of the single unit both proximal and distal to the region of compression, so that control recordings from the proximal electrodes could be obtained. Recordings were taken only from large myelinated fibers conducting between 30 and 50 m/sec. The temperature in the oil baths was not controlled, so slowing of conduction velocity owing to lowered temperature undoubtedly occurred.

RESULTS

After each single unit was identified by a sharp threshold to increasing stimulus strength, the stimulus was set to at least $1\frac{1}{2}$ times the threshold value. Stimulation at the proximal electrode determined the maximum frequency that could be transmitted along the axon up to and including any damaged region at the recording electrode. After application of pressure, effects on trains of impulses from the distal electrode were not immediately apparent but were detected within 10 to 30 minutes. In no case did full conduction block occur, despite periods of compression up to 2 hours; thus the pressures applied to the nerve were presumably less than the 50 to 300 mm Hg pressure range over which conduction block has been found to occur in mammalian nerves.[2-4]

The effect of compression was to decrease the ability of the axon to conduct high-frequency impulse trains. For example, in Fig. 20-3 there is a conducted action potential for each distal stimulus at rates up to 135 Hz. At a frequency of 165 Hz, some impulses after the fourth are missing from the train. At 295 Hz only the first and third impulses in the train traverse the compressed region, and at 360 Hz only the first impulse in the train is conducted. However, at that time the first 12 impulses at 360 Hz were conducted over the nerve proximal to the compression. The difference between the proximal and distal stimulations indicates the degree of conduction impairment caused by compression between the pairs of stimulating electrodes. The inability to transmit all the proximal stimuli is probably related to mechanical injury near the recording electrodes owing to the nerve splitting necessary to record the single unit.

Fig. 20-3 also demonstrates that there can be a mixture of both trains block and alternating block at some train frequencies, as shown in the second, third, and fourth tracings from the top.

The development of the impulse blockade during continuous application of pressure is shown in Fig. 20-4. After only 3 minutes of pressure, the stimulation at the distal electrodes could transmit at least nine consecutive impulses at 340 Hz. After 22 minutes of pressure only four impulses were transmitted before alternating block occurred (spike height is down as a result of changed conditions at the recording electrodes). However, at nearly the same time (third tracing) the compressed axon was still capable of trans-

mitting each impulse at 260 Hz. However, after another 16 minutes the axon could not transmit all impulses at 260 Hz and after yet another 3 minutes shows complete trains block (except for the first impulse of the train) at 340 Hz (bottom tracing). Thus acute compression gradually impairs the ability of the axon to conduct trains of impulses: the longer the compression, the lower the frequency of impulses that still can be transmitted through the region without dropout.

After prolonged compression, recovery was either slow or not observed during the time the single units were recorded. Fig. 20-3 shows the results 1 hour after cessation of $1\frac{1}{2}$ hours of compression. With shorter durations of pressure, recovery of function could be observed (Fig. 20-5). In Fig. 20-5 the small spikes are those of a stimulated axon, while the large spikes are those of a

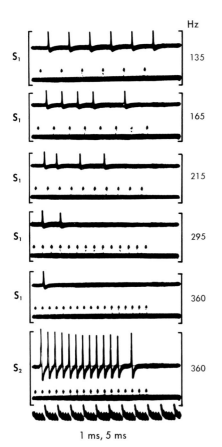

Fig. 20-3. Single unit recordings taken 1.5 hours after 1 hour of compression at differing train stimulus rates as indicated on right of each tracing. In each recording lower trace shows pattern and rate of stimulus presentation, while upper trace shows single unit response. Note that as train rate is increased, fewer impulses are transmitted through compressed region from S_1 stimulating electrodes; both trains block and alternate block occur; first action potential is always transmitted at this level of compression. Control stimulation at S_2 (bottom tracing) shows ability to follow 360 Hz much in excess of that which can traverse compressed region from S_1 (second tracing from bottom).

1 ms, 5 ms

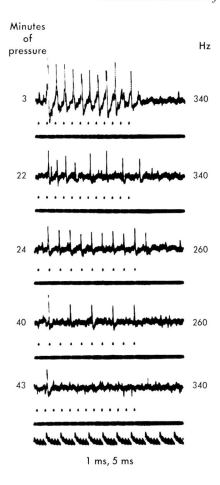

Minutes
of
pressure

Hz

1 ms, 5 ms

Fig. 20-4. Development of blockade during application of continuous compression, as shown by times to left of tracings. Note that top and bottom traces show stimulation at same frequency, differing only by amount of time nerve is compressed; some decrease in action potential heights occurs during sequence as a result of changes at recording electrodes, but control recording from S_2 taken after last tracing showed following at greater than 300 Hz.

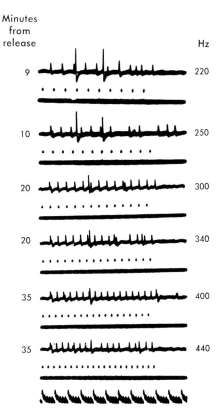

Minutes
from
release

Hz

1 ms, 5 ms

Fig. 20-5. Recovery of blockade after short (11 min) compression. Time after release of compression is shown on left, train frequency on right. Note that large single unit was firing spontaneously, and stimulated unit has smaller spike. At each time highest frequency at which all impulses conduct through compressed region is shown, together with higher frequency at which blockade occurs in latter part of impulse train.

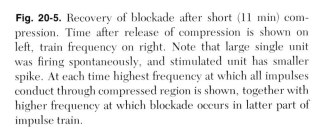

spontaneously firing, unstimulated unit in the same nerve twig. It can be seen in Fig. 20-5 that about 10 minutes after release of 11 minutes of pressure the unit could transmit at about 220 Hz but had some interference with trains of impulses at rates above 250 Hz. Twenty minutes after release the axon could transmit at 300 Hz but not at 340 Hz. At 35 minutes it could transmit at 400 Hz but not at 440 Hz.

When there was interference with trains of impulses, the pattern of those impulses of the train that were conducted was not constant. As shown in Fig. 20-6, the pattern of the single impaired train is not consistent when multiple sweeps are overlaid. Thus, for similar sensory inputs, there may be different patterns transmitted to the central nervous system. Furthermore, if computer averaging techniques are used when detecting skin surface potentials, the dropouts may occur dispersed throughout the train.

Fast oscilloscope sweeps (not shown) were analyzed for comparison between the latency of the action potentials before and after compression. There was a reduction in conduction velocity from about 35 to 50 m/sec to less than 10 m/sec in the compressed region if one ascribes all slowing to the 5 mm length of the compression device. This implies that com-

pound action potentials may have increased temporal dispersion, and hence lowered heights, even when no impulses are blocked. To correct for this it would be necessary to record the area under the monophasic action potential (see Chapter 15).

DISCUSSION

The mechanism of conduction impairment caused by acute compression in these experiments is unknown. Hemostasis undoubtedly occurred, but by the indirect evidence noted in the results, arterial blockage is less likely to have occurred. Intussusception may have occurred, but in those cases where compression was for a short time and recovery occurred, one would have to postulate a reversible intussusception (see Chapter 4). Certainly there was not enough time for demyelination to occur, although prolonged compression might ultimately give such a histological picture (assuming that recovery does not occur within a few hours). The 10- to 30-minute period needed to affect conduction in the compressed region would be compatible with physical changes in axonal size in the compressed region owing to slow movement of the viscous axoplasm to noncompressed regions of the axon. Such diameter change might account for the blockades seen since

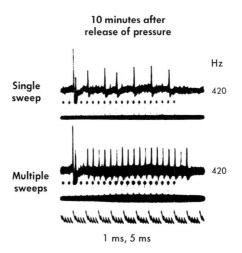

Fig. 20-6. Comparison of blockade pattern of single train with overlapped multiple stimulations. Note that except for period just after first impulse pattern of activity is variable but still time-locked to stimuli from S_I.

smaller diameter fibers are less able to transmit high frequencies of nerve impulses than larger fibers.[5,8-10] If this were the mechanism, then when an axon tapers distal to a nerve repair or has multiple branches that are smaller than the main axon, centrifugal conduction would be affected, with possible trains block at the region of axonal narrowing (see Chapter 9). Irrespective of the mechanism of trains block that results from acute compression, it seems reasonable to assume that impaired axonal conduction from a variety of different mechanisms can lead to the same functional result of dropout or complete block of trains of nerve impulses.

There are a number of clinical implications of these findings. The possible effects on tapered nerve fibers arising from repaired nerves has already been mentioned. In the anterior compartment syndrome increased pressure may lead to progressive loss of motor power in the following sequence: (1) muscle weakness, (2) a flick of contraction at the start of each voluntary effort, and finally (3) paralysis of the involved muscle. One can hypothesize that if the loss is due to a pressure block on the axon, then the weakness corresponds to a time when action potentials are dropping out of the continuous barrage of impulses being generated by the CNS; the flick of contraction may represent blockade of impulse trains with only the first few impulses in a train able to traverse the compressed region; and the paralysis indicates a complete conduction block.

Many of the characteristics of first degree lesions (also termed "neurapraxia"[11]) are consistent with the idea of blockade of impulse trains. Momentary compression can be one of the causes of neurapraxia.[11] The period of functional loss can be variable. It is much shorter than in more severe forms of nerve injury. There may be no significant demyelination, just as we have postulated for the acute compressions reported here. If an injured nerve has impaired conduction that would lead to either trains block or alternating block, then we would expect that the axons normally having the fastest firing rates might be those that are most affected,

namely, motor nerves, proprioceptive fibers, and those serving transient touch. These are the modalities most often involved in neurapraxia. Slower firing, smaller fibers, such as autonomic axons, would be less affected, as is also the case in neurapraxia. (This explanation presumes that there is a differential effect on larger fibers, although this effect has not been experimentally verified.) It should be noted that in the clinical evaluation of touch one often uses a pin to detect sensation. This could stimulate only a few action potentials, the first of which could be transmitted through a region that would block a train of impulses. On the other hand, rapid impulse trains, such as those that occur when attempting maximal muscle contractions, would be blocked; hence there would be a more severe functional loss in a motor fiber than in a sensory fiber of similar diameter. Thus this might be the explanation for the clinical observation that motor function is affected more than sensory function. Another possibility is that trains block may occur where there was a continuous barrage of activity associated with muscle stretch receptors; this in turn might change spinal cord excitability at an unconscious level and thus affect the motor power in this manner.

With chronic compression, such as might occur with localized inflammatory response around an injury, it is possible that large fibers may be selectively affected mechanically, as compared with smaller fibers.[12]

Compound action potentials to trains of stimuli have been recorded in normal human median nerves[1] and ulnar nerves.[7,14] In recordings in the carpal tunnel syndrome, trains of impulses have been shown to be a more sensitive objective measure than the EMG or sensory conduction studies.[6] Compound action potential recordings such as these demonstrate the usefulness of trains of impulses in the analysis of human nerve function but must be interpreted with care, since changes in the height of the compound action potential can be due to a number of different causes as follows: (1) a change in the height of the individual action potentials in the later part of the train (see bottom trace of Fig.

20-3), (2) a temporal dispersion of the action potentials either by decreased conduction in the impaired region or by differential effects on conduction related to differing axonal size,[12] or (3) the change in the number of axons contributing action potentials to the compound potential. Thus small changes in the height of the compound action potential may be due to either of the first two mechanisms. However, the changes observed in the reference literature just cited are sufficiently great to indicate that some dropout of action potentials must be occurring under the conditions observed.

Many variables remain to be investigated, such as the interaction between the amount and duration of compression, the effect of the length of axon compressed, and the potentiating effects of factors like inflammation, anoxia, and drugs. However, it seems reasonably safe to prognosticate that trains of impulses are likely to be a better measure of impaired conduction than complete axonal block in milder forms of nerve injury. Similarly, trains of impulses may be important in evaluating the time course of functional recovery as regrowing axons mature and enlarge. Permanent impairment of train conduction may still result after nerve repair if the distal axons do not recover their full diameters.

REFERENCES

1. Buchthal, F., and Rosenfalck, A.: Evoked action potentials and conduction velocity in human sensory nerves, Brain Res. **3:**1, 1966.
2. Causey, G.: The effect of pressure on nerve fibers, J. Anat. **82:**262, 1948.
3. Causey, G., and Palmer, E.: The effect of pressure on nerve conduction and nerve-fiber size, J. Physiol. (Lond) **109:**220, 1949.
4. Denny-Brown, D., and Brenner, C.: Paralysis of nerve induced by direct pressure and by tourniquet, Arch. Neurol. Psychiatry **51:**1, 1944.
5. Franz, D. N., and Iggo, A.: Conduction failure in myelinated and non-myelinated axons at low temperatures, J. Physiol. (Lond) **199:**319, 1968.
6. Lehmann, H. J., and Tackmann, W.: Neurographic analysis of trains of frequent electric stimuli in the diagnosis of peripheral nerve diseases: investigations in the carpal tunnel syndrome, Eur. Neurol. **12:**293, 1974.
7. Lowitzsch, K., and Hopf, H. C.: Refraktärperiode and Übermittlung frequenter Reizserien im gemischten peripheren Nerven des Menschen, J. Neurol. Sci. **17:**255, 1972.
8. Paintal, A. S.: The influence of diameter of medullated nerve fibers of cats on the rising and falling phases of the spike and its recovery, J. Physiol. (Lond) **184:**791, 1966.
9. Paintal, A. S.: A comparison of the nerve impulses of mammalian non-medullated nerve fibres with those of the smallest diameter medullated fibres, J. Physiol. (Lond) **193:**523, 1967.
10. Paintal, A. S.: Conduction in mammalian nerve fibres. In Desmedt, J. E., ed.: New developments in electromyography and clinical neurophysiology, vol. 2, Basel, 1973, Karger, p. 19.
11. Seddon, H.: Surgical disorders of the peripheral nerves, Edinburgh, 1975, Chruchill Livingstone.
12. Strain, R. E., Jr., and Olson, W. H.: Selective damage of large diameter peripheral nerve fibers by compression: an application of Laplace's law, Exp. Neurol. **47:**68, 1975.
13. Sunderland, S., Sir: Nerves and nerve injuries, ed 2, Edinburgh, 1978, Churchill Livingstone.
14. Tackmann, W., Ullerich, D., and Lehmann, H. J.: Transmission of frequent impulse series in human sensory nerve fibres, Eur. Neurol. **12:**261, 1974.

DISCUSSION

W. Newmar (San Francisco): In the carpal tunnel syndrome, we see sensory dropout before motor dropout. How do we explain this?

Jewett: First of all clinical tests of both sensation and motor power are relatively coarse, so that there may be physiological impairment of maximum performance before clinical manifestations are apparent. The degree of impairment will relate to the diameters of the axons as well as the firing frequencies, so it is conceivable that either motor dropout or sensory dropout could be affected first. Finally, there is no single unit data on chronic compression comparable to what I showed with respect to acute compression. All the chronic data are based on compound potentials. Perhaps the relationship of affected firing frequency and diameter may be different in the chronic case, although there is no question that in chronic compression there is decreased function.

Newmar: With a compartment syndrome, isn't it a good possibility that it is the muscle that is affected before the nerve?

Jewett: I have no data on muscle action potentials. It would be of considerable interest to see if muscle were affected as well. In the compartment syndrome the muscle would be under uniform pressure throughout its length. The experiments in which nerves were placed in hyperbaric chambers indicate that high pressure can be tolerated if the pressure is uniformly distributed. As Dr. Waxman has indicated in this volume, it is the transition areas in nerve where conduction failure is likely. Therefore in compartment syndromes one would suspect the region of nerve as it entered the high-pressure region as being the most susceptible. This is theoretical, of course, and needs experimental verification.

Roger Crumly (San Francisco): In Bell's palsy, it has been shown that patients that have lower function of the involved submaxillary gland and lacrimal gland tend to have poorer results in regard to regeneration. Yet we have been shown by Dr. Sunderland that the facial nerve is a monofunicular nerve throughout the temporal bone, so that if this is a compressive lesion, why are these smaller nerves prognostic indicators? Dr. Jewett's data suggest that the large motor fibers going to the facial muscles should be the most sensitive to compression. Are the poorer results evidence that there is an increased pressure in those patients that have secretomotor nerve involvement?

Jewett: The presence of a palsy implies complete conduction block, a first degree lesion. I agree that smaller fiber involvement may well indicate the severity of the compressive lesion. This is reasonable since large fibers are compressed proportionally more than small fibers.

Sunderland: The facial nerve in Bell's palsy is actually analogous to the median nerve in the carpal tunnel syndrome, hence we must consider it a conduction block injury. Clearly we are beginning to broaden our classification and understanding of conduction block lesions. There are many factors that we do not yet understand about them. I wish to emphasize the importance of an adequate blood supply. The nodes must be oxygen sensitive, and impairment of blood supply must clearly have significant effects on conduction properties.

Ochoa: On the use of the term "neurapraxia," I quite agree with Sir Sidney that we had better drop it because it is confusing. Neurapraxia has been used interchangeably to express two totally different concepts. One is the immediately reversible block that is ischemic, and the other one is

207

a prolonged demyelinating block. Now what are we going to do with the term? We must drop it because it is confusing, but we have to replace it with something else, and I would suggest that we expand the nerve injury classification in order to accomodate the main concept of neurapraxia, which is primarily a myelin and a Schwann cell lesion. I would suggest that we incorporate, in agreement with Dr. Jewett, a "zero degree" classification to bring in the demyelinating block. We probably even need a "zero-zero degree" to avoid the confusion of the demyelinating block with the purely ischemic block.

Sunderland: I think that is most helpful and certainly in conduction block, we now need subgrades of a first degree lesion.

Editor: Readers may also find the following reference of interest. Smith, D. O., and Hatt, H.: Axon conduction block in a region of dense connective tissue in crayfish, J. Neurophysiol. **39:**794, 1976.

21

Clinical usefulness of EMG and nerve conduction tests in nerve injury and repair

Kenneth C. Archibald

Clinical electromyography, using appropriate audio and visual instrumentation, can be extremely helpful in depicting the changes that occur in denervated muscles and during progressive regeneration following nerve injury and repair. A small (25 to 27 gauge) monopolar or coaxial (bipolar) needle electrode is inserted into the muscle belly for pickup of electrical activity. After a relative period of electrical silence for about 5 to 7 days following injury, small spontaneously occurring potentials called fibrillations (Fig. 21-1, A) begin appearing. In a completely severed nerve these usually become abundant and continuously active from 10 days to 2 weeks onward in the muscles supplied by that nerve. In addition, small, predominantly monophasic, potentials called positive sharp waves (Fig. 21-1, B) may appear with the fibrillations, usually briefly following needle insertion or movement. Obviously no voluntary motor unit potentials are obtainable from completely denervated muscles, nor can any response be elicited to stimulation of the nerve above the site of injury, although stimulation below the injury would continue to produce a gradually diminishing response for about 4 to 5 days with complete loss of response after that time. The full manifestations of electrical RD (reaction of degeneration) should be present by 3 weeks following injury. By that time, a fully severed nerve would not respond to electrical stimulation either above or below the injury site, and de-

nervated muscles would produce frequent (4+) fibrillation potentials electromyographically.

Following nerve repair and subsequent nerve regeneration down to the muscle, a few low-amplitude, short-duration, often highly polyphasic motor unit potentials appear during attempted voluntary muscle contraction (Fig. 21-2), usually preceding palpable muscle contraction by several months. As reinnervation continues, progressively larger (higher amplitude, longer duration) polyphasic as well as bi- and triphasic motor units appear, with a progressive decrease in the number of fibrillation potentials and positive sharp waves noted at rest. Although regeneration can continue sometimes for more than 4 or 5 years, a relative plateau is usually reached within 2 to 3 years. However, fibrillation potentials may occasionally linger for many years. Also the percentage of polyphasic motor units may remain elevated even with apparent full clinical recovery. Conduction down the nerve gradually improves with recovery, with gradual increase in the amplitude of response to nerve stimulation as well as in the speed of conduction.

In practice, nerve injuries, of course, vary considerably from complete nerve division to a relatively minor compression or stretch type of injury. Rodriquez and Oester[4] have classified the electrical abnormalities into mild, moderate, and severe physiological blocks, partial and complete axonal degener-

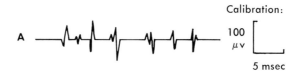

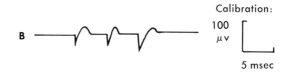

Fig. 21-1. Spontaneously occurring potentials in denervated muscle. **A,** Fibrillation potentials. **B,** Positive sharp waves.

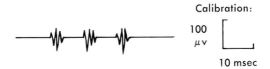

Fig. 21-2. Small, polyphasic, voluntary motor unit potentials in early reinnervation.

ation, and nerve trunk severance; they attempt to correlate electrical function with five pathological classifications of nerve injury described by Sunderland[6] and three by Seddon[5]. In addition to the relative presence of fibrillation potentials as correlated with decreased or absent motor units during voluntary contraction, responses to electrical stimulation are utilized. In reality, however, it may be extremely difficult to grade or evaluate such differences. In a compressive or stretch type of injury, electromyography can be helpful in localizing the area of involvement to those muscles supplied by the injured nerve, although possible anomalous innervation may complicate the picture. Briefly, in a physiological block (neurapraxia), electromyography would show very rare fibrillation potentials or none, whereas with axonal degeneration (axonotmesis) more frequent fibrillation potentials are readily noted in almost all samplings. Serial chronaxy determinations may supplement EMG findings in appraising injury and recovery,

with a fall in chronaxy as reinnervation progresses.

Nerve conduction time measurements can be helpful in localization as well as determining degree of involvement. Nerve conduction velocities between two points of stimulation can be determined in meters per second when the distance between them is divided by the differences in conduction times measured in milliseconds to a peripheral innervated muscle. The most accessible nerves for clinical study have classically been the median and ulnar nerves in the upper extremities and the peroneal and posterior tibial nerves in the lower extremities. For example, delays in ulnar conduction across the elbow may be indicated by a significantly slower velocity from above than from below the elbow to the wrist; delays in median motor and/or sensory nerve conduction times across the wrist may localize a median nerve compression at this point as in carpal tunnel syndrome. In the leg, peroneal nerve conduction delay across the head of the fibula or posterior tibial conduction delay at the ankle may localize compression at such a site. Conduction times can also be determined for the suprascapular, axillary, and musculocutaneous nerves, with stimulation from Erb's point to the supraspinatus, infraspinatus, deltoid, and biceps muscles, respectively; also facial, radial, femoral, and sural nerves can be studied. Techniques with some of the latter nerves vary and need further standardization. Also, sources of error in technique of electrode placement and stimulation as well as measurement must be reduced to a minimum in order to avoid misinterpretation. Such sources and some of their remedies are well described by Goodgold and Eberstein.[2] Comparison with the contralateral side may be helpful in this regard, particularly in a borderline situation, or where a coexisting metabolic neuropathy is suspected, inasmuch as there is some variation in the accepted normal limits, especially in the less frequently studied nerves. Also, one must always be cognizant of such anomalies as the Martin-Gruber median-ulnar anastomosis when axons descending in the median nerve cross through the forearm to join the ulnar nerve, ultimately innervating intrinsic hand muscles; in such a situation stimulation of the median nerve at the elbow may evoke a response in the first dorsal interosseous and/or abductor digiti quinti, whereas stimulation of the median nerve at the wrist will not.[3]

Detailed discussion of the potential sites and causes of peripheral nerve entrapment, however, is beyond the scope of this volume; a recently published review of this subject included a description of electrodiagnostic techniques helpful in their evaluation.[1]

SUMMARY

In summary, EMG and nerve conduction testing can be extremely useful adjuncts in the evaluation of nerve injury and repair, as long as such studies are performed and interpreted carefully and appropriately. The timing and frequency of repeat studies should be aimed at obtaining maximum pertinent information, depending on the clinical course of recovery or lack thereof, or if surgical intervention is contemplated. It should be emphasized that an accurate baseline for future comparison cannot be established until 3 weeks after injury although earlier electrical studies may be useful if clinically warranted. Most well-motivated patients accept EMG and nerve conduction testing with stoicism and resignation when the procedures are described concisely before and during an efficient, yet thorough, examination performed by a competently trained and experienced physician-electromyographer with a practical clinical background and understanding of neuromuscular function and dysfunction.

REFERENCES

1. Cracchiolo, A., III, et al.: Peripheral nerve entrapments. Interdepartmental Clinical Case Conference, University of California, Los Angeles (Specialty Conference), West. J. Med. **127**:299, 1977.
2. Goodgold, J., and Eberstein, A.: Motor and sensory nerve conduction measurements. In Electrodiagnosis of neuromuscular diseases, Baltimore, 1972, The Williams & Wilkins Co., Chap. 7.
3. Gutman, L.: Important anomalous innervations of the extremities, American Association of Electromyography and Electrodiagnosis, Minimonograph No. 2, 1976.
4. Rodriquez, A. A., and Oester, Y. T.: Fundamentals of electromyography. In Licht, S., ed.: Electrodiagnosis and electromyography, New Haven, Conn., 1961, E. Licht, Chap. 12.
5. Seddon, J. H.: Three types of nerve injury, Brain **66**:237, 1943.
6. Sunderland, S.: A classification of peripheral nerve injuries producing a loss of function, Brain **74**:491, 1951.

22

Action potentials from sensory nerves in man in nerve damage and during recovery

Annelise Rosenfalck

In nerve damage and during nerve repair the recording of action potentials from sensory nerves can give an estimate of the number of nerve fibers that can be activated and their ability to conduct at normal or reduced rates. Since percutaneous recording allows recording of a potential in only half the patients, Buchthal's group has improved the recording conditions. A large needle electrode with a recording surface about two times greater than the cross section of the nerve is positioned near the nerve[7,8,11,12] (Fig. 22-1). By averaging the responses to 500 to 4000 stimuli, components of 0.03 μV can be distinguished from noise. This allows detection of a response at distal and proximal sites in nearly all diseased nerves even when only a few fibers can be activated.

SENSORY POTENTIAL OF NORMAL NERVES

Since all findings in diseased nerves are compared to recordings from normal nerves, the method of recording and the findings in normal nerve are summarized. (For review of the literature see Buchthal and co-workers.[8])

Stimulus

Sensory nerves were stimulated by electrical stimuli at sites where only sensory fibers can be activated (Fig. 22-2). The electric stimulus was constant current and floating; activation of all fibers in diseased nerves may

require up to 80 ma with surface stimulus electrodes.

The *recording electrode* was a macroelectrode positioned at a distance of 0.5 to 1 mm from the nerve (Fig. 22-1). Fibers from the total cross section of the nerve then contributed about equally to the compound potential. We could not use a selective microelectrode inserted into the nerve close to individual fibers because the information about most of the fiber population then was lost. The distance between the electrode and the nerve was standardized. The electrode was used for stimulation and adjusted in position until the threshold of an evoked muscle or nerve potential was less than 1 ma and more than 0.5 ma. When the electrode was placed at a shorter distance from the nerve (threshold less than 0.5 ma), small displacements of the electrode caused large variations in amplitude. The action potential was recorded between the near-nerve electrode and a remote electrode placed at a distance of 3 to 4 cm from the nerve (Fig. 22-2).

The *maximum sensory velocity* determined to the first positive peak of the triphasic action potential was 60 to 70 m/sec. In the sural nerve, conduction velocity and distribution of fiber diameters from nerve biopsies have been determined in the same nerves.[1,2,3,5] The main phases of the potential originated from about 1400 nerve fibers, 9 to 14 μm in diameter; they represent 60% of all

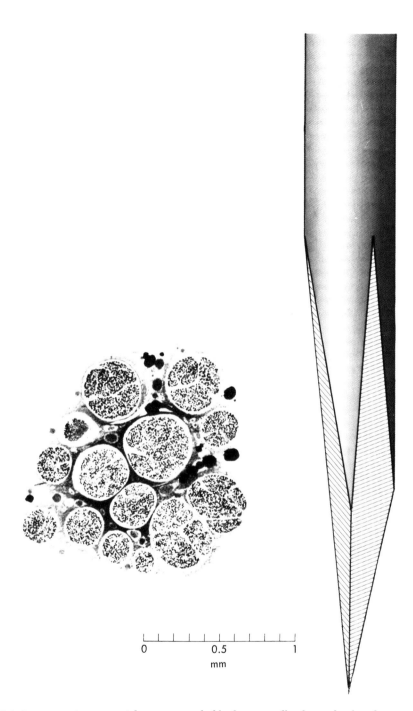

Fig. 22-1. Sensory action potentials were recorded by large needle electrode placed near nerve. Cross section of biopsy is taken from sural nerve at lateral malleolus. Stainless steel needle, 0.6 mm, was insulated except for 3 mm bared tip. It was positioned 0.5 to 1 mm from nerve. Large electrode has several advantages over smaller electrode: (1) all fibers in nerve contribute about equally to potential; (2) small variations in distance between electrode and nerve give less rise to variations in amplitude; and (3) large electrode is less noisy than small electrode.

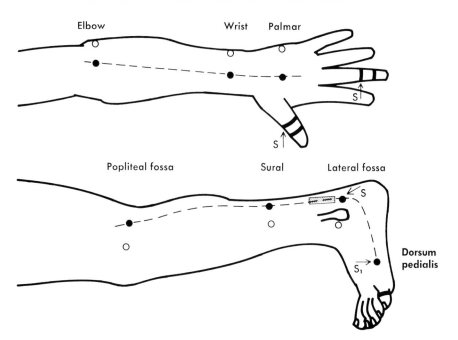

Fig. 22-2. Placement of the "near-nerve," ●, and remote, ○, needle electrodes to record from different segments of median and sural nerves. S, Stimulating cathode (surface or needle); S_1, cathode to stimulate distal segment of sural nerve. Shaded area shows 3 cm segment taken in toto as biopsy. (From Buchthal, F., Rosenfalck, A., and Behse, F. In Dyck, P., Thomas, P. K., and Lambert, E., eds.: Peripheral neuropathy, vol. II, Philadelphia, 1975, W. B. Saunders Co., Chap. 21, p. 442.)

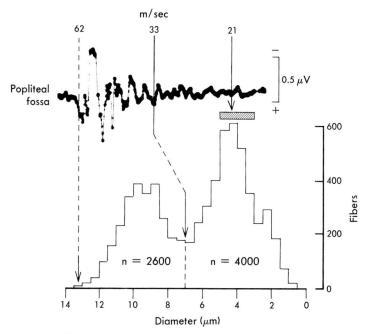

Fig. 22-3. Components of sensory potential as related to diameters of myelinated fibers in normal sural nerve (male, 14 years old). Above, nerve was stimulated maximally at lateral malleolus; potential was recorded in popliteal fossa (electronic averaging of 200 responses). Temperature near nerve was 36° to 37° C. Below, distribution of diameters of all myelinated fibers (n = 6600) obtained from biopsy of same nerve 2 cm proximal to lateral malleolus. Ratio between conduction velocity (62 m/sec) and diameter (13 to 13.5 μm) of largest fibers was 4.7; components of potential that were conducted at 33 and 21 m/sec (arrows) corresponded to fibers of 7 and 5—3 μm (hatched bar) in diameter. (From Buchthal, F., Rosenfalck, A., and Behse, F. In Dyck, P., Thomas, P. K., and Lambert, E., eds.: Peripheral neuropathy, vol. II, Philadelphia, 1975, W. B. Saunders Co., Chap. 21, p. 442.)

myelinated fibers 7 μm or more in diameter (Fig. 22-3). The slower components in the potential derived from the large group of myelinated fibers 7 μm or less in diameter.

The *minimum sensory velocity* was determined from the latency to the last of these components of the average response. When the action potential was recorded 15 to 20 cm from the point of stimulation, the minimum velocity was about 15 m/sec for the median, ulnar, and sural nerves.

Shape and amplitude

The volume-conducted action potential had a triphasic main component followed by four or five small components (Fig. 22-4). When all fibers were stimulated at the digits, the peak-to-peak amplitude recorded at the wrist ranged from 10 to 50 μV. With a larger distance of conduction the amplitude was smaller owing to temporal dispersion of the components. The amplitude of the potential recorded in the leg, at the ankle, and in the popliteal fossa was 5% to 10% of that recorded at the wrist and at the elbow.

Normal values

When conduction along an abnormal nerve is evaluated, it is important that findings in patients are compared to those in normal subjects of the same age because maximum velocity and amplitude in normal adult nerves decrease with age.[13] It is also important to control the temperature of the nerve, since conduction velocity decreases 2 m/sec/°C.

There is a large scatter in amplitude of the sensory potential from subject to subject (standard deviation: 40%). In experiments repeated on the same subjects the variation in amplitude was 20% to 30%, indicating that

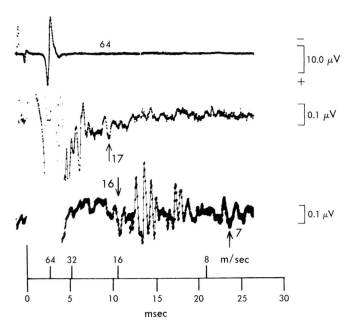

Fig. 22-4. Sensory potentials recorded in normal median nerve and in patient with carpal tunnel syndrome. Above, normal nerve potential recorded at low gain. Middle, same potential as above at 80 times higher gain (1000 responses). Below, potential in carpal tunnel syndrome recorded at high gain (1000 responses). Normal subject (E. B.), 28-year-old male. Patient (E. E. P.), 69-year-old woman. Stimulus to digit III, recording at wrist. Figures above traces give maximum velocities; figures below traces give minimum velocities (m/sec). Lower scale, conduction time. Upper scale, conduction velocity. (From Buchthal, F., Rosenfalck, A., and Trojaborg, W.: J. Neurol. Neurosurg. Psychiatry **37:**340, 1974.)

the variation in amplitude caused by different electrode positions is less than the interindividual differences.

SENSORY POTENTIAL IN DISEASED NERVES

Abnormal shape and diminished amplitude, with or without a reduction in conduction, are the main indicators of nerve damage (Figs. 22-4 and 22-5). These parameters help to elucidate the cause of nerve damage and to follow nerve repair. A reduced amplitude, with or without slight reduction in conduction, is a sign of axonal loss. A severe decrease in conduction velocity indicates that the split-up potential originates from demyelinated, remyelinated, or regenerating fibers.

This was confirmed by Buchthal and Behse[1,2,3,5] from investigations of the sural nerve in normal man and in patients with polyneuropathy. The sensory potentials were recorded and compared to findings in biopsies from the same nerve. In nerves with axonal loss and without demyelination the decrease from normal conduction velocity could be predicted from the diameter of the largest myelinated fibers found in the nerve biopsy. In demyelinated nerves conduction was lower than expected from the diameter of the largest nerve fibers.

The amplitude of the main component of the sensory potential decreased with decreasing numbers of fibers, 9 μm or more in diameter.[5]

Conduction after complete transection of a nerve

In regeneration after complete transection of the nerve, the sensory potential was ex-

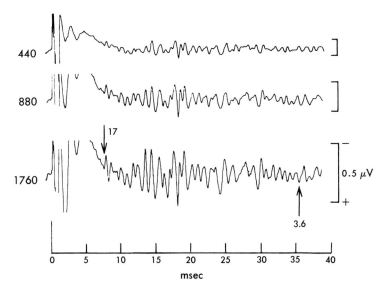

Fig. 22-5. Sensory potentials in regenerating fibers after wallerian degeneration. Responses were evoked by stimulation of proximal phalanx of digit III and recorded at wrist 9 months after suture of completely divided median nerve. Fastest (17 m/sec) and slowest (3.6 m/sec) components in averaged responses were identified by their increase in amplitude in three consecutive averages of increasing number (n) of responses. Subject was 20-year-old woman (B. M.) with complicated fracture at wrist. Three centimeters of median nerve were removed and stumps reunited by suture. Four months later there was no motor or sensory response in median nerve. Nine months after suture distal motor latency was 9 m/sec (distance, 6 cm). Sensitivity to touch was present on volar surface of proximal phalanx of digit III and absent distal to it. Temperature near nerve was 35° to 37° C. (From Buchthal, F., Rosenfalck, A., and Behse, F. In Dyck, P., Thomas, P. K., and Lambert, E., eds.: Peripheral neuropathy, vol. II, Philadelphia, 1975, W. B. Saunders Co., Chap. 21, p. 442.)

tremely small in amplitude (0.1 to 0.2 μV, less than 1% of normal.)[6] The minimum velocity was less than 3 m/sec. The potential was extremely split up and contained many more components than a potential recorded from normal nerve at the same resolution. An example of the potentials recorded from the median nerve 9 months after suture is shown in Fig. 22-5. When the same patient was reinvestigated 26 months later,[4,6] the main component of the potential was 10 times larger, the maximum velocity was 28 m/sec, and the main component was followed by 20 to 30 components indicating that recovery was still proceeding. The peak-to-peak amplitude of such split-up potentials is a poor indicator of the number of active fibers. In follow-up studies the amplitude of the individual components was therefore measured and added to a cumulative amplitude. Even this is a rough estimate, since the amplitude of the action potentials from immature regenerating fibers may be smaller than those from normal nerve fibers.

Three patients with total transection of the nerve were followed up to 3 years after suture. The amplitude and conduction velocity increased to more than 50% of normal but was still not complete. The rate of recovery was faster in children than in adults.

Conduction in localized traumatic lesions and entrapment of peripheral nerves

For lesions in the ulnar nerve at the elbow and the median nerve in the carpal tunnel, the diagnostic yield by recording sensory conduction was found to be greater than for motor conduction.[8,9] This was also true when conduction studies were used to establish whether a peroneal palsy was due to compression of the nerve in the region of capitulum fibulae.[14]

To localize the lesions, sensory potentials were recorded distal and proximal to the lesion. The method was a sensitive gauge in early recognition of pressure lesions. In 25% of 111 patients with carpal tunnel syndrome the distal motor latency from the wrist to the abductor pollicis brevis was normal, and slowing in the sensory fibers established the site of the lesion. In patients with slight or borderline slowing from digits to wrist, slowing became significant when determined between recording electrodes at the palm and the wrist (Figs. 22-2 and 22-6). This was because velocity was determined solely along the abnormal stretch of the nerve. Conduction from digit to palm was normal or less slowed than conduction across the flexor retinaculum. Across the region of compression the maximum velocity was as slow as 20 m/sec, and the minimum velocity was as slow as 5 m/sec.

In all patients with carpal tunnel syndrome the *same* fibers in which conduction was severely slowed across the flexor retinaculum conducted at a normal rate from the wrist to the elbow. This indicates that the slowing is caused by demyelination of the fibers and not by loss of the largest fibers.

In most patients the amplitude recorded at the wrist was less than 10% of normal, indicating that there was, in addition, loss or block of many fibers.

The number of slow components in the potential was much greater than normal, and they often occurred in bursts indicating that some fibers have degenerated from the compression.[10]

Some patients were followed after surgical division of the flexor retinaculum at the wrist (Fig. 22-6). The signs of recovery were increase in maximal velocity and increase in amplitude of the main component. In addition, there were more slow components and they had longer latencies and higher amplitudes 15 to 30 days after decompression, compatible with remyelination as the main factor during recovery.

The change in the shape of the sensory potential and the presence of slow components were often the earliest signs of a pressure palsy. The detection of the responses from a few slowly conducting nerve fibers may, in the future, prove to be a more sensitive gauge than most clinical tests for recognition of the first signs of recovery after a nerve suture. Repeated recordings during nerve re-

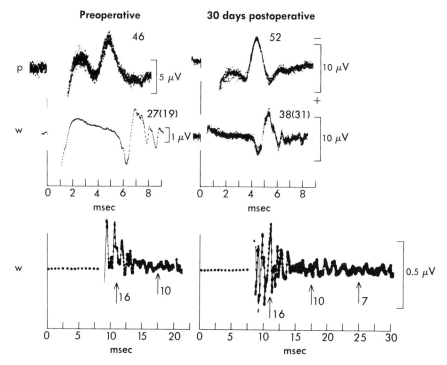

Fig. 22-6. Recovery of maximum and minimum sensory conduction 30 days after surgical division of flexor retinaculum. Increase in amplitude of sensory potential at palm, *p*, and at wrist, *w;* increase in maximum sensory velocity from digit III to palm and from digit III to wrist. Below, potentials at wrist recorded with high gain (500 responses). Slow components had longer latencies after than before decompression. Figures above traces give velocities in m/sec distal to site of recording. Numbers in parentheses indicate velocity from palm to wrist. Dotted lines indicate delay before sampling. Arrows below averaged responses indicate average minimum velocity in normal nerve (16 m/sec), minimum velocity before (10 m/sec) and after (7 m/sec) decompression. Note two bursts of slow components after decompression. Twenty-one-year-old woman (B. L. J.) with carpal tunnel syndrome. (From Buchthal, F., Rosenfalck, A., and Trojaborg, W.: J. Neurol. Neurosurg. Psychiatry **37:**340, 1974.)

pair may indicate the state of the nerve during recovery.

CONCLUSION

A method for the recording of sensory action potentials by a gross needle electrode placed near the nerve in man is reviewed. It allows the detection of responses from a small number of nerve fibers. Change in the shape of the response indicates nerve damage. The amplitude of the response gives an estimate of the number of nerve fibers that can be activated. A decreased velocity and the appearance of low-amplitude slow components indicates that the response originates from demyelinated, remyelinated, or regenerating fibers.

REFERENCES

1. Behse, F., and Buchthal, F.: Peroneal muscular atrophy (PMA) and related disorders. II. Histological findings in sural nerves, Brain **100:**67, 1977.
2. Behse, F., and Buchthal, F.: Alcoholic neuropathy: clinical, electrophysiological, and biopsy findings, Ann. Neurol. **2:**95, 1977.
3. Behse, F., Buchthal, F., and Rosenfalck, A.: Sensory conduction and quantitation of biopsy findings in the sural nerve. In Kunze, K., and Desmedt, J. E., eds.: Studies of neuromuscular diseases, Basel, 1975, Karger, p. 229.

4. Buchthal, F.: The spectrum of sensory conduction velocities during degeneration after suture of a nerve in man. Abstracts of communications. Fifth International Congress of Electromyography, Rochester, Minnesota, 1975.

5. Buchthal, F., and Behse, F.: Peroneal muscular atrophy (PMA) and related disorders. I. Clinical manifestations as related to biopsy findings, nerve conduction and electromyography, Brain **100**:41, 1977.

6. Buchthal, F., and Kühl, V.: Nerve conduction, tactile sensibility, and the electromyogram after suture or compression of peripheral nerve: a longitudinal study in man, J. Neurol. Neurosurg. Psychiatry **42**:436, 1979.

7. Buchthal, F., and Rosenfalck, A.: Evoked action potentials and conduction velocity in human sensory nerves, Brain Res. **3**:1, 1966.

8. Buchthal, F., Rosenfalck, A., and Behse, F.: Sensory potentials of normal and diseased nerves. In Dyck, P., Thomas, P. K., and Lambert, E., eds.: Peripheral neuropathy, vol. II, Philadelphia, 1975, W. B. Saunders Co., Chap. 21, p. 442.

9. Buchthal, F., Rosenfalck, A., and Trojaborg, W.: Electrophysiological findings in entrapment of the median nerve at wrist and elbow, J. Neurol. Neurosurg. Psychiatry **37**:340, 1974.

10. Le Quesne, P. M., and Casey, E. B.: Recovery of conduction velocity distal to a compressive lesion, J. Neurol. Neurosurg. Psychiatry **37**:1346, 1974.

11. Rosenfalck, A.: Technique for recording of action potentials from sensory nerve. Proceedings of III Nordic Meeting on Medical and Biological Engineering, Tampere, 15-18.1.1975. p. 15.1-15.3.

12. Rosenfalck, A.: Early recognition of nerve disorders by near-nerve recording of sensory action potentials. Muscle and Nerve **1**:360, 1978.

13. Rosenfalck, A., and Rosenfalck, P.: Electromyography—sensory and motor conduction. Findings in normal subjects, Laboratory of Clinical Neurophysiology, Rigshospitalet, Copenhagen, 1975, 1-49.

14. Singh, N., Behse, F., and Buchthal, F.: Physiological study of peroneal palsy, J. Nuerol. Neurosurg. Psychiatry **37**:1202, 1974.

23

Axonal growth at the suture line

Alan R. Hudson, David Kline, Bert Bratton, and Daniel Hunter

A sequence of electron photomicrographs has been chosen to illustrate axonal growth from the proximal to the distal stumps in a sutured nerve.

Fig. 23-1. *Proximal stump transverse section* ($\times 10,500$).

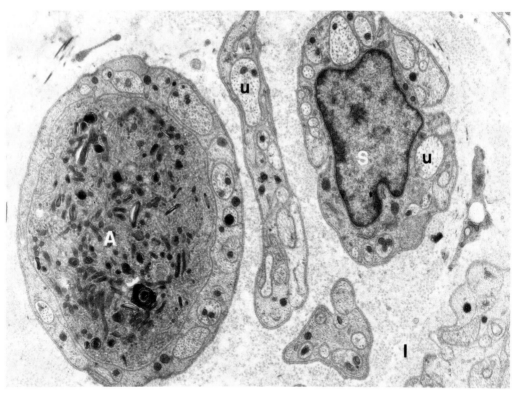

Following injury, nerve fibers in the proximal stump pass through the phase of traumatic degeneration.[8] This is followed by the phase of active regeneration that is illustrated here. The unmyelinated collateral and terminal sprouts, *u*, derived from nodes of Ranvier proximal to the site of injury, are supported by reduplicating Schwann cells, *S. A*, Greatly distended axon packed with organelles. *I*, Interfiber ground substance and collagen fibrils.

Fig. 23-2. *Distal stump transverse section* (×6500).

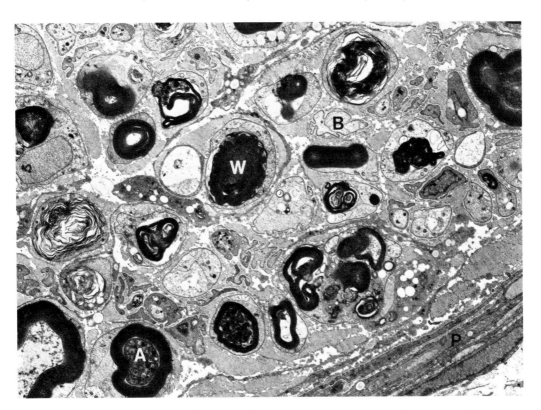

The nerve fibers enclosed within the perineurium, *P*, are undergoing wallerian degeneration. Axonal degeneration, *A*, appears to signal the Schwann cell to commence digesting its myelin. This process is seen at a further stage at the fiber marked *W*. Eventually, myelin lamellae are all that remain of the original structure. Finally, when all the myelin is digested or fragments have been removed by macrophages, the end stage is a basement membrane system containing finger processes of reduplicated Schwann cells, the band of Büngner, *B*.

Fig. 23-3. *Distal stump transverse section* (×4500)

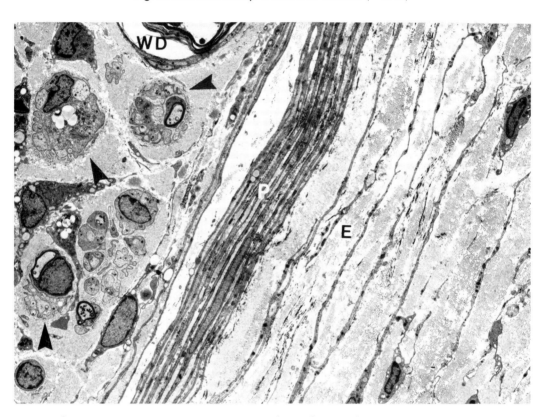

The regenerating units must grow into the endoneurial environment of the distal fascicles if they are to be transmitted to the periphery. This section illustrates three regenerative units (◀) that have successfully negotiated the suture line. The regenerative units are growing between the fibers undergoing wallerian degeneration, *WD*. Regenerating axon sprouts are supported by the columns of Schwann cells in the denervated bands of the distal stump. *P*, Perineurium; *E*, epineurium.[6]

Fig. 23-4. *Suture line transverse section* ($\times 8120$).

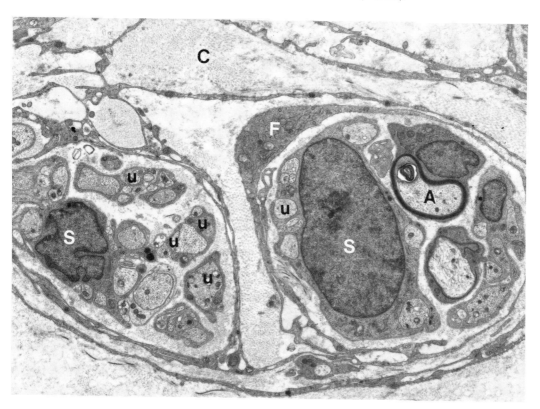

The regenerative units are separated one from another in their passage through the anastomotic scar by fibroblasts. If this pattern of compartmentation becomes more dense, the regenerating axon units are obstructed and will either be blocked in their progress or turned aside into the epineurial tissues.[2,5,7] *C*, Collagen; *F*, fibroblast; *S*, Schwann cell nucleus; *A*, myelinated axon; and, *u*, unmyelinated axons in two regenerative clusters.

Fig. 23-5. *Distal stump transverse section* ($\times 400$).

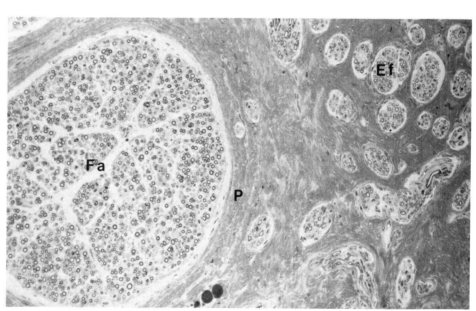

A fascicle, *Fa*, of the distal stump has been well reinnervated. Unfortunately, some groups of regenerating axon sprouts have not gained the favorable environment of the fascicle and are growing in epineurial tissues as extrafascicular axons, *Ef*. These fibers contribute to the neuroma at the suture line but are not transmitted to the periphery and, therefore, do not assume a useful function.[4] *P*, Perineurial boundary of fascicle.

Fig. 23-6. *Suture line transverse section* ($\times 15,070$). *Interfascicular suture.*

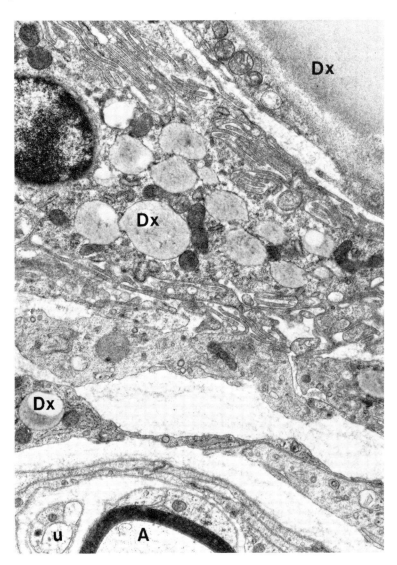

The suture material selected must have sufficient strength to maintain the fascicles in apposition and must cause minimal reaction in the conducting tissues. A polyglycolic acid suture filament, *Dx*, is surrounded by a macrophage that is absorbing fragments of the polymer, *Dx*. Myelinated, *A*, and unmyelinated, *u*, fibers immediately adjacent to the suture material are completely unaffected by the suture material.[1,3]

Fig. 23-7. *Suture line transverse section* (×400).

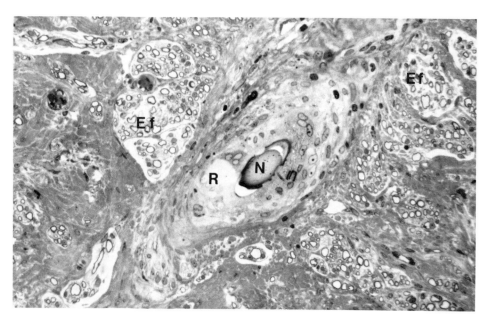

If a grouped fascicular or fascicular repair is performed, the suture material will eventually be incorporated within the nerve trunk as a whole. *N*, Nylon suture; *R*, reactive macrophages and fibroblasts; *Ef*, extrafascicular axons that have not gained the main fascicles and are contributing to the formation of the neuroma at the suture line.

On the basis of these examples, it would seem evident that the surgeon should design his repair in such a way as to minimize suture line scarring and to maximize the capture of regenerating axon units by the fascicles of the distal stump.

REFERENCES

1. Hudson, A., and Hunter, D.: Polyglycolic acid suture in peripheral nerve II: sutured sciatic nerve, Can. J. Neurol. Sci. **3**:69, 1976.
2. Hudson, A., and Kline, D.: Progression of partial experimental injury to peripheral nerve, part 2: light and electron microscopic studies, J. Neurosurg. **42**:15, 1975.
3. Hudson, A., Bilbao, J., and Hunter, D.: Polyglycolic acid suture in peripheral nerve: an electronmicroscopic study, Can. J. Neurol. Sci. **2**:17, 1975.
4. Hudson, A., et al.: Peripheral nerve autografts, J. Surg. Res. **12**:267, 1972.
5. Kline, D., Hudson, A.: Surgical repair of acute peripheral nerve injuries: timing and technique. In Morley, T. P., ed.: Current controversies in neurosurgery, Philadelphia, 1976, W. B. Saunders Co. p. 184.
6. Kline, D., and Nulsen, F.: Acute injuries of peripheral nerves. In Youmans, J., ed.: Neurological surgery, ed. 2. In press.
7. Kline, D., et al.: Progression of partial experimental injury to peripheral nerve, part 1: periodic measurements of muscle contraction strength, J. Neurosurg. **42**:1, 1975.
8. Morris, J., Hudson, A., and Weddell, G.: A study of degeneration and regeneration in the divided rat sciatic nerve based on electronmicroscopy, Z. Zellforsch, Mikrosk, Anat. **124**:76, 1972.

DISCUSSION

Rosen: Dr. Hudson, do you have any data comparing the proximal axon counts to see whether they change differentially between different repair techniques?

Hudson: We are doing these counts now, but I don't have any figures available. We have done counts on grafted rabbit nerves, comparing normal counts at the site where the procedure was done, and peripheral counts both within and beyond the grafts. Our conclusion was that there was an enormous amount of sprouting at the first suture line and that although you could lose an enormous amount of axonal material at the first suture line, there seemed to be so much sprouting that maybe it did not matter. Our conclusion with regard to the second suture line was that there was very much less sprouting, so that the safety factor was much less.

Rosen: Proximal to the lesion, perhaps 1 cm proximal to the lesion, is the axon population normal or is that population abnormal? How far back do you see retrograde degeneration and regeneration?

Hudson: What we have observed is that they will usually degenerate back two, three, or four internodes, something of that nature. Further back the impression is that the numbers are unchanged, but we have not counted that far from the lesion.

Rosen: Is the fiber diameter histogram also unchanged?

Hudson: Our impression is that it is unchanged.

24

Results of suture of cat ulnar nerves: a comparison of surgical techniques*

H. Relton McCarroll, Jr., William G. Rodkey, and H. Edward Cabaud

With the availability of the operating microscope in the last decade, there has been considerable attention directed to advanced microsurgical techniques and their possible application to peripheral nerve repair. The magnification provided by the operating microscope has made possible a more detailed subdivision of the nerve, which can then be sutured either in small bundles of fascicles or by single individual fascicles. Although interest in this type of approach to nerve suture began in the early part of the 20th century, only with practical methods of higher magnification has its application been possible.

The use of the operating microscope has also made possible revision of the older techniques of nerve grafting. With magnification it has become possible to use an "interfascicular graft" technique as described by Millesi and co-workers in 1972, with results reported to be superior to those obtained with the older "cable graft" technique.[3]

Now that these new techniques are available, it is important to compare them with each other and with older techniques to determine whether one is clearly superior. Although the clinician's primary concern is with the results obtained by suture of human nerve injuries, it is very difficult to obtain a large series of similar, much less identical, injuries that permits statistical analysis. By studying the results of nerve repair in an experimental animal, the investigator can create a large series of similar nerve lesions suitable for statistical comparisons.

Animal experiments have a number of advantages in addition to providing a large number of similar lesions for study. It is possible to study muscle recovery using quantitative tests rather than the semiquantitative, functional tests permissible with human subjects.[5] With a strain gauge, the tension provided by a stimulated muscle can be measured and graphed. This is in contrast to the visual and palpable estimation of the return of function in a muscle used to evaluate humans. After an animal experiment, the whole muscle is available for weighing and histological study. Indeed, the repaired nerve itself is available for study. This can include neurophysiologic measurements by either single axon studies or whole nerve studies using the compound action potential (see Chapters 11 and 15). The nerve is also available for histological study of the repair site and axon counts above and below the repair.

A final major advantage to animal experiments occurs if the model is such that bilateral lesions are well tolerated. In this case, two techniques of repair can be performed in

*In conducting the research described in this report, the investigators adhered to the *Guide for Laboratory Animal Facilities and Care*, as promulgated by the Committee on the Guide for Laboratory Animal Resources, National Academy of Sciences, National Research Council. The opinions or assertions contained herein are the private views of the authors and are not to be construed as official or as reflecting the views of the Department of the Army or the Department of Defense.

a single animal, with each animal serving as its own control. This advantage has probably been underestimated; as our work suggests there is more variation between cats than between the right and left limbs of one animal.

Animal experiments do, however, have two major drawbacks. The surgeon is interested in extrapolating any conclusions to human nerve problems; this final step may or may not be justified. The second drawback is the difficulty in studying sensory return in animals. Although it is possible to study reinnervation of individual receptors, it is not possible to study the sensation that results centrally from all the information provided by those receptors.[2]

THE CAT EXPERIMENTAL MODEL

For our experimental model, we chose the ulnar nerve in the forelimb of the domestic house cat.[1] The ulnar nerve is quite suitable for study of suture techniques as it is a mixed motor and sensory major peripheral nerve that is easily approached. In the cat the ulnar nerve comes much closer to the axis of the elbow joint and is not affected by flexion and extension of the joint as much as it is in primates and humans. The nerve is fairly loose and can easily be sutured without tension being placed on the repair by motion of the elbow. Thus the model permits elimination of tension as a factor that could influence regeneration of the nerve.

Because the ulnar nerve routinely supplies all of the flexor carpi ulnaris muscle belly, there is a good forearm flexor muscle available for evaluation. In the postoperative period, a postural deformity is easily noted in the upper extremities, with a J-shape to the forearm-paw junction caused by the weakness of the wrist flexors in contrast to the sharp angle usually seen as the cat stands on its metacarpal heads. This is the only functional deficit observed. The cat tolerates acute bilateral ulnar nerve palsies quite well, so contrasting types of nerve suture can be performed in the right and left upper extremities.

EPINEURIAL vs. PERINEURIAL REPAIR

In our first study we performed sharp lacerations of both ulnar nerves 2 cm above the medial epicondyle.[1] At that level the nerve consists of between three and six fascicles. One nerve of each cat was repaired by epineurial suture and the other by perineurial fascicular suture, using microsurgical technique for both repairs. The evaluation at 4 months consisted of both subjective and objective observations as well as gross and microscopical inspection of the neuromas. Of particular interest was the fact that there was more variation between the individual animals as far as neuroma size and fibrosis than there was between the right and left forelimbs of an individual cat. Approximately two thirds of the animals had equal size neuromas on both ulnar nerves. In the remaining one-third, there was a discrepancy in neuroma size, but there was no preference for one type of repair to be larger.

Subjective evaluation consisted of gross grading on a 0 to 4+ scale of withdrawal of the upper extremity from pinprick, fanning of the claws, and resolution of the J-shape postural deformity of the upper extremities with walking. In none of these three techniques of evaluation was a significant difference observed between the two suture techniques.

Objective evaluation consisted of quantitative measurement of: (1) forearm flexor muscle tension produced by tetanic stimulation, (2) muscle efficiency, and (3) weight of the dissected flexor carpi ulnaris muscle. Axon counts of myelinated fibers of the repaired ulnar nerves were performed on cross sections obtained 1.5 cm above and below each suture line. Results were expressed as the percentage of myelinated fibers crossing each suture line. Comparison of the objective measurements resulting from epineurial and perineurial fascicular suture showed no statistically significant difference using Student's paired t test.

We concluded that in our experimental model there is no difference between repair of a clean, acute nerve laceration by epineurial or by fascicular techniques.

EPINEURIAL REPAIR UNDER TENSION vs. SURAL NERVE GRAFTS

Our most recent series of animals has involved repair of the ulnar nerves after removal of a 2 cm section in each forelimb.[4] The cat's nerve is quite pliable and elastic, and it is possible to pull the two nerve ends together and do an epineurial suture even after resection of what represents a significant portion of the nerve in the length of the limb. To prevent dehiscence of the epineurial repairs, that extremity was immobilized in a body wrap for 3 weeks. This was well tolerated by the animals.

An epineurial repair was performed on one ulnar nerve of each animal using the operating microscope. In the contralateral extremity of each animal, the 2 cm gap in the ulnar nerve was closed with multiple segments of caudal cutaneous sural nerve free grafts obtained from both lower extremities. At the level of the proximal division of the ulnar nerve, the internal architecture usually consists of one single very large fascicle and most of the time a very tiny second fascicle. At the proximal end, therefore, the nerve grafts were sutured about the perimeter of the large fascicle and one graft was sutured to the smaller fascicle, if present. Distally, a fascicular-type graft repair was performed. If there was a large fascicle present distally, two sural nerve grafts were frequently sutured to that fascicle.

The animals were allowed free ambulation and exercise after the 3-week period of protection of the epineurial repair. They were evaluated at 6 months using the subjective and objective criteria as outlined. Of the subjective criteria, only gait analysis showed a statistically significant difference between the two types of repair, favoring epineurial repair slightly. Using the objective measurements, no statistically significant difference could be demonstrated between the two methods of nerve suture.

The fact that no difference was found between epineurial repair under tension and repair of an identical gap by nerve grafts is moderately surprising. Tension is presently considered one of the major causes of failure of human peripheral nerve repairs.[3] The elimination of tension possible with nerve grafts is thought to be a desirable feature of that suture technique.[3] The repairs we performed under tension could, in the human, be expected to fail and produce no functional regeneration. Although cats' nerves may handle tension better than human nerves, it is interesting that the two repair techniques produced such similar results. There are two different ways of viewing these data.

Tension at the suture line probably prejudices the result of an epineurial suture. The fact that nerve grafts require two suture lines and interpose a dead segment of nerve probably limits the regeneration observed after that technique. Perhaps with 2 cm defects in cat ulnar nerves, these factors affect regeneration equally, but with other lengths of deficit one repair might be superior. Thus with a nerve loss of only 1 cm the diminished tension across the epineurial suture might improve the results of that repair more than the decreased nerve graft length would benefit the results of that technique.

There is, however, a second possible interpretation to be considered. Perhaps the loss of a 2 cm segment of nerve limits the potential regeneration of the nerve regardless of the technique of suture employed. Thus the amount of nerve lost would be more important than the surgical technique used to repair it. If this experiment were repeated but only 1 cm of nerve was removed, this would suggest that the two suture techniques would again produce similar regeneration. Further experimentation using different lengths of nerve loss should help to choose between these two interpretations.

COMPARISON OF THE TWO CAT STUDIES

The two studies reported demonstrate no significant difference between the suture techniques employed within each study. The major difference in the experimental conditions of the two studies is the amount of nerve resected. In the first study no nerve was resected, and in the second study 2 cm of nerve were removed. We have compared all nerve repairs in the first study with all nerve repairs in the second study using Student's paired t test. Of the subjective and objective factors studied only a comparison of flexor carpi ulnaris muscle weights showed a statistically significant difference (P < 0.02). Muscles from cats with a segment of nerve resected had smaller weights than those with no nerve resected, suggesting that the amount of nerve substance lost is an important determinant of the functional return observed after nerve repair. It is apparent that in this comparison a number of uncontrolled factors, such as the size of the animals, could be important.

Two experimental approaches are suggested to investigate further the effect of loss of nerve substance. Using an epineurial suture technique, repairs after removal of 0, $1/2$, and 1 cm of nerve could be contrasted. We have not investigated $1/2$- or 1-cm defects and do not know whether the tension produced could be expected to affect regeneration.

A second possibility would be to eliminate tension by performing nerve graft repairs. A nerve with a 1 cm defect and a nerve that is simply lacerated could both be repaired using nerve grafts. Unless another suitable donor nerve can be identified, the defect will have to be 1 cm or less, as repair of the 2 cm defects required all of both sural nerves. Either approach should provide further insight into the effect of a lost nerve segment.

CONCLUSION

Using the cat ulnar nerve as an experimental model, we have found no statistically significant difference between epineurial and perineurial fascicular repairs of acute, sharp nerve lacerations. In addition, epineurial repairs under tension and nerve graft repairs give similar results after resection of 2 cm segments of nerve.

The results of our two studies suggest that in the cat the loss of nerve substance may be a major determinant of the functional regeneration obtained with any technique of nerve suture.

REFERENCES

1. Cabaud, H. E., et al.: Epineurial and perineurial fascicular nerve repairs: a critical comparison, J. Hand Surg. **1**:131, 1976
2. Dellon, A. L.: Rennervation of denervated Meissner corpuscles, J. Hand Surg. **1**:98, 1976
3. Millesi, H., Meissl, G., and Berger, A.: Interfascicular nerve grafting of the median and ulnar nerves, J. Bone Joint Surg. **54A**:727, 1972
4. Rodkey, W. G., et al.: Neurorrhaphy after loss of a nerve segment. J. Hand Surg. In press.
5. Seddon, H.: Surgical disorders of the peripheral nerves, Baltimore, 1972, The Williams & Wilkins Co.

DISCUSSION

Stein (Edmonton): As a complete outsider, can I play the devil's advocate and ask whether I understood the conclusions correctly from the comments I have heard? Is it correct or is it not that experimentally with these elegant techniques no one has been able to demonstrate any advantage statistically of one repair method to another, but yet surgically you are going to go on doing exactly the same things that you have been doing before?

McCarroll: When faced with a fresh, clean nerve laceration like those studied in the experimental animal, many of us would do what our studies suggest, an epineural repair. The problem is that many clinical situations are very complicated. There are many factors involved, especially with secondary repairs, that have been eliminated in the experimental studies. If you must repair a nerve that was cut by a Skill saw, I would agree that you have to debride a lot of nerve until you get back to where it even approaches looking normal. I usually cannot get those together again unless I put grafts in them. If I am faced with a clinical situation that is different from the clean, sharp lacerations of the experimental studies, I use my best judgment to determine what will work best.

Julia Terzis (Montreal): Adding to what Dr. Stein has said, unfortunately, with these animal models, significant differences were not seen between different repair methods. I think a significant point in our study was that even when the epineurial repairs were done under high magnification utilizing microsurgical techniques, there was a tendency throughout the whole study for fascicular repairs to be superior. I think what we are seeing, at least in that study, are the tremendous limitations of the rabbit model as compared to the primate.

The work of Sunderland has shown the tremendous difference between the connective tissue component of a cut fascicle in the primate vs. other animals. Klein has demonstrated the differences in neuroma size by making cross-species comparisons. Thus the comparison of epineurial and perineurial repairs will have to be tested in a high primate model. Then we might be able to find some difference.

What is disturbing to me in Dr. McCarroll's work was the effect of tension. In a series of animal experiments we did a couple of years ago, we saw objectively that the effect of tension was detrimental. It really bothers me that taking out 2-cm segments showed no difference. It bothers me because in all our studies, over 50 animals, we saw a tremendous difference when there was severe tension. We got absolutely no regeneration. Regardless of the type of repair, I would hate to see surgeons go home and apply a lot of tension between two nerve ends.

Millesi: We must be very careful in applying the results of animal experimentation to human practice. Many animal experiments have a clinical background, but we must go back a few years to understand this clinical background. Ten years ago epineurial nerve repair was the clinical technique. Perineurial nerve repair was tried but was condemned. Perineurial repair was tried because it seemed that with a nerve like the median nerve with its multifascicular pattern of sensory and motor fascicles there would be a better chance for regrowth of the motor fibers into the distal stump if fascicular alignment were achieved. Ten years or more ago nerve grafting was condemned completely, and it was evident that a graft with its two suture lines should be much inferior to an end-to-end nerve repair.

Now when animal experiments show no difference between epineurial and fascicular types of repair, this means that the nerve grafts were as good as the end-to-end nerve repairs. Both Dr. Hudson and Dr. McCarroll concluded that the epineurial repair should not be abandoned. We have come to the point where the authors feel they must defend the epineurial nerve repair, but no one has ever attacked the epineurial nerve repair. These different techniques are not in competition. If you are dealing with a multifascicular nerve without any group arrangement or a monofascicular or oligofascicular nerve, you will do an epineurial nerve repair if there is no loss of substance. If you are suturing a multifascicular nerve with group arrangement, you will try to do an interfascicular type of repair, and if there is a gap, you will use nerve grafts.

Animal experiments cannot be applied directly to clinical practice. Primates are very similar to humans, but there is still a small but significant difference. Years ago I tried to produce a scar contracture in the finger of a monkey by a longitudinal incision crossing all the transverse creases, but I didn't succeed. The monkey did not develop the flexion contracture that we would expect in humans. So, there is still a little difference.

Finally, turning to the experiments in which the cat was used as an experimental model, the cat is an animal that has a very good potential for regeneration, better than some others, perhaps. If you analyze the results more carefully, what have you done? You have produced a high ulnar nerve lesion and repaired it. You have measured return by studying the flexor carpi ulnaris muscle. From human practice we know that good function of this proximal muscle returns in nearly all the patients. By Highet's scheme for evaluation, this would be an M2 result, but an M2 result is not considered a useful result. To get a useful result in a human patient there must be good intrinsic muscle function. You cannot tell very much about intrinsic

muscle function in the cat. You should have good adduction of the thumb, but you cannot test this in your model. You should have good stabilization of the metacarpophalangeal joint of the thumb, but you also cannot test this. You should have good two-point discrimination and good sensibility. This is very difficult to study in cats. So I would warn against applying such results directly to human patients.

Sunderland: I would like to comment on these issues by endorsing what Dr. Millesi has said in this regard. This is a situation where animal experiments can be very misleading indeed. If you visualize the complexity of the internal anatomy of human nerve trunks, you will appreciate how significantly different they are from the animal situation, in which the internal anatomy of the nerves usually used for experimentation is of the simplest variety, either a single funiculus or at most three major funiculi. In any event, there is usually no significant change in the funicular patterns of the nerve ends. So we are dealing here with an oversimplified situation. We are dealing with a situation where epineurial suture is almost a perineurial suture. Hence there is practically no difference between them, except in instances where comparison is made of suture material going through the epineurium (where it should be going) and going through the perineurium (which you attempt to avoid). Regardless of the suture you do or the graft that you put in, you still have a situation that is going to favor the entry of regenerating axons into the distal stump, whether it's across an end-to-end union or across two graft unions.

Now there is one further point and that is in the end result evaluations. I think we want to be careful about this question of axon regeneration and axon conducting properties and the restoration of function. In this regard it's the recovery of muscle function, in terms of what the muscle will do, that I'd attach greatest value to. I can create a situation for you in which you can get 100% axon regeneration and no recovery. That can happen in the sciatic nerve. The proof of the pudding is in the eating here. It's what the patient finishes up with in terms of function that's all important.

I think that what this animal experimental work does do is to direct attention to such factors as tension at suture lines and the question of the reaction to suture materials. We should be looking for biodegradable membranes or sutures, be-cause even 10-0 nylon will cause a considerable degree of obstructive fibrosis over the long term. So, this is interesting. Please don't misunderstand me and get the impression that I regard this as unimportant. I do regard it as important, but I think we want to exercise great caution in transferring these results directly to human situations. That's the point that Dr. Millesi has made and I wanted to endorse.

25

Suture and sutureless methods of repairing experimental nerve injuries

Joseph M. Rosen, E. N. Kaplan, and Don L. Jewett

The primary objective of the surgeon is to repair the injured nerve with a technique that has the greatest probability of providing maximum functional recovery to the patient. The surgeon with a knowledge of the conditions of the injury must choose between various alternative repair methods: primary or secondary, graft or tension, epineurial or fascicular (or grouped fascicular), and suture or sutureless. Many of these choices are clearly indicated by the specific conditions of the clinical nerve injury. In other cases animal experimentation may help the surgeon to decide between two alternatives.

There still exists an active controversy as to whether fascicular suture repair results in a better functional recovery than epineurial suture repair. Experimental studies of fascicular and epineurial suture repair have been unable to resolve this controversy.* Methodological problems with both the experimental models and the evaluation methods have led to inconclusive results in many of these studies (see Chapter 15). Yet the failure to find a statistically significant difference between different repair methods may only reflect the limitations of the evaluation technique or some unique aspect of the animal model.

Despite the inconclusive animal studies, some clinical studies have reported fascicular suture repair resulting in improved func-

tional results compared with epineurial repair.[14,16,21,26,34] Sunderland states that there is no controversy between epineurial and fascicular repair, only specific indications for each type of repair (see Chapter 37). Epineurial and fascicular repair have advantages and disadvantages for a specific nerve injury, depending on the following conditions at the site of injury: (1) the correspondence of the funicular pattern of the two nerve ends, (2) the amount of intervening epineurial tissue, and (3) the branch fiber localization (see Chapter 37).

However, up to now no studies have combined the advantages of fascicular repair with those of sutureless technique, as we report later in this chapter. First we will review the more important sutureless repair techniques.

ADHESIVE REPAIR

Adhesives can act as a glue to hold the two severed ends of a nerve in close apposition. Synthetic adhesives such as acyl-cyanoacrylate have resulted in severe tissue reactions and necrosis.[15,20] Heterologous and homologous clotting substances have been studied for nerve anastomosis.[11,22,33] A study by the authors[31] of clot, suture, and tubulization repair in a single fascicular rat model evaluated by measuring the area under the monophasic compound action potential demonstrated (1) no statistically significant difference between suture and clot and (2) tubulization to be superior to both suture and clot (see the following).

---

*See references 2, 5, 12, 13, 27, 28, 38, and 40.

TUBULIZATION REPAIR

Tubulization techniques hold the two ends of the nerve in close apposition either by wrapping a membrane around the site of discontinuity or by passing a preformed tube over the two ends of the nerve (Fig. 25-1). The first successful tubulization repair was achieved by von Bungner in 1891.[4] He reported histological evidence of nerve regeneration between the stumps. Since that time, many different tubulization materials have been used for nerve repairs; decalcified bone, arteries, veins, fascia lata, fat, muscle, parchment, gelatin, rubber, and various metals were all tried before World War II.[35,36] These substances demonstrated an improved longitudinal orientation of fibers across the nerve anastomosis; however, long-term evaluations of these tubulization techniques failed to show a functional improvement over conventional suture techniques, possibly as a result of limitations of the evaluation methods (see Chapter 15).

There are numerous reasons for many of the observed failures of some tubulization techniques. Many tubulization materials have resulted in inflammatory and fibrous reactions because of tissue incompatibility, liberation of irritating substances, or simple mechanical irritation. Other tubes were placed over epineurial suture repairs, which limited the advantages of tubulization repair and introduced the disadvantages of suture repair.

Weiss in 1944 reviewed previous repair techniques and summarized the basic principles of nerve repair for optimal regeneration.[35] In nerve repair by tubulization, Weiss stated that an orderly regeneration results from the longitudinal stress pattern that guides the regenerating axons, Schwann cells, fibroblasts, and blood vessels. The disorganized "suture line" normally seen in nerve repair is replaced by an organized "union tissue" that spans the anastomosis. This should improve functional recovery by maximizing the number of nerve fibers that cross the anastomosis and by preserving their fascicular topography.

Weiss believed that prior attempts had failed because of the "current form of its application," rather than the principles of the suture technique. He stated that a continued search should be made for a material that would fulfill the demands required for a successful tubulization without the disadvantages of previous tubulization materials.[35]

Epineurial tubulization

Elastic cuffs of tantalum were used in clinical epineurial nerve repairs during World War II. Clinical evaluation of their results did *not* demonstrate a statistically significant improvement of function compared with nerve

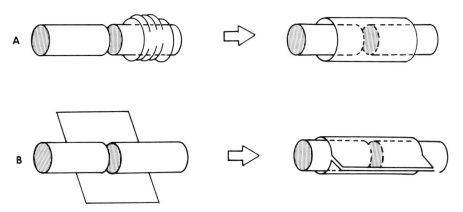

Fig. 25-1. Tubulization nerve repair. **A,** Sleeve method: a preformed tube is passed over one end of nerve (above left) and is then pulled over anastomosis (above right). **B,** Single leaf method: membrane is passed under nerve (below left) and then wrapped around nerve to form a tube (below right).

repairs without tantalum.[39] It was also shown that tantalum eventually fragmented, leading to a foreign body reaction and calcification, often requiring a second operation to remove the tube. After World War II, Millipore and Micropore were both experimented with for tubulization.[6,9] These materials had the same problems seen with tantalum tubes. More recently, silicone tubes have been used for nerve repair;[8] initial testing of thick Silastic tubes results in fibrosis and proximal neuroma formation, secondary to stiff, ill-fitting tubes.[7] Further refinements in Silastic that use thin, elastic tubes have shown better anatomical results.[8] When compared with conventional epineural suture repair in animals, however, crude functional evaluation has demonstrated no significant statistical difference (see below), although clinical studies have reported a more rapid return of function.[24] A study comparing epineural suture repairs with and without polyglycolic tubes demonstrated no statistically significant difference in nerve conduction velocities or EMG results.[30] The authors suggested that this may only reflect the insensitivity of the evaluation methods used.

Many workers[3,8,17,37] have attempted to use collagen membranes to overcome the problem of excessive tissue reaction found in previous materials. Weiss and Taylor in 1946[37] used reconstituted bovine collagen. They experimented with both tanned and untanned collagen tubes, and they found the untanned ones more suitable for tubulization because of the elasticity of the material. Evaluation by nonquantitative histological and physiological methods showed reinnervation, but their experiments did not compare these results with conventional suture techniques.

Working with chimpanzees, Kline and Hayes in 1964[17] compared peroneal nerves *repaired by epineural suture* wrapped with a variety of reconstituted, irradiated bovine collagen films and epineural suture with no wrapper. The untanned collagen films produced a notable tissue reaction. They found that the lightly tanned collagen film resulted in the least tissue reaction and also reduced

the disorganization and neuroma formation found in the repairs without the wrapper. Determination of threshold of the muscular response to stimulation showed no statistically significant difference.

In 1966 Braun[3] also used reconstituted collagen films to repair the sciatic nerves of rats and rabbits. The collagen films *were applied over sutured nerves*. The histological results of epineural tubulization with the collagen film demonstrated excellent longitudinal orientation of the anastomosis and minimal tissue reaction. Although the histological results of tubulization were better than either standard or microsurgical epineural suture, evaluation of muscle contraction responses to stimulation showed no significant difference between suture methods and tubulization.

Ducker and Hayes in 1968[8] compared the following five epineural nerve repair techniques in chimpanzees: standard epineural suture, irradiated bovine collagen wrap, Millipore wrap, Silastic wrap, and thin and thick Silastic tubes. The wraps and tubes *were applied over sutured anastomoses*. The repairs were evaluated from between the sixth and twelfth month by histological and physiological methods. The tubulization repairs all showed an improved histological pattern when compared with the standard epineural suture technique. No significant difference was seen by EMG and nerve conduction evaluation between any of the tubulization techniques and the standard epineural suture technique.

Recent studies with collagen wraps have reconfirmed the above results.[1,23,25] In 1972 Millesi and co-workers[25] studied a number of materials (Millipore membrane, collagen sheath, and silicone) for epineural tubulization. They concluded that there was no advantage in using epineural sutureless techniques with these materials compared with epineural suture techniques.

Evaluation of tubulization techniques has thus indicated that epineural tubulization results in better longitudinal orientation of the anastomosis but has not shown a statistically significant improvement in physiological results over conventional epineural su-

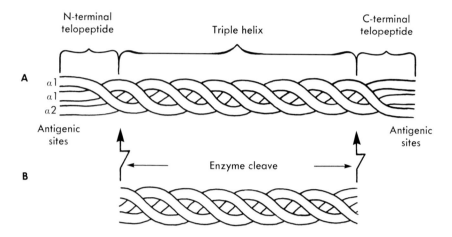

Fig. 25-2. Hypoantigenic collagen. Enzyme cleavage of telopeptides. **A,** Collagen molecule before removal of terminal telopeptides has antigenic sites at either end. **B,** Collagen molecule after removal of terminal telopeptides is hypoantigenic.

ture techniques. Yet this lack of improvement might be the result of insufficiently sensitive quantitative methods used for comparison (see Chapter 15). Furthermore, the common use of tubulization *in addition to suture* could obscure the benefits of tubulization if suturing is itself disruptive to axonal regrowth.

Fascicular tubulization

The aim of our recent study[31] was to evaluate a *fascicular technique* of sutureless repair done with a new hypoantigenic collagen membrane. The collagen membrane used in this study is composed of dermal calf collagen that has been solubilized and purified by limited pepsin digestion.* The collagen is then reassembled into macroscopic fibers, which are utilized as starting material to form the membrane.

The major antigenic sites of the collagen molecule reside in the nonhelical amino terminal and carboxyl terminal molecular extensions (the telopeptides).[10] Removal of the telopeptides by pepsin digestion results in reduced immunogenicity (see Fig. 25-2). It has been demonstrated that collagen that has

been altered in this way may be implanted in a xenogenic recipient without provoking a rejection response. The implanted collagen persists as an implant that is vascularized and colonized by recipient fibroblasts.[18,19] We refer to this collagen as hypoantigenic.

In our experimental model a single fascicular nerve in the rat was transected and repaired by tubulization on one side and suture on the opposite side (Fig. 25-3). Histological evaluation of the repair site demonstrated a more orderly regeneration in the tubulization repairs compared with the sutured repairs.[31]

Quantitative population physiological evaluation (described in Chapter 15) was done in 10 animals in which the nerve was transected and repaired by tubulization on one side and suture on the opposite side. These results are presented in Table 25-1. In five of the ten animals the nerve of the tubulized repair was found to have elongated, curving back across the accompanying artery and vein. The results for these nerves did not differ from the rest and are included in Table 25-1. The area of the compound action potential recorded from the distal stimulator is expressed as a percentage of the compound action potential recorded from the proximal stimulator. The area ratios indicate

---

*Developed and supplied by Collagen Corporation of Palo Alto, California.

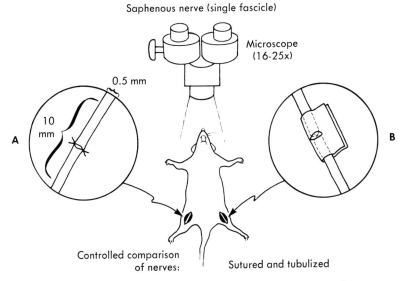

Fig. 25-3. Rat experimental model. Microsurgical nerve repair. **A,** Fascicular suture. **B,** Fascicular tubulization.

Table 25-1. Experimental data from perineurial tubulization and suture nerve repairs

Date of repair (month)	Area (IMCAP) (percent)		Myelinated axon count (percent)	
	Tube	Suture	Tube	Suture
3	83*	46	145	123
3	84*	10	156	164
3	77	61	136	165
6	74*	24	129	133
6	86	44	104	174
6	89	79	139	143
6	88	45	180	160
6	86	39	167	159
6	83*	39	177	139
6	70*	29	140	129

*Nerves that appeared to have elongated, having bowed out of the natural bed in the region of the repair.

that in all 10 animals the nerve with the sutureless repair had a greater proportion of proximal myelinated axons conducting across the anastomosis than did the contralateral suture side. The nerve repairs were symmetrical matched pairs; the difference in area ratios is statistically significant (P < 0.005 using nonparametric statistics).

However, we saw no significant difference between tubulized and sutured nerves by histological count ratios that were determined by dividing the proximal myelinated count by the distal count (P > 0.10) (Table 25-1). Histological count ratios cannot indicate how many of the proximal fibers are capable of conducting action potentials, nor how many fibers are not connected across the anastomosis, that is, end in the scar (see Chapter 15).

Our results in monofascicular tensionless primary nerve repairs demonstrated by quantitative physiological methods that fascicular tubulization with hypoantigenic collagen results in greater regeneration compared with fascicular suture in the rat (fascicular) model. In this same study[31] the authors demonstrated that tubulization repairs were statistically superior to fibrin blood clot repairs (P < 0.001), and there was no statistical difference between fibrin blood clot and suture repair by area of the compound action potential (P > 0.3).

These results argue that although histological methods may demonstrate no difference between repair techniques, there may still be differences that can be detected using our physiological method (see Chapter 15). Thus

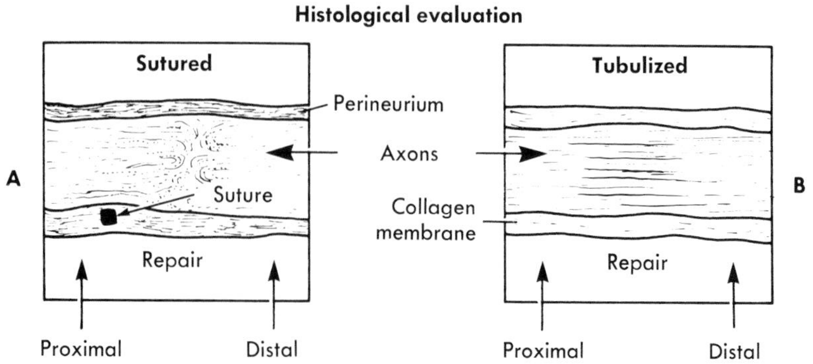

Histological evaluation

Fig. 25-4. Pattern of regeneration. Schematic longitudinal sections of repair site. **A,** Suture repair demonstrating disorganized pattern of regeneration, which is also seen in clot repair. **B,** Tubulization repair demonstrating longitudinally organized pattern of regeneration at repair site.

it will probably be necessary to use such evaluation methods to avoid discarding better repair techniques on the basis of insufficiently sensitive histological analysis.

The following alternatives can account for our success in showing superiority of tubulization repair over suture.

1. Our physiological testing method is sufficiently sensitive to detect differences that might have been found in tubulization experiments with other materials if the same testing method had been used.
2. It is necessary to use hypoantigenic collagen to achieve the differences observed.
3. The rat saphenous nerve model is sufficiently different (that is, monofascicular) that our results are applicable only to this specific location.

Obviously, further experimentation will be needed to distinguish between the alternatives of evaluation method, repair material, and animal model, as described in the foregoing sections. But our results may be sufficient to encourage further experimentation with sutureless techniques, which have a number of theoretical advantages, as will be described in the remainder of this chapter.

In tubulization the nerve ends are brought loosely together and a blood clot forms between the two ends of the transected nerve. Weiss proposed that the shrinkage or "syn-

eresis" of the blood clot may lead to longitudinal tension on the fibrin structure connecting the two ends of the nerve when the repair site is enclosed in a tube without sutures.[35] Orientation of the fibrin matrix may then influence the outgrowing nerve fibers into uninterrupted parallel bundles of fibers that grow across the anastomosis (Fig. 25-4). The orderly regeneration that results from tubulization may in part explain the increased axonal regeneration we observed. In both fascicular suture and fibrin blood clot repairs, a disorderly array of regenerating axons develops at the site of repair (see Fig. 25-4).

Inside the epineurium each fascicle is surrounded by perineurium, a unique structure composed of perineurial cells and collagenous support.[32] The collagen fibers of the perineurium are finer than those of the epineurium, and there is a relative absence of the elastic fibers found in the epineurium. The epineurium functions as a blood-nerve barrier isolating the enclosed nerve fibers from the outside environment.[29] The perineurium must be intact for normal axonal flow (see Chapter 7).

In fascicular suture and fibrin blood clot repair the anastomosis is not protected from the invasion of the epineurial connective tissue and does not prevent the escape of regenerating axons and Schwann cells. In addition, the space around the sutures also acts as

Histological evaluation

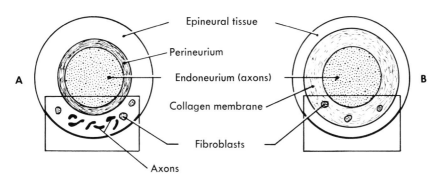

Fig. 25-5. Protective barrier. Schematic transverse sections of repair site just distal to anastomosis. **A,** Suture repair demonstrating axons outside of perineurium in epineurial tissue, which is also seen in clot repair. **B,** Tubulization repair demonstrating protective barrier of collagen membrane preventing escape of axons into epineurial tissue.

a pathway for invasion and escape of these elements (Fig. 25-5). By contrast, in fascicular tubulization the tube of collagen may act as a protective barrier isolating the enclosed nerve fibers from the extraneural mesodermal environment (see Fig. 25-5). The tube may provide a barrier to prevent axons and Schwann cells from escaping and may act to protect the gap between the proximal and distal stumps from the ingrowth of the epineurial mesenchymal connective tissue elements, which are prone to fibrosis and may block the path of regenerating nerve fibers.

REFERENCES

1. Berger, A., Meissl, G., and Samii, M.: Experimentelle Erfahrungen mit Kollagenfolien uber nahtlose Nerven-Anastomosen, Acta Neurochir. (Wien) **23:** 141, 1970.
2. Bora, F. W., Pleasure, D. E., and Didzian, N. A.: A study of nerve regeneration and neuroma formation after nerve suture by various techniques, J. Hand Surg. **1:**138, 1976.
3. Braun, R. M.: Comparative studies of neurorrhaphy and sutureless peripheral nerve repair, Surg. Gynecol. Obstet. **122:**15, 1966.
4. Bungner, v. O.: Ueber die degenerations—and regenerations—vorange am nerven nach cerletzungen, Beitr. Pathol. **10:**321, 1891.
5. Cabaud, H. E., et al.: Epineurial and perineurial fascicular nerve repairs: a critical comparison, J. Hand Surg. **1:**131, 1976.
6. Campbell, J., et al.: Microfilter sheaths in peripheral nerve surgery, J. Trauma **1:**139, 1961.
7. Ducker, T. B.: Personal communication, 1977.
8. Ducker, T. B., and Hayes, G. J.: Peripheral nerve injuries: a comparative study of the anatomical and functional results following primary nerve repair in chimpanzees, Milit. Med. **133:**298, 1968.
9. Freeman, B. S.: Adhesive anastomosis technique for fine nerves: experimental and chemical techniques, Am. J. Surg. **108:**529, 1964.
10. Furthmayr, H., and Timpl, R.: Immunochemistry of collagens and procollagens, Int. Rev. Connect. Tissue Res. **7:**61, 1976.
11. Goldfarb, A., et al.: Plasma clot tensile strength measurement: its relation to plasma fibrinogen, J. Clin. Invest. **22:**183, 1943.
12. Goto, Y.: Experimental study of nerve autografting by funicular suture, Arch. Jpn. Chir. **36:**478, 1967.
13. Grabb, W. C., et al.: Comparison of methods of peripheral nerve suturing in monkeys, Plast. Reconstr. Surg. **46:**31, 1970.
14. Hakstian, R. W.: Funicular orientation by direct stimulation, J. Bone Joint Surg. **50A:**1178, 1968.
15. Hurwitz, P. J., et al.: Microsurgical techniques and the use of tissue adhesive in the repair of peripheral nerves, J. Surg. Res. **17:**245, 1974.
16. Ito, T., Hirotani, H., and Yanamoto, K.: Peripheral nerve repairs by the funicular suture technique, Acta Orthop. Scand. **47:**283, 1974.
17. Kline, D. G., and Hayes, G. J.: The use of a resorbable wrapper for peripheral nerve repair, J. Neurosurg. **21:**737, 1964.
18. Knapp, T. R., Kaplan, E. N., and Daniels, J. R.: Injectable collagen for soft tissue augmentation, Plast. Reconstr. Surg. **60:**398, 1977.

19. Knapp, T. R., Luck, E., and Daniels, J. R.: Behavior of solubilized collagen as a bioimplant, J. Surg. Res. **23**:96, 1977.

20. Lehman, R. A. W., Hayes, G. J., and Leonard, F.: Toxicity of alkyl 2—cyanoacrylates I, peripheral nerve, Arch. Surg. **93**:441, 1966.

21. Levinthal, R., Brown, W. J., and Rand, R. W.: Comparison of fascicular, interfascicular and epineurial suture techniques in the repair of simple nerve lacerations, J. Neurosurg. **47**:744, 1977.

22. Matras, H., et al.: Plasma clot welding of nerves, J. Maxillofac. Surg. **1**:236, 1973.

23. Metz, R., and Seeger, W.: Collagen wrapping of nerve homotransplants in dogs, Eur. Surg. Res. **1**:157, 1969.

24. Midgley, R. D., and Woolhouse, F. M.: Silicone rubber sheathing as an adjunct to neural anastomosis, Surg. Clin. North Am. **48**:1149, 1968.

25. Millesi, H., Berger, A., and Meissl, G.: Experimentelle Untersuchungen zur Heilung durchtrennter peripherer Nerven, Chir. Plast. (Berl) **1**:174, 1972.

26. Millesi, H., Meissl, G., and Berger, A.: The interfascicular nerve grafting of the median and ulnar nerves, J. Bone Joint Surg. **54**:727, 1972.

27. O'Brien, B.: Microvascular reconstructive surgery, New York, 1977, Churchill Livingstone, Chap. 16.

28. Orgel, M. G., and Terzis, J. K.: Epineurial vs. Perineurial repair. An ultrastructural and electrophysiological study of nerve regeneration, Plast. Reconstr. Surg. **60**:80, 1977.

29. Peters, A., Sanford, P., and Webster, H.: The fine structure of nervous system; the neurons and supporting cells, Philadelphia, 1976, W. B. Saunders Co.

30. Reid, R. L., Cutright, D. E., and Garrison, J. S.: Biodegradable cuff an adjunct to peripheral nerve repair; a study in dogs, Government Report 35762775A825, August 29, 1977.

31. Rosen, J. M., et al.: Fascicular sutureless and suture repair of the peripheral nerves. A comparison study in laboratory animals, Orthop. Rev. **8**(4):85, 1979.

32. Shantahveerappa, T., and Bourne, G.: Perineurial epithelium: a new concept of its role in the integrity of the peripheral nervous system, Science **154**:1464, 1966.

33. Tarlov, I. M., et al.: Plasma clot suture of nerves, Arch. Surg. **47**:44, 1943.

34. Usbeck, W.: Nerve suture without tension, a method for repairing transected peripheral nerves, Acta Neurochir. (Wien) **34**:215, 1976.

35. Weiss, P. A.: Sutureless reunion of severed nerves with elastic cuffs of Tantalum, J. Neurosurg. **1**:370, 1944.

36. Weiss, P. A.: From cell research to nerve repair: articles illustrating the transition from biological experience to medical practice, New York, 1976, Futura Publishing Co., Inc., p. 315.

37. Weiss, P. A., and Taylor, A. C.: Guides for nerve regeneration across gaps, J. Neurosurg. **3**:400, 1946.

38. Wise, A. J., et al.: A comparative analysis of macro and microsurgical neurorrhaphy techniques, Am. J. Surg. **117**:566, 1969.

39. Woodhall, B., and Beebe, G., eds.: Peripheral nerve regeneration—a follow-up study of 3,656 World War II injuries, VA Medical Monograph, 1956.

40. Yanamoto, K.: A comparative analysis of the process of nerve regeneration following funicular and epineurial suture for peripheral nerve repair, Arch. Jpn. Chir. **43**:276, 1974.

DISCUSSION

Clayton Wiley (San Diego): When Wendell used this technique with spinal cords, I believe he had the problem that movement of the spinal cord caused separation to a larger gap. Have you solved this problem by immobilizing the limbs used?

Kaplan: First of all, the collagen in his study was not the hypoantigenic collagen. Second, I'm not sure that a slight distraction of the nerve ends is a disadvantage in peripheral nerve repair. I can't really comment on whether it makes a difference within the spinal cord, but a slight distraction of the nerve ends in peripheral nerve may not be of any significance. Perhaps as long as the nerve ends lie within the tube, you still have the same situation for regrowth of the axon. Thus the answer to your question is no; there has been no attempt to immobilize the limb. None of our repairs pulled apart.

Anonymous: I'd just like to comment on this beautiful work. It's really stimulated my excitement to feel that in any of our evaluations for the future, this method probably should be tried as a third group.

Dick Braun (San Diego): I can answer your question because we have done it. It was published in 1965. You do have more failures with the collagen film wraparound tubulization technique, because you can't control the nerves pulling apart inside the tube once you close up the animal. So you have several choices, one is to gimmick the study. You put a suture at the end of the tube, so that the nerve won't pull pack on you. You use some sort of stay-suture technique. With this variation you can usually produce a better repair pattern with the tubulization technique, using a model exactly like this. That's the good news. The bad news is that you can produce the same result in this model, in a rat, by putting the piece of nerve down on a piece of tape, putting them down in a block of Silastic that has been carved to create a trough, putting them inside an artery, putting them inside a vein, and probably just letting them lie there. The problem is that the rat is going to really try to repair that nerve. So I don't think this is a great model to live with for very long, once you get your feet on the ground and start working.

Kaplan: What we're comparing is sutures with a sutureless method. Point No. 1 is should we be using sutures at all? What you're saying is that tubulization methods, regardless of what kind of tube you're using, are better than sutures, and I would agree with that. The problem with all of the prior sutureless, tubed methods was that eventually there was a problem with the material you were using for the tube. With silicone, it kinked; it caused compression when there was swelling, and the tube didn't expand. The tube that we're using does not have those disadvantages. I'm not claiming that the results are, in the long run, going to be applied to human or clinical situations, but I think that conceptually I see no theoretical disadvantage to what I am proposing.

Edshage: I would like to know if you have made any studies on the tensile strength during the first week after repair by this method. This is most essential when you try to apply this to human material. This was the crucial point with the attempt to use tantalum. It was very promising, but then, we all know the story.

Kaplan: No, we have not measured the tensile strength.

26

Experience with clinical methods of testing sensation after peripheral nerve surgery

Svante Edshage

Regeneration after peripheral nerve surgery follows a pattern schematically drawn in Fig. 26-1. Before surgery has been performed there is no sensory function below the point of the lesion in the area supplied by the nerve. When axons have crossed the suture line, a Tinel's sign can be elicited over the advancing axons. The Tinel's sign proceeds along the nerve until the target for the axons in the skin is reached. In the area of innervation the newly arrived axons give rise to paresthesias. This means that light stroking of the skin elicits a tingling sensation. From this point on two possible courses seem to exist. There is a normal route by which protective sensory function develops in the skin or an abnormal route in which the paresthesias progress to a pathological stage of painful sensation, hyperesthesia, on touching the skin. The latter is particularly the case when the skin is not used or trained to sensory stimuli but voluntarily or involuntarily protected. In the normal situation protective sensory function is followed by a state characterized by increasing two-point discrimination until tactile gnosis is present.

TESTS FOR SENSORY FUNCTION

It is necessary to establish what we do want to measure clinically and when. In my opinion the only thing that is of real interest is measurement of the progress of improved sensibility from protective sensation to tactile gnosis. As the von Frey test, the temperature test, the pinprick test, and even the vibration test are positive both with protective sensory function and with painful hyperesthesias, there is very little use for these tests.[3] The fact that the axons have reached the skin is shown by the presence of paresthesias, and to show this no real test is necessary. To follow the regeneration of sensory function from the state of protective sensation to the state of tactile gnosis we presently use the two-point discrimination test and the pickup test.

Two-point discrimination test

The two-point discrimination test is performed by pressing two blunt tips with decreasing distance between the tips against the skin to find the shortest distance that is felt as two points by the patient. The touch should be very light and only permit the skin to blanch in a limited area. The tips should not rest on the skin but merely touch it. The skin is touched either with one or both tips and the patient should report whether he feels one or two. The one-two variation should be without any pattern. For the best results it is necessary to perform 10 tests with each distance between the tips, preferably every millimeter. Five of these tests should be performed, with tests two and five having one tip touching the skin. The limit for two-point discrimination is found when less than seven of the answers are correct. Such a test will be very time consuming and is almost

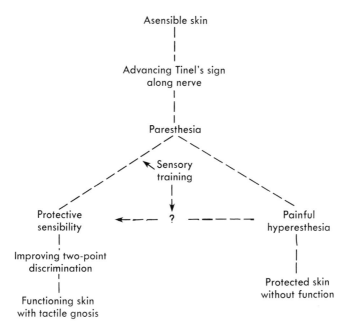

Fig. 26-1. Schematic illustration of returning sensibility after peripheral nerve surgery.

impossible in daily clinical work. In the clinic we prefer to perform the test in this way: we vary the stimuli as suggested above, and from the speed with which the answers are given, we can decide fairly exactly whether the patient is truly feeling one or two points. As soon as the patient starts to hesitate, we know that we are under the limit of his two-point discrimination. This means that only four or five tests with every distance are necessary.

There are several ways to misuse the two-point discrimination test. One way is to press too hard; this causes a spread of the stimuli to distant parts of the skin. Another way is to permit the patient to move his finger during the test; this gives a value lower than what is correct. The same is true if the two points are wiggled against the skin. The tips must not be sharp, as this will elicit painful stimuli and disturb the patient. The cooperation and concentration of the patient are necessary. The patient must be in a relaxed position and be able to concentrate on his fingertip while the test is performed. Of course, the test should be performed with the patient blindfolded.

If the test is performed correctly, it can give very accurate answers, and a decreasing two-point discrimination can be found after peripheral nerve surgery until the stage of tactile gnosis. On the fingertips this means a value below 10 mm and sometimes even down to the normal value of 3 to 4 mm.

Pickup test

When this test is first performed, the patient is allowed to view 10 small objects laying on a cloth surface near a box. He is asked to pick up the objects as quickly as possible and put them in the box. After this he is asked to perform the same test blindfolded. It is of course possible to measure the time required, but there are several factors that may influence the result. The motor function of the hand is highly involved in the test, so a better pickup test may be found not as a result of better sensory function but as a result of better motor function. Therefore we rarely rely on the time required, but instead judge the skill with which the patient performs the test. This test may be made a little more difficult by adding pieces like bolts and nuts of different sizes and by asking the patient to screw a nut onto a bolt that is held by the investigator.

Arrow test

In our clinic we have worked with a new test, which is called the arrow test. The blindfolded patient is asked to point out the direction in which a slightly elevated arrow is pointing. The arrows have different sizes, and we try to find the smallest arrow that can be correctly identified. This test, however, does not give as reproducible results as we initially thought, and we are presently trying to construct a better test of this type.

Test for sweat secretion

In the literature the sweat secretion tests are often mentioned as tests for sensory function. Some comments on the sweat secretion test therefore seem to be necessary.

Testing sweat secretion from the skin can be performed either by a starch-iodine test or the Ninhydrin test. First of all, one must be aware that these tests are not tests for sensory function. Returning sweat secretion after peripheral nerve surgery is not to be equated with returning sensibility. There is no relationship whatsoever between these two functions.

After an injury to a peripheral nerve, loss of sweat secretion is the rule. An absence of sweat secretion in a skin area will then be an objective sign of loss of sensory function. After a time period of up to 6 months, there may be returning sweat secretion without any sensory function, and there may also be some sensory function without sweat secretion. The later, though, is very unusual. The same is true after peripheral nerve surgery, especially nerve suture. Here the rule is that sweat secretion is found long before sensory function has returned, especially sensory function with the quality of tactile gnosis.

SUMMARY

The drawbacks of the tests that we find of value in evaluating our cases of peripheral nerve suture are numerous. The two-point discrimination test is a very difficult test to

perform. It must be performed by a skilled investigator. Rarely is it possible to use a physical therapist or an occupational therapist to perform this test without very thorough instructions. In the follow-up of a patient the same investigator must perform all the tests, as variations caused by the investigator's technique are frequent. Therefore most of the time it is necessary for the surgeon to perform the tests himself. The tests are time consuming and necessitate a certain intelligence from the patient. They are very difficult to use in children, especially small children. Sometimes we have found that the two-point discrimination test gives us values that indicate that tactile gnosis is present, but functional tests will not confirm this. This may be due either to deficient motor function or to the patient having developed a technique for differentiating one from two stimuli. In other words he has become a good two-point discriminator. We also find the opposite, where two-point discrimination is above the value of tactile gnosis but the patient has functional sensibility that enables him to perform even rather delicate work with the previously denervated fingertips without the aid of vision.

The pickup test is a very good functional test but has previously mentioned limits, as motor function must be almost intact or at least in a steady state so that it does not influence the results of tests made in a series. When time is not used to quantitate the pickup test, there is only the possibility of subjective evaluation of the test with all the usual errors of such an evaluation, especially when performed by the operating surgeon.

When the two-point discrimination test and the pickup test are combined, we may find four different situations.

1. The two-point discrimination is good and there is a good pickup test. Tactile gnosis is present, and regeneration has reached a functional level.
2. There is a poor two-point discrimination but a good pickup test. The functional sensibility has been regained, even if we are not able to measure it. In

these cases we tend to disregard the two-point discrimination and classify our results as good.

3. There is good two-point discrimination and a poor pickup test. The result of the peripheral nerve surgery is questionable.

4. Both tests are negative. The bad result is obvious.

Interpretation of the inconsistencies between the two tests and the poor correlation between electrophysiological tests and functional tests sometimes seen may be facilitated by discussing perception of the sensory stimuli we get from the surrounding world.

PERCEPTION

Generally speaking one may say that feeling, like hearing or seeing, cannot be equated with understanding. One may think of hearing or seeing a foreign word without knowing the language. It is necessary to understand the message that is brought from the periphery in order to interpret it correctly. It is very probable that after a peripheral nerve suture the impulses coming into the brain are no longer recognized by the brain and thus the patient has to relearn in order to interpret the incoming new impulses correctly. This cannot be directly compared with learning a new language. It is partly due to the fact that after a peripheral nerve suture the patient is in a situation where an object is sending out a different message when touched with the right hand as compared to the left hand. In that situation the patient must be able to interpret differently the signal coming from one or the other hand. To understand the difficulties one may think of the difficulty that would ensue if the picture we saw with one eye differed in shape and form from the same picture viewed with the other eye. Our brain is not constructed for such a situation, and this may be partly responsible for the difficulty faced after a peripheral nerve suture. I have tried to elucidate what I mean by a sketch (Fig. 26-2). Interpretation in the brain is generally believed to be achieved by bringing out of memory different patterns that are compared with the incoming signals. The closest match is accepted as the correct one, and the incoming signal is interpreted as being one of that kind. In the depicted case when the eye sees the nut, the nut pattern is brought forward from memory and is matched with the information coming from the eye. When the normal hand is handling the nut and the patient is blindfolded, the nut pattern is once more brought forward from memory and is found to fit with the incoming information. The hand has recognized a nut. When the injured hand handles the nut, memory does not find anything that matches the incoming signals, and the patient does not recognize the nut. After comparing the visual and palpable images for a shorter or longer time period, the memory may store the new form produced by the injured hand and interpret this as a nut. The next time that particular information is produced by the injured hand it will be interpreted as a nut. This means that one model must be stored by memory for the injured side and another for the normal side, both being interpreted as the same thing by the eye.

This mode of action in perception is probably one of the causes for the much better results after peripheral nerve surgery in children. Their brain is able to accomodate much better to new circumstances. One may just think of how easily a child picks up a new language when stimulated in the right way. The same is probably true for a changed sensory situation.

TRAINING AND REEDUCATION

A definite necessity can be pointed out for training and reeducation after peripheral nerve surgery. It is not only that the new information coming in must be interpreted differently, but also that this information must be able to start the appropriate motor responses in the brain. Much of what we regard as voluntary movements are actually unconscious movements started by a certain sensory stimulus. When a new kind of stimulus comes in after a peripheral nerve injury,

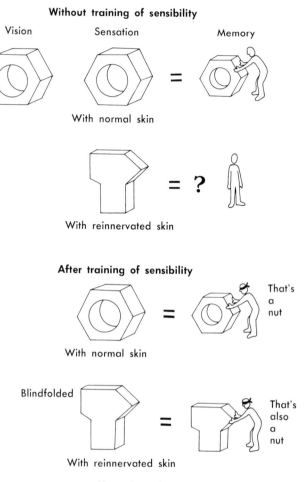

Fig. 26-2. Schematic presentation of hypothesis for interpretation of incoming sensory signals in brain.

training is necessary to start the appropriate motor response.

Wynn-Parry[4] has stressed the value of sensory training in rehabilitation of the hand, and Dellon[2] and his collaborators have shown that it is possible to improve the functional results by training. That an intensified training of sensation results in better sensory function is shown by the findings of Almquist[1] who found that blind people reading braille had a significantly lowered two-point discrimination as compared to seeing people.

FOR THE FUTURE

For the future we could wish for a better scientific test of returning sensibility than what we have presently, a test that is objective and quantitative and not influenced by motor function. Such a test should enable us to compare results in cases from different parts of the world and thus make it possible for us to collect a sufficiently large series of cases so that single changes in the operative technique could be evaluated correctly. At the same time we want to develop a clinical test that is easy to perform yet will give correct and reliable results in different situations. Such a test should enable us to evaluate cases with peripheral nerve injuries better, and, after peripheral nerve surgery, help and stimulate our patients to improve their results by training and reeducation.

SUMMARY

The techniques for sensory testing used clinically are described as used in our unit. The advantages and disadvantages of the tests are discussed and also the discrepancies between the results. A hypothetical explanation for the discrepancies is advanced.

REFERENCES

1. Almquist, E. E.: The effect of training on sensory function. Traumatic nerve lesions of the upper limb. In Michon, J., and Moberg, E., eds.: G.E.M. Monograph 2 London, 1975, Churchill Livingstone.
2. Dellon, A. L., Curtis, R. M., and Edgerton, K. E.: Reeducation of sensation in the hand after nerve injury and repair, Plast. Reconstr. Surg. **53:**297, 1974.
3. Moberg, E.: Objective methods of determining the functional value of sensibility of the hand, J. Bone Joint Surg. **40B:**454, 1958.
4. Wynn-Parry, C. B.: Rehabilitation of the hand, London, 1966, Butterworth & Co.

27

Sensory evaluation by the pickup test

George E. Omer, Jr.

In 1958, Moberg published the pickup test as a technique for determining the functional value of sensibility in the hand: ". . . pick up a number of small objects on a table and put them as quickly as he can into a small box, first with one hand and then with the other. After he has done this a few times he is asked to do the same thing blindfolded. It is then studied how rapidly and efficiently he picks up the objects; comparison is made between his right and left hands. The test with blindfolding can be made harder by asking him to identify the objects as he picks them up."[1] Moberg demonstrated the abnormal functional pattern in a hand with median cutaneous sensibility loss: the finger-chuck for picking up changes from the thumb–index finger to the thumb–ring finger for improved tactile gnosis. The pickup test is used only in patients with median or combined median and ulnar nerve injuries.

Seddon states that the precursor of the pickup test is the coin test, as described by Riddoch in 1940.[5] The patient, whose eyes must be closed, is given a coin and asked to identify it.

The pickup test was quantitated in the mid-1960's at Brooke Army Medical Center. We stated: "The test is measured by time required to pick up nine objects of different size and shape. The injured hand is checked against the uninjured hand, but a normal result is considered to be five to eight seconds."[3] This "normal" is for young adult males, and a better normal is the time required by the contralateral hand. At Moberg's suggestion, we used a piece of chalk as one of the nine objects because chalk would leave an obvious trail of functional surfaces.

At Brooke Army Medical Center we performed daily pickup tests for patients with traumatic nerve injuries over periods of many months. Our experience suggests that the pickup test improves with homeostasis of the hand.[4] Each patient performing the pickup test at regular intervals improved as the fibrosis of injury subsided and physical medicine treatment mobilized the injured hand. Another operation with subsequent immobilization of the hand always increased the pickup test time. At the end of the initial hospitalization the majority of the patients could perform the test at least twice as fast as they had done initially.

Moberg stated that tactile gnosis varies directly with the sudomotor function in the hand.[1] Gross sudomotor activity returns in the young individual in 9 to 12 months after injury without recovery of normal two-point discrimination distance.[2]

Moberg also stated that the hand must have sufficient motor function to make its sensibility of use.[1] The pickup test was utilized at Brooke Army Medical Center in a series of patients with high median nerve palsy that received neurovascular cutaneous island pedicle transfers to provide sensibility.[4] In spite of the area of normal two-point discrimination, the pickup test was slow in these patients; subsequently, there was a gradual loss of sensibility in the neurovascular cutaneous island pedicle to merely protective sensation. This gradual loss of sensibility was related to the associated motor loss for the radial side of the hand, and without adequate motion and power for tactile gnosis, the sensibility for precise prehension must be lost.

We noted that patients without good recovery of the nerve lesion could learn to recognize the majority of objects used in a given pickup test administered daily over a period of several months but would fail to recognize new objects introduced into the pickup test. This experience sensibility will disappear in the adult if the extremity is immobilized, as in a plaster cast, and must be relearned when activity is resumed.[2]

The pickup test will demonstrate abnormal functional patterns in hands with median or median and ulnar nerve injuries. The test is not static and will change with the level of homeostasis of the tissues, sensibility recovery, and motor function capability. Patients can improve results with experience with the test. The pickup test is a study of coordination involving sensory and motor function and is a good quantitative test of function.

REFERENCES

1. Moberg, E.: Objective methods for determining the functional value of sensibility in the hand, J. Bone Joint Surg. **40B:**454, 1958.
2. Omer, G. E. Jr.: Sensation and sensibility in the upper extremity, Clin. Orthop. **104:**30, 1974.
3. Omer, G. E. Jr.: Evaluation and reconstruction of the forearm and hand after acute treatment peripheral nerve injuries, J. Bone Joint Surg. **50A:**1454, 1968.
4. Omer, G. E. Jr., et al.: Neurovascular cutaneous island pedicles for deficient median nerve sensibility, J. Bone Joint Surg. **52A:**1181, 1970.
5. Seddon, H.: Surgical disorders of the peripheral nerves, ed. 2, New York, 1975, Churchill Livingstone, p. 53.

28

Clinical evaluation of the von Frey and two-point discrimination tests and correlation with a dynamic test of sensibility

Norman K. Poppen

The profound disability and loss of function following peripheral nerve injury was noted by Sterling Bunnell[3] in a report of the results of sutured nerves in the hand more than 50 years ago. Since that time, efforts to describe the return of sensation after nerve suture have led to the distinction between "academic recovery" (the response to conventional tests for touch and pain) and "functional recovery" (the ability to do work with the injured hand).[16]

This chapter presents an evaluation of three sensory testing methods used to assess the recovery of sensation following suture of 97 nerves in the hand in a group of 63 patients (49 patients had digital nerve injuries).

The three tests evaluated were: (1) the von Frey[22] plastic filaments test,[17] (2) the two-point discrimination test,[24] and (3) the ridge device test.[14,15]

SINGLE DIGITAL NERVE DEFICIT

In a series of 36 single digital nerve injuries, the area of sensory deficit was determined by "geographical mapping." This technique uses the end of a paper clip (or preferably a 3 gm von Frey filament) to map out the area of decreased sensation. Starting on the normal side of the digit, the end of the paper clip is lightly moved across the finger, and the patient asked to report changes in sensation. This is repeated at different areas until the whole area of deficit is outlined.

Fig. 28-1, *A*, shows a representative index finger with a single digital nerve injury after repair at the metacarpophalangeal level. There are usually two zones of deficit: an outer zone, where sensation changes from normal to altered, and an inner zone of worst sensation. Note that the zone of worst sensation is located on the axial third of the volar pulp. In the lateral view of the same injured index finger (Fig. 28-1, *B*), the area of worst sensation covers the entire axial surface of the volar pulp.

The volar digital nerve commonly gives off a dorsal branch distal to the metacarpophalangeal joint and proximal to the proximal finger crease.[23] More distal lesions may therefore produce a much smaller area of deficit. Fig. 28-2 shows the deficit after suture of a lesion at the distal joint level, a small area at the corner of the fingernail, and a small adjoining axial strip.

Two-point discrimination testing after digital nerve injuries at the distal interphalangeal or thumb interphalangeal joint level may be unreliable owing to the small area of the deficit, which may be smaller than the size of the appropriate two-point discrimination. Moberg[7] described similar limitation of two-point discrimination testing when applying

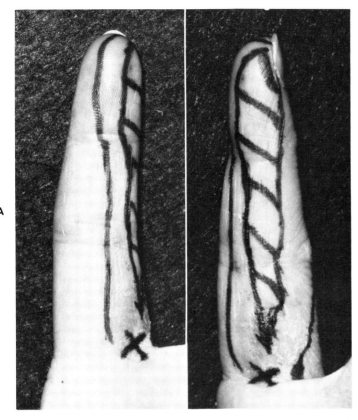

A

B

Fig. 28-1. Deficit area in single volar digital nerve injury at meta-carpophalangeal joint level. **A,** Volar view—maximal deficit area is located on axial third of distal phalanx. **B,** Lateral view.

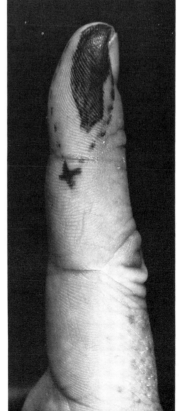

Fig. 28-2. Deficit area in single digital nerve injury at distal interphalangeal joint level.

the Weber compass to the narrow border zones of the fingertips.

Knowing the area of deficit, we can address the problem of where in the finger to test for recovery of sensation in single digital nerve injuries to avoid overlap sensation. Onnë[12] approached the problem by testing both sides of fingers with double digital nerve injuries and then averaging the two results.

We approached the problem of overlap sensation by blocking the common digital nerve supplying the uninjured side of the finger. A web space approach was used. By blocking the common digital nerve at the level of the midpalmar crease with 0.5 ml of lidocaine, we were able to confine the block to the uninjured nerve. The dorsum of the digit was blocked at metacarpal neck level through a separate injection site.

Sensory testing, both prior to and following lidocaine block of the uninjured nerve, was performed in 26 of 35 digits with single digital nerve injuries. von Frey plastic filaments (Semmes-Weinstein), a new two-point discrimination device, and a dynamic testing device, the plastic ridge, were employed. The end point was taken as eight correct responses out of ten trials.[1,2]

In those 26 nerves tested after block, no significant change occurred in the results as long as testing was carried out within the zone of worst sensation as previously determine by geographical mapping. Changes did, however, occasionally occur in the peripheral zone of altered sensation. Changes in this peripheral zone may account for the changes in tested value following nerve block noted in an earlier study by Honner and co-workers.[5] In their study the injured side of the finger in 28 of the 32 single digital nerve injuries tested was found to lose sensation following metacarpal level block.

PROBLEMS AND PITFALLS OF SENSORY TESTING

Almost innumerable factors can influence the results of sensory testing using von Frey plastic filaments. These include environmental factors (temperature, noise, stress), physiological factors (skin thickness, spotty mosaic reinnervation, hyperesthesia), testing technique, and fatigue. Patient and examiner bias is never completely eliminated. To obtain reproducible results, accurate sensory testing requires: a single examiner, an intelligent cooperative patient, sufficient time, and perfect technique (see Chapter 26).

The technique of performing the von Frey test is demanding. The filament must be applied perpendicular to the skin surface to maintain constant pressure.[18,20] We have found that percussion of the filament on the skin or sliding of the filament across the skin surface markedly lowers threshold values. Threshold of sensation has been found to change as a result of vibratory stimulation.[4,25] If less than 5 to 7 seconds is allowed between individual trials, a stimulus otherwise perceived as above threshold level may not be detected.[19,21] If the probit method is used and tests are performed at threshold, one level above threshold, and one level below threshold, then 30 tests are required for each digital nerve. To test both sides of the injured digit and contralateral digit, 120 tests and about 1 hour of time are required.

Even when correctly performed, the von Frey test measures only a threshold level of static touch. It is an "academic test" of recovery that is poorly correlated with functional sensibility.[8,16]

In addition to the preceding, two-point discrimination testing has unique problems of its own. Simultaneous application of the two points maintaining equal, constant pressure is difficult using one of the standard techniques and instruments. The two points must be applied simultaneously and with equal pressure to avoid inhibition of perception of one of the two points.[20] Care must be taken to apply the points longitudinally along the volar axial border of the finger or autonomous zone of the digital nerve to avoid crossover sensation from the other digital nerve.

The use of the Weber compass to measure two-point discrimination has an inherent error, as the angle of application of the tips decreases from the perpendicular with spreading of the tips and the applied pressure changes. The other common two-point discrimination device, the paper clip, requires application of "pressure to blanching."

In experiments using von Frey plastic filaments, a pressure of 8 to 15 gm was required to produce blanching equivalent to that of a 0.9 mm diameter paper clip at the point of minimal pressure to blanching. Since threshold after nerve repair uncommonly exceeds 3.63 gm,[13] this is an excessive amount of pressure. Even when using a rounded tip vernier caliper, maintaining a uniform, reproducible pressure with each individual test is most difficult. The Semmes-Weinstein Aesthesiometer[17] was used for the von Frey values in this study. Each instrument is labeled with a modified log value ($4 + \log_{10}$ gm). The range of forces available is from 0.0045 to 447.0 gm: therefore the modified log value of 4.56 corresponds to 3.63 gm.

To standardize the applied pressure, a new device was fabricated* (Fig. 28-3). This con-

*Two-Point Pressure Aesthesiometer, Research Design Incorporated, 9881 E. Harwin Drive, Houston, Texas 77036.

sisted of two parallel von Frey plastic filaments, each delivering a uniform pressure at bending of 3.6 gm. This pressure was above threshold for the injured nerves tested. A set of these devices with the interval between filaments ranging from 2 mm to 30 mm was used.

When correctly performed, two-point discrimination correlates better with functional sensibility than the von Frey test. Tactile gnosis is not present with two-point discrimination values exceeding 10 to 12 mm.[9,11] But this is not a test that corresponds to the way we identify objects, that is, by motion of a digit over a surface such as the thumb-forefinger motion used to ascertain the texture of a fabric. As Katz has pointed out: "The touch organ when at rest relative to external objects is beset with a partial anesthesia. Movement is as indispensable to touch as light is to vision."[6]

In an effort to find a dynamic test, a number of devices were evaluated. A plastic device that we call the ridge (Fig. 28-4) gave

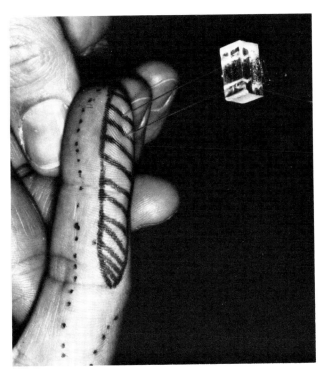

Fig. 28-3. Modified Weber two-point discrimination device—blunt points are applied in longitudinal axis of digit within deficit area determined by geographical mapping.

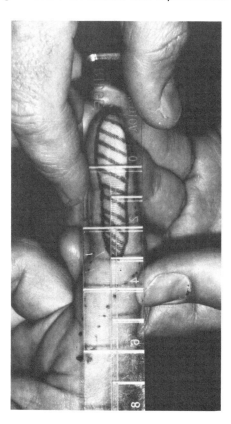

Fig. 28-4. Ridge device. With finger gently supported by examiner, device is moved from proximal to distal over area of maximal sensory deficit until patient declares that he feels ridge on a "not smooth" surface.

the most reproducible results. This device consists of a 10×1.5 cm rectangular block of plastic. It is smooth at one end, and there is a narrow central ridge that rises from the smooth end to attain a height of 1.5 mm at the opposite end. The transverse lines, located on the back side of the device, are at 1 cm intervals. Our device is a modification of a similar device used in Great Britian.[14,15] However, the British device is shorter and the maximum height of the ridge is 1 mm.

With the finger supported by the examiner, the smooth end of the device is touched to the area of sensory deficit. The slide is moved past the finger bringing increasing depths of the ridge into contact with the skin. Care must be taken to avoid contact with skin outside the area of sensory deficit. The slide is moved at a rate of 10 cm in approximately 10 seconds. On a normal finger, the ridge will be felt at or before the first 1 cm division. On the injured finger with poor sensory return, the ridge may not be felt at all. In contrast to testing with the von Frey plastic filaments and the two-point discrimination device, which may require 40 to 60 minutes each using the probit method, both nerves of the injured digit and the corresponding nerves of the contralateral digit may be evaluated in 5 minutes using the ridge device.

In a study group of 63 patients, the autonomous sensory area of 97 injured nerves in the hand and the 97 matching uninjured nerves was studied. Normal values for the von Frey test were less than or equal to 1 gm. A group of hardworking patients with heavy callosities had values in the 1.2 to 2 gm

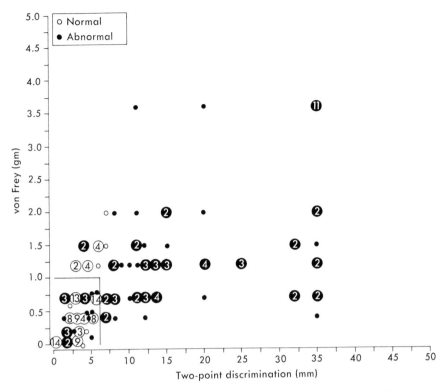

Fig. 28-5. Relationship between threshold for von Frey values and two-point discrimination. For sutured nerves, 97 injured nerves are plotted in black o and 97 uninjured nerves in white o. (Same convention is used for Figs. 28-6 and 28-7). For uninjured nerves, normal values correspond to von Frey less than or equal to 1 gm and two-point discrimination less than or equal to 6 mm.

range. There is considerable overlap of the von Frey values for injured nerves with the normal values, especially in the gray zone of 1.2 to 2 gm (Fig. 28-5). Normal values for two-point discrimination were less than or equal to 6 mm.

For the injured nerves, there is a general trend correlating increasing values for von Frey and two-point discrimination tests. This correlation is highly significant, but the correlation coefficient is only 0.7. This is in general agreement with Onnë's findings.[12] In both studies, there is a considerable spread of the plotted values. This means you cannot predict von Frey values from two-point discrimination test results, and you cannot predict two-point discrimination values from von Frey test results.

Normal values of sensation tested with the

plastic ridge were less than or equal to 1.5 cm. Test results from injured nerves show that inability to feel the ridge was arbitrarily correlated with the von Frey test results (Fig. 28-6).

The most interesting comparison is that between values obtained for two-point discrimination and values obtained with the plastic ridge (Fig. 28-7). A ridge value of less than 2 cm was found to correspond to a two-point discrimination of less than 10 mm. It should be noted that the American Society for Surgery of the Hand considers two-point discrimination greater than 10 mm as poor. In any area of sensation where the two-point discrimination exceeded 12 mm, the plastic ridge could not be felt. All patients who could not feel the plastic ridge had two-point discrimination values greater than or equal to 8

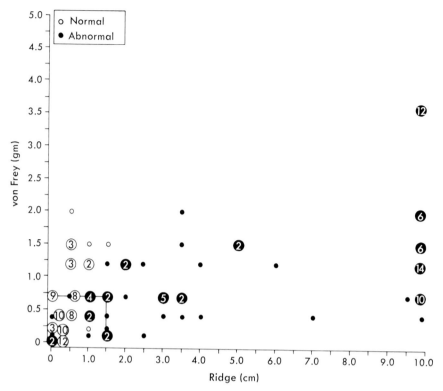

Fig. 28-6. Relationship between threshold for ridge and von Frey values. For uninjured nerves, normal values correspond to von Frey less than or equal to 1 gm and ridge less than or equal to 1.5 cm.

mm. Moberg[10] states that tactile gnosis is hardly present with two-point discrimination values exceeding 8 mm. Two-point discrimination values between 8 and 12 mm would seem to be of dubious significance, since some of these patients are unable to feel a 1.5 mm ridge on a smooth slab of plastic. In such a situation, it seems unreasonable to consider tactile gnosis to be present.

Results corresponding to two-point discrimination values can be approximated by use of the plastic ridge. Testing with the plastic ridge is, however, more reproducible and quicker than two-point discrimination testing.

SUMMARY

1. There are definable patterns of sensory return after suture of a digital nerve that vary with the level of injury. This results in an autonomous zone of sensation for an individual digital nerve. In this zone, accurate evaluation of sensory return after nerve suture is possible.

2. In many cases the von Frey test is not sensitive enough to discriminate between injured and uninjured nerves.

3. Two-point discrimination is a better test than the von Frey, but correlation with tactile gnosis is difficult in the range between 8 and 12 mm.

4. Results of sensory testing with a plastic ridge device are presented. Only those patients whose two-point discrimination values indicate usable sensation by the American Society for Surgery of the Hand criteria can feel the ridge. More importantly, the ridge detects the presence or absence of tactile

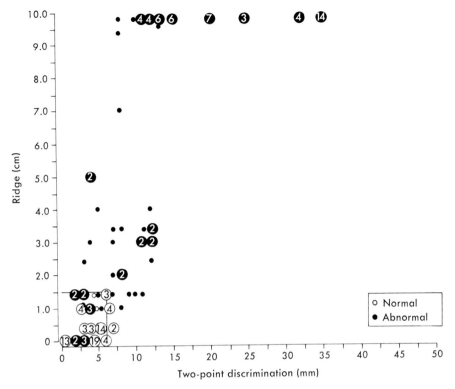

Fig. 28-7. Relationship between threshold for ridge and two-point discrimination. For uninjured nerves, normal values correspond to ridge less than or equal to 1.5 cm and two-point discrimination less than or equal to 6 mm.

gnosis in patients with two-point discrimination in the intermediate range between 8 and 12 mm.

ACKNOWLEDGMENT

I would like to express my appreciation to Drs. John J. Niebauer, Robert L. Brown, and James R. Doyle for permission to examine their patients and to Ms. Barbara Kamm for the computer analysis of the data.

REFERENCES

1. Bliss, C.: The method of probits, Science **79**:38, 1934.
2. Bliss, C.: The method of probits—a correction, Science **79**:409, 1934.
3. Bunnell, S.: Surgery of the nerves of the hand, Surg. Gynecol. Obstet. **44**:145, 1927.
4. Cohen, L. H., and Lindley, S. B.: Studies in vibratory sensibility, Am. J. Psychol. **51**:44, 1938.
5. Honner, R., Fragiadakis, E. G., and Lamb, D. W.: An investigation of the factors affecting the results of digital nerve divisions, The Hand **2**:21, 1970.
6. Katz, D.: Der Aufbau de Tastwelt. Zeitschrift für Psychologie, 1925. In Kruegar, L.: David Katz's Der Aufbau der Tastwelt (The world of touch): a synopsis, Percept. Psychopsych. **7**:337, 1970.
7. Moberg, E.: Objective methods for determining the functional value of sensibility in the hand, J. Bone Joint Surg. **40B**:454, 1958.
8. Moberg, E.: Criticism and study of methods for examining sensibility in the hand, Neurology **12**:8, 1962.
9. Moberg, E.: Evaluation and management of nerve injuries in the hand, Surg. Clin. North Am. **44**:1019, 1964.
10. Moberg, E.: Methods for examining sensibility of the hand. In Flynn, J. E., ed.: Hand surgery, ed. 2, Baltimore, 1975, The Williams & Wilkins Co.
11. Moberg, E.: Reconstructive hand surgery in tetraplegia, stroke and cerebral palsy: some basic concepts in physiology and neurology, J. Hand Surg. **1**:29, 1976.
12. Onnë, L.: Recovery of sensibility and sudomotor activity in the hand after nerve suture, Acta Chir. Scand. Suppl. **300**:1, 1962.

13. Poppen, N., et al.: Recovery of sensibility after suture of digital nerves, J. Hand Surg. **4:**212, 1979.
14. Renfrew, S.: Aesthiometers, Lancet **1:**1011, 1960.
15. Renfrew, S.: Fingertip sensation, a routine neurological test, Lancet **1:**396, 1969.
16. Seddon, H. J., ed.: Peripheral nerve injuries, London, 1954, Her Majesty's Stationery Office, p. 1.
17. Semmes, J., et al.: Somatosensory changes after penetrating brain wounds in man, Cambridge, 1960, Harvard University Press.
18. von Békésy, G.: The neural terminations responding to stimulation of pressure and vibration, J. Exp. Psychol. **26:**514, 1940.
19. von Békésy, G.: Neural volleys and the similarity between some sensations produced by tones and skin vibrations, J. Acoust. Soc. Am. **29:**1059, 1957.
20. von Békésy, G.: Neural funnelling along the skin and between the inner and outer hair cells of the cochlea, J. Acoust. Soc. Am. **31:**1236, 1959.
21. von Békésy, G.: Sensory inhibition, Princeton, 1975, Princeton University Press.
22. von Frey, M.: Beitrage zur Physiologic des Schmesinns, Ber Sachs Ges Wissench. **46:**283, 1894.
23. Wallace, W. A., and Coupland, R. E.: Variations in the nerves of the thumb and index finger, J. Bone Joint Surg. **57B:**491, 1975.
24. Weber, E. H.: Ueber den Tastsinn, Arch. Anat. Physiol. Wissench. Med. p. 152, 1835.
25. Weddell, C. H., and Cumming, S. B.: Fatigue of vibratory sense, J. Exp. Psychol. **22:**429, 1938.

DISCUSSION

Doyle: We spent quite a bit of time discussing techniques for evaluating sensibility. I want to ask Dr. O'Brien to come forward and answer this question: Just how important is sensibility to function? Do you think it's really important? Have we been wasting our time talking about sensibility?

B. O'Brien (Melbourne): Two-point discrimination is not always a reliable assessment of work performance. For instance, the radial digital nerve may be divided cleanly and an excellent microneural union carried out. For a long time the patient will use his other normal fingers in preference to this index finger until the level of sensibility reached on the radial aspect of the index finger is of sufficient quality to enable him to use that aspect of the digit with precision. Indeed, for the finest tasks, even after years, the patient may prefer to use the normal adjacent middle finger in preference to the index finger where, although the two-point discrimination may be less than 10 mm, the quality of sensibility has not reached a sufficiently precise level.

When the number of normal digits is greatly reduced or even completely absent, we see a different situation. These mutilated hands can be reconstructed by the use of toe transfers or iliac crest bone grafts with neurovascular free flaps from the first web of the foot wrapped around them or with cross-hand, ring finger transfers. We have not seen the two-point discrimination reach a level better than existed on the donor foot or hand, and, usually, the two-point discrimination was less than in the donor site. Yet, there has been a significant upgrading of the function of these mutilated hands by these rather sophisticated microvascular transfers. The patients will use digits with two-point discrimination of 15 mm or more with a good work performance. They simply do not have any other digit to use. The value of the nerve repairs must be related to the work performance, and the two-point discrimination may be only a rough guide to the level of that performance. Too much emphasis has been placed on two-point discrimination and not enough on the capacity of the patient to use the affected parts. More and more I rely on the patient's description of his work performance and my own observations of his work capacity.

Doyle: Thank you very much for that delightful perspective on this interesting problem, Dr. O'Brien. Dr. Jack Tupper, I'd like to ask you a question. You and I don't have time to do 30,000 separate tests. We do not have all the time that Dr. Edshage has told us it takes to get some really useful information about sensibility. In your office when those patients are in the waiting room and you want to evaluate your nerve repair, how do you do it? Have you got any tricks to tell us about, Jack?

Tupper: I think the main trick is that the medic or the therapist does the major portion of our evaluation for us. I would agree with most of what has been said this morning. I think, however, one additional point should be emphasized. I keep hearing the word normal or near-normal sensation used. I don't think I have a single digital nerve repair in a postepiphyseal closure adult that has normal sensation. I don't think these patients have even a percentage of normal sensation. These people do not have normal sensation diminished. They have different sensation; they have paresthesias, and this changes a great deal. This means that the patient who is extremely clever, who is adaptable and so forth, is able to use his hand extremely well. Some people have a neurosensory stupidity that precludes them ever using anything. We have all seen the index

261

finger with a little hypesthesia that has become an emotional amputation.

I would like to mention one other detail. My therapist has developed a chart sheet with a hand diagram on it to document the area used for testing. Therefore two-point testing is always done in the same place. I think this is of some importance as it provides some consistency.

Niebauer: I think we should keep in mind the fact that peripheral nerve lesions also disrupt the sympathetic nerves. With loss of sympathetic tone, sweating stops within 30 minutes. This can be detected by feeling the affected finger pulp and comparing the wetness with an uninvolved pulp. I find this is particularly useful in young children when cooperation after an acute injury is poor.

When the injury is long-standing, the skin is not only dry but also very smooth and soft. This change from normal can be seen as well as palpated, and thus it is a good objective test.

Doyle: Yes, I agree. The third gentleman that we would like to help us in this discussion is Dr. Dykes.

Robert Dykes (Halifax): We're faced with a very serious problem of having, as we all heard, no adequate way to test sensibility. Most of the procedures that we use, in fact, for testing sensibility were developed as neurological tests before the turn of the century, and, with the single and major contribution of Dr. Moberg, I believe that is still the state of the art. There is nothing existing that is comparable to the Snellen eye chart for testing visual acuity, and something like this I'm sure must be developed. We can't say "Well, these tests aren't good enough, let's not do them." We have to find a better way to do it.

29

Factors affecting clinical results of nerve suture

James R. Doyle

The results following nerve suture are often inconsistent, unpredictable, and variable. The experienced nerve surgeon has long recognized this enigma. It is important, therefore, to look at some factors that might affect the outcome of nerve suture. It must be understood, however, that multiple factors are involved and that each of these factors is subject to a wide range of variation. Furthermore, it is the variation and complex interplay of these factors that make it exceedingly difficult to evaluate the effect of any single factor in a given case. Certain factors, however, lend themselves to discussion and include the age of the patient, nature of the injury, size of the defect, level of the injury, time from injury to suture, type of nerve, and surgical or technical factors.

Age

In the adult group the age of the patient as an isolated factor has no apparent effect on the rate of regeneration or quality of the end result. In contrast, all other factors being equal, the rate and quality of recovery in children are faster and better.[9] Although retrograde neuronal degeneration following injury is more severe in children than in adults, this does not overbalance the superior recovery noted in children.[9]

It must also be appreciated that children are capable of central reorganization,[9] which makes it possible for them to sometimes achieve astounding function in a part that has been partially or even completely denervated. It is well known that children are quite capable of establishing substitution patterns in use and function of a part that will often circumvent or bypass an area of poor motor function or poor sensibility.

In regard to an age limit after which nerve suture should not be performed, Elkington[2] stated that it was doubtful that nerve suture was of real value after age 50. This statement is in contrast to that of Marble and others who noted good results in patients over 50 years of age.[3,4,8] It is unlikely that an experienced nerve surgeon would deny surgery to a patient with an injured peripheral nerve based solely on the factor of advanced age.

Nature of injury

The greater the violence to the axon, the greater the retrograde reaction and neuronal death. The intensity of the reaction is also increased with the length of the nerve destroyed.[9] Significant neuronal death and incomplete recovery of the neuron from these retrograde effects would, of course, limit axonal regeneration and subsequently the quality of recovery. A crush or other such injury is usually associated with poorer recovery than a clean laceration because of several other factors including: (1) increased dissimilarity of funicular pattern at the suture line owing to loss of nerve substance and consequent funicular mismatch; (2) union under tension because of loss of nerve substance; (3) associated tissue injuries including bone, muscle, and vascular supply; (4) infection; and (5) prolonged delay in nerve repair secondary to associated tissue injuries.

Size of defect

As previously noted, the intensity of the proximal neuronal reaction increases with the length of nerve destroyed. Zachary found that the greater the gap, the worse the prognosis.[10] Nicholson and Seddon[6] found that in reference to epineurial repair of the median nerve defects or gaps of less than 2.5 cm resulted in grade M3 or better in 70%, whereas gaps of 2.6 cm to 5 cm resulted in a grade of M3 or better in 50%. These preceding comments are in reference to epineurial or similar-type sutures. Milessi, in reference to his experience with nerve grafting, noted that 12 of 15 median nerves with defects of 5 cm or less gained M4 function or better, in contrast to 5 of 13 nerves with defects greater than 5 cm. Ten of twenty-four nerves with defects of 5 cm or less regained a level of S3+, while only 5 of 14 nerves with defects greater than 5 cm regained S3+ level.[5]

Large defects make end-to-end suture difficult and introduce the hazards of tension at the repair site and, secondarily, postoperative stretching of the nerve when the joint is mobilized. Loss of significant portions of nerve result in loss of axial relationships and, therefore, funicular pattern. It must also be observed that large gaps in nerves are more often than not associated with more severe injuries, which may result in delays in nerve suture.[9] In general, the greater the gap the worse the prognosis.

Level of injury

Generally, the more proximal the lesion, the worse the prognosis.[10] Retrograde neuronal reaction, a factor that influences regeneration, varies inversely with the distance from the site of injury to cell.[9] However, this factor of increased neuronal reaction in high lesions cannot be a very significant factor in view of the usually good recovery in proximal muscles after high sutures. In terms of terminal recovery in the hand or foot, however, the results with high lesions are much poorer than with low lesions. At proximal levels the sensory and motor fibers are thoroughly scattered and mixed in contrast to more distal levels where localization of motor and sen-

sory fibers has occurred. Finally, the greater distance the regenerating axons must grow and the slower rate of growth at the distal levels mean that distal muscles must remain in a denervated state for longer periods and, consequently, limits the quality of recovery after reinnervation.[9]

Time from injury to repair

Almost all nerve surgeons agree that delay in suture of a nerve is to be avoided. Seddon[7] believed that the element of urgency in nerve suture is especially important in high nerve lesions in terms of "axonal exhaustion."[7] Zachary[10] noted that the quality of recovery was better in sutures performed within 6 months of injury than after 6 months.

Is there a critical delay period beyond which nerve suture should not be attempted? The answer, of course, depends on the nature of the injury, level of injury, age of patient, type of nerve, and whether the lost function could be regained by other means such as tendon transfer. It is generally believed that the quality of the end result declines as the interval between injury and suture increases. It must be appreciated, however, that early suture is usually associated with clean lacerations or noncrushing injuries in contrast to more serious injuries that, because of extensive wounding and side-effects, are associated with delayed nerve suture. Specifically, the harmful effects of delay in nerve suture may not be the delay itself but rather the secondary effects of the wound including a scarred vascular bed, infection, or loss of muscle substance. Sunderland has concluded that within 12 months of injury the capacity for the central nerve stump to regenerate is fully retained and the rate of growth is not affected. Secondly, he concluded that the distal stump will receive and transmit axons in a manner that does not significantly differ from early repairs. Thirdly, good restoration of muscle function may occur following denervation of this duration provided axons can be directed in sufficient numbers to their original or functionally similar end-organs and that muscle has been maintained in good condition by appropriate therapy.[9]

Although a time limit has not been established beyond which nerve suture would be useless, it is significant to note that Bowden and Guttman[1] found irreversible changes in human muscle incompatible with recovery at 3 years of denervation.

Type of nerve

The relative mixture of motor and sensory fibers in a nerve has much to do with the results following nerve suture. Nerves in which one group of fibers predominate demonstrate a predictably better end result. This is easily understood on the basis of random selection of opposing nerve fibers. If the nerve is predominately motor or sensory, it is likely that similar fibers would be reunited. A useful example in this regard is to contrast the median nerve above the elbow and at the wrist. Above the elbow this nerve is 66% sensory and 4% terminal motor (the remainder of the fibers being motor branches to the proximal forearm). Unfortunately for the nerve surgeon, these fibers are intermingled rather than localized above the level of the elbow. In contrast, at the wrist, the median nerve is 94% sensory and only 6% motor with relatively good localization.[9] In general then it can be concluded that mixed nerves do not carry as favorable a prognosis after suture as do nerves that are predominately motor or sensory.

The nerve surgeon and technical aspects

It is obvious that restoration of function after nerve severance involves more than restoration of continuity of nerve ends. However, the attempted restoration of anatomical continuity is the first step in a series of complex processes. The challenge in nerve surgery is to promote and assist these processes and above all to "do no harm."

This is no field for the casual or novice surgeon. His early experience with nerve suture should be learned by well-directed laboratory exposure followed by appropriate observation and assisting in the operating room.

Certain factors are incumbent on the surgeon: (1) to achieve and maintain skills; (2) to adopt a system or philosophy of treatment that encompasses all the aspects of the problem including joints, muscles, circulation, skin coverage, and psychological factors; and (3) to know when nerve surgery is *not* the best solution to a particular patient's problem and to proceed rapidly to tendon transfers, amputation, or arthrodesis as indicated.

Nerve suture requires detailed knowledge of intraneural anatomy, skill, and experience. Atraumatic technique is required along with familiarity in the use of special instruments and sutures designed for nerve work. Nerves should be handled in a gentle fashion, since rough manipulation may result in further retrograde neuronal effects. Most surgeons agree that nerve suture under tension is to be avoided and that significant gaps in nerves should be overcome by other means including nerve grafting. A surgeon must remember that there is no automatic or selective reunion at the suture line to promote regrowth of axons into their original endoneurial tubes; therefore close funicular reapproximation is important.

SUMMARY

This chapter has reviewed several of the many factors that relate to the end result following nerve injury and suture. A great majority of these factors are beyond the control of the surgeon; but the assimilation of these factors in each case is important in reference to choosing the most appropriate therapy for the patient. The surgeon must carefully assess the apparent effect of any particular factor in the framework of current available knowledge. None of these factors should be taken as an isolated entity in choosing a particular course of management or in the assessment of quality of recovery.

REFERENCES

1. Bowden, R. E. M., and Gutmann, E.: Denervation and re-innervation of human voluntary muscle, Brain **67**:273, 1944.
2. Elkington, J. St. C.: Prognosis of peripheral nerve injuries, Proc. R. Soc. Med. **37**:547, 1944.
3. Hamlin, E., and Watkins, A. L.: Regeneration in

the ulnar, median and radial nerves, Surg. Clin. North Am. **27:**1052, 1947.

4. Marble, H. C., Hamlin, E., Jr., and Watkins, A. L.: Regeneration in the ulnar, median and radial nerves, Am. J. Surg. **55:**274, 1942.

5. Milessi, H., Meissl, G., and Berger, A.: Further experience with interfascicular grafting of the median, ulnar and radial nerves, J. Bone Joint Surg. **58A:**209, 1976.

6. Nicholson, O. R., and Seddon, H. J.: Nerve repair in civil practice, result of treatment of median and ulnar nerve lesions, Br. Med. J. **2:**1065, 1957.

7. Seddon, H. J.: Surgical disorders of the peripheral nerves, ed. 2, Edinburgh, 1975, Churchill Livingstone, pp. 9 and 242.

8. Sunderland, S.: Observations on the course of recovery and late end results in a series of cases of peripheral nerve suture, Aust. N. Z. J. Surg. **18:**264, 1949.

9. Sunderland, S.: Nerves and nerve injuries, ed. 1, Edinburgh, 1968, E. and S. Livingstone, Ltd.

10. Zachary, R. B.: Peripheral nerve injuries, Medical Research Council Special Report Series, No. 282, London, 1954, Her Majesty's Stationery Office.

30

Past experience with epineurial repair: primary, secondary, and grafts

George E. Omer, Jr.

Procedure

Flourens (1828) and Baudens (1836)* are credited as the earliest surgeons to utilize the epineurial technique for the suture of peripheral nerves.[18] The basic procedure is closure of the divided nerve at the epineurial layer to contain circumferentially the regenerating fasciculi. The technique was standardized during World War II.[27]

The nerve is exposed through an appropriate longitudinal incision. A "guide suture" is placed in the epineurium proximal to the injury, and a second "guide suture" is placed distal to the injury in precise longitudinal alignment. These sutures are alignment markers after the nerve has been freed from scar and the neuroma and glioma (distal fibroma) have been resected. Without extensive dissection, the nerve should be mobilized until there is a generous overlap of proximal and distal stumps in order to decrease longitudinal tension at the suture line. The neuroma is resected by wrapping the proximal stump with a strip of sterile glove paper and cutting across the nerve with a superior grade safety razor blade. An alternate instrument is a neurectotome, which resembles a miter box, and produces a plane surface.

An identical technique is used with the distal fibroma, which is more difficult to

evaluate because there may be collagenization within the distal funiculi. One should err on the generous side when resecting the distal fibroma. There should be no surface incongruity when the two cut surfaces are matched; this is the most demanding technical step in the epineurial repair. The tourniquet is released and all bleeding is arrested, particularly from the cut ends of the nerve. If the extremity incision is extensive, it should be closed except in the area of nerve suture. This will decrease post nerve repair handling of the extremity with potential disruption of the suture site.

The nerve is now carefully inspected to obtain precise longitudinal alignment. The "guide sutures," any longitudinal blood vessels within the epineurium, and the funicular pattern on each of the cut surfaces are all matched as accurately as possible, while the first two sutures are placed 180 degrees around the circumference (9 o'clock and 3 o'clock) of the epineurium. The ends of the first sutures are left long. The suture is fine nylon material (8-0 to 10-0) and is placed only in the epineurial layer. The aligned anterior arc of epineurium is repaired with interrupted sutures. It is important to match the caliber of the proximal and distal ends to maintain the surface congruity at the suture line. The nerve is then rotated 180 degrees by passing one of the initial coaptation sutures posteriorly and rotating the unrepaired posterior epineurium into view. If this maneuver distorts the nerve, it should be

---

*Baudens was a French army surgeon serving in Algiers, who sutured the median and ulnar nerves in the axilla. He sutured adjoining tissues and thus avoided contact of the nerve with the suture material.[8]

mobilized until there is no resistance. The interrupted sutures in the posterior epineurium must be as neat as the anterior portion. A running suture is not used because a tight knot at the end of the suture line would constrict the circumference of the nerve. The "guide sutures" are removed, and the wound is closed. The limb is immobilized for 3 weeks in a plaster bandage and then gradually full active motion is allowed.

Historically, the epineurial repair has been performed without magnification and with heavy reactive suture material. In addition, it is common to mobilize the nerve to close the gap found at surgery. Circumferential tension, with decrease in the cross-sectional area, causes deflection of the funicular alignment with many regenerating axons ending blindly against the perineurium.[34] Longitudinal tension may result in subepineurial and intrafunicular hemorrhage with subsequent fibrosis.[10] Histological examination of epineurial repairs done without magnification and fine suture material demonstrates funicular malalignment with gaps, overriding, buckling, and straddling.[7] Past experience has reflected these problems.

The use of magnification has stimulated better techniques for funicular alignment with minimal tension, both circumferential and longitudinal. Extensive mobilization of the nerve for approximation, such as 14 to 20 cm, may result in the nerve acting as a free graft.[29] Particular attention must be paid to the cut surface of the nerve.[7,14] Special techniques have developed a combined epineurial and perineurial interrupted suture to accurately align the funiculi and close the epineurium with a single stitch.[1,9,14] Instruments and suture material have been adapted to the more precise techniques utilized with magnification.[9,14]

Definition of a successful result

A major problem in evaluating the nerve repair is the definition of a successful clinical result. Seddon[27] has modified the grading systems introduced by the British Medical Research Council report of 1954[25] and the United States Veterans Administration monograph of 1956[38]:

Motor recovery

M0	No contraction
M1	Perceptible contraction in proximal muscles
M2	Return of perceptible contraction in both proximal and distal muscles
M3	Functional return of such degree that all important muscles are acting against resistance
M4	All synergistic and independent movements are possible
M5	Normal

Sensory recovery

S0	Absence of sensibility in autonomous area
S1	Deep pain sensibility within autonomous area
S2	Some degree of superficial pain and tactile sensibility
S3	Superficial pain and tactile sensibility throughout the autonomous area with disappearance of any overreaction
S3+	Some recovery of two-point discrimination within the autonomous area
S4	Normal

In addition, Seddon[27] would adjust the motor and sensory findings according to which nerve is under consideration:

Median nerve

Good	S4 or S3+	:M3
Fair	S3	:M2
Bad	S1 or S2	:M1 or M0

Ulnar nerve

Good	S3	:M4
Fair	S2	:M3
Bad	S1 or S0	:M2 or M1

Radial nerve

Good		:M4
Fair		:M3
Bad		:M2 or M1

Digital nerve

Good	S4 or S3+
Fair	S3
Bad	S2 or S1

These ratings are not as specific as Moberg's[15] evaluation of sensibility in the autonomous areas of the median and ulnar nerves:

Median and ulnar sensibility

Two-point discrimination distance

Good	<12 mm
Fair	<20 mm
Bad	>20 mm

Moberg states that a two-point discrimination distance greater than 12 mm provides only protective sensibility, and the patient must utilize visual control of hand function.[15]

In 1908, Sherron reported 50 cases of nerve suture and analyzed the return of function.[8] It was reported that pain sensibility returned in 5 to 25 weeks, touch sensibility was intact in 19 to 46 weeks, and tactile sensibility was near complete in 2 years. Motor return occurred after 1 year for lacerations at the wrist and 2 years for lacerations at the elbow level. Zachary's studies in 1954 indicate that regeneration takes place mainly during the first 3 years; the next 2 years yield a small but definite improvement.[25] Sunderland[33] noted that after the repair of the median and ulnar nerves, signs of cutaneous sensory recovery usually appear in the hand before the return of voluntary contractions in the intrinsic muscles, and motor recovery also occurs on many occasions within 2 years of suture.

An appropriate clinical study to evaluate the results of suture would be (1) 3 to 5 years after suture, (2) two-point discrimination distance for sensibility, (3) voluntary muscle test for motor function, and (4) a continuing interval study of coordination and self-education, such as the pickup test.

PRIMARY AND SECONDARY SUTURE

Sherron[8,27] reported that primary suture gave the best results in his 50 cases. Thorburn, in the history of British surgery during World War I, regarded primary suture as the better procedure.[27,37] In 1928, Gonzalez and Aguilar advocated suture soon after myelin remains had been removed from the distal stump by maximal Schwann cell activity, about 30 days after nerve division.[8] In 1937, Platt and Bristow studied primary and secondary nerve sutures and advocated primary repair for small clean wounds but secondary suture on bruised or infected wounds.[8] During World War II, the British school clearly favored secondary suture.[27] Following that conflict, Rank, Wakefield, and Hueston[21] were strongly in favor of primary suture, but they also were very clear about the importance of a clean surgical field.[27]

The largest clinical series prior to routine magnification were the military injuries in World War II. An extensive review of World War II peripheral injuries was recorded by Woodhall and Beebe: 3415 definite procedures were performed on 3656 nerve lesions.[38] This study was compared with similar cases in the British review of World War II[25] (Table 30-1). This study indicates that the potential for a "good clinical result" (Sed-

Table 30-1 Recovery following complete suture (percentage—5 year results)*

Code		Median		Ulnar		Radial	
U.S.	British	U.S.	British	U.S.	British	U.S.	British
M0-1	M0-1	10.7	3.8	8.8	0.0	12.7	10.5
	S0-1	23.0	0.0	28.5	0.0		
M2-3	M(1+)-2	38.2	63.5	43.7	80.8	41.6	28.0
	S2-(2+)	45.4	61.9	40.1	69.2		
M4	M3	29.6	14.1	34.6	14.3	24.4	24.6
	S3	13.9	29.5	18.9	28.2		
M5-6	M4-5	21.5	18.6	12.9	4.9	21.3	36.9
	S(3+)-4	17.6	8.6	12.5	2.6		
TOTAL NERVES —M†		233	290	433	384	197	114
+S‡		244	278	441	390		

*From Woodhall, B., and Beebe, G. W., eds.: Peripheral nerve regeneration, Veterans Administration Medical Monograph, Washington, D.C., 1956, U.S. Government Printing Office.
†Number of motor studies.
‡Number of sensory studies.

don[27]) 5 years after a secondary suture in a severe injury is as follows:

Nerve (British code)	U.S.	British
Radial—M4-M5 plus	21.3	36.9
Median—M4-S3+ plus	M 51.1	M 32.7
	S 17.6	S 8.6
Ulnar—M4-S3 plus	M 12.9	M 4.9
	S 31.4	S 30.8

This prognosis for a good result in approximately one in five nerves needs to consider that many of these lesions were above the elbow, and most resulted from gunshot wounds or similar severe trauma.

Later studies of delayed suture involve military injuries during the Vietnam War. During this period, the use of magnification,

Table 30-2. Vietnam neurorrhaphy secondary suture—specific nerves*

Nerve	Number repaired	No return (percent)	Some return (percent
Ulnar	68	44 (65)	24 (35)
Median	38	19 (50)	19 (50)
Radial	5	3 (60)	2 (40)
Digital	24	10 (40)	14 (60)
TOTAL	135	76 (56)	59 (44)

*From Brown, P. W.: Clin. Orthop. **68:**14, 1970.

delicate instruments, and finer less reactive suture material improved the technique of nerve suture. In addition, there was better battle area evacuation time, and the majority of sutures were performed within the first 3 months after injury. An effort was made to perform suture as early as possible, and 70% of the successful anastomoses were performed within 6 weeks of injury.[17] I reported the results of 143 epineural sutures of upper extremity nerves followed for at least 12 months,[17] and Brown recorded the results of 135 epineural sutures followed 6 to 24 months[4] (Tables 30-2 and 30-3). Neither study had adequate follow-up, and the results are not fully graded. Brown states "some return," and I have two criteria for "clinical return": for the above-elbow lesion—progressive motor return with independent movement and point localization of 3.84 von Frey filament without overresponse (M3-S3); for the below-elbow lesion—progressive motor return with independent movement and two-point discrimination of 20 mm (M3-S3+). In addition, I noted that none of my patients with above-elbow neurorrhaphy had recovery of the intrinsic muscles of the hand during the period of study. The results of the two Vietnam series were very similar and only indicated that 40% to 45% of sutured nerves result in progressive functional re-

Table 30-3. Vietnam neurorrhaphy related to etiology and level of injury*

Etiology	Adequate follow-up	Clinical return	Percentage
Lacerations			
9 above elbow	8	3	37
90 below elbow	67	30	45
High-velocity gunshot			
24 above elbow	21	6	28
24 below elbow	14	6	43
Low-velocity gunshot			
19 above elbow	18	9	50
16 below elbow	14	6	43
Fracture-dislocations			
1 above elbow	1	0	0
1 below elbow	0	0	0
184 TOTAL	143	60	42

*From Omer, G. E., Jr.: J. Bone Joint Surg. **56A:**1615, 1974.

turn; final recovery was not complete and therefore not evaluated.

The "civilian" injury is considered the more likely candidate for immediate suture, although the individual problem may be severe in either circumstance.

Sakellarides[22] evaluated 205 sutures of 172 nerves in 149 patients. Secondary suture gave better results than primary suture in the median and ulnar nerve. In this series sensory recovery had a higher percentage than motor recovery (Table 30-4). The prognosis for recovery was best for radial nerve lesions and poorest for the ulnar nerve suture. All patients had been followed for at least 2 years at the Massachusetts General Hospital.

Another series prior to routine magnification was reported by Stromberg and co-authors in 1961.[32] In a series of 150 cases distal to the mid-third of the forearm with minimal extremity destruction, they found that the patient's own evaluation was a good indicator of functional activity. The patients were followed between 1 and 24 years. Sweating returned in 7 to 12 months. Weber two-point discrimination distance was 20 mm or less in 13 patients (9%). A similar study was done by Boswick and co-authors in 1965,[2] with two-point discrimination recovery in 11 patients (13%) of 82 cases (Table 30-5).

Onnë[19] reported on 32 median and 17 ulnar nerve sutures. The patients were examined not less than 3 years after the suture. When sensibility was measured with the two-point discrimination test, the value in millimeters was the same as the age of the patient up to 20 years. Digital nerve sutures, however, showed a good result up to the age of 50 years.

Seddon makes the point that the "civilian" injury that produces a distal lesion in a child has the best prognosis for functional recovery. He refers to McEwan's study[12] that demonstrates a decline with age in the quality of recovery, but he firmly adheres to secondary suture as the procedure of choice (Table 30-6) because it is the best method to determine the extent of the longitudinal injury to the internal structures of the nerve.[16]

Buncke[5] reported his results in 20 digital

Table 30-4. Results in civilian injuries

	Median				Ulnar				Radial			
	High		Low		High		Low		High		Low	
	Primary	Secondary	Primary	Secondary	Primary	Secondary	Primary	Secondary	Primary	Secondary	Primary	Secondary
M0-1	2	2	15	13	3	3	13	12	2	1	0	0
S0-1	2	2	13	6	3	3	13	8	1	1	0	1
M2-3	1	3	5	8	4	4	24	30	1	0	2	2
S2-(2+)	1	3	19	21	6	6	16	24				
M3	0	1	14	8	2	4	2	3	1	0	2	2
S3	0	1	5	9	0	2	9	10				
M4-5	0	0	4	5	0	0	0	1	0	0	1	1
S(3+)-4	0	0	2	1	0	0	2	5				
TOTAL*	3	6	39	37	9	11	40	47	4	2	3	4

*Totals include resuture and reevaluations.

Table 30-5. Peripheral nerve repairs below elbow

Nerves	Primary	Secondary	Patients under age 12	Subjective good result*		Age (sweating)	Age (two-point discrimination)
Digital	17	6	1	14P	5S	2-21-23	21-23-30
Median	17	9	9	14P	6S	5-9-11-17	5-9-11
Ulnar	14	5	7	12P	3S	7-8-10	7-8-9-10
Median-ulnar	9	2	5	3P		6-9	6
Radial	2	1					
TOTAL	59	23	22	57	(72%)	12 (15%)	11 (13%)
		82					

*P = primary; S = secondary.

Table 30-6. Median and ulnar nerves at the wrist (percentage of recovery)*

	Median		Ulnar	
Series	M3	S3+	M4	S3
A[25]	39.8	11	16	38
B[16]	65.4	24.6	35	68.5
C[12]				
Adult	60	67	23	84
Child	92	93	71	100

*From Seddon, H. J.: Surgical disorders of the peripheral nerves, ed. 2, Edinburgh, 1975, Churchill Livingstone.

Table 30-7. Digital nerve recovery (microsurgical technique)

Patients	Age	Repair		Two-point discrimination	
		Primary	Secondary	<10 mm	>10 mm
4	20 or less	1		1	
			3	3	
15	20 to 50	6		5	1 (24 mm)
			8	8	
			1 (graft)		1 (20 mm)
1	Over 50		1		1 (24 mm)

nerves in which microsurgical techniques were utilized (Table 30-7). Two-point discrimination under 10 mm was demonstrated in 17 of 20 patients.

The past experience with epineurial repairs would indicate a primary suture in: (1) a "tidy" wound, (2) a distal lesion, and (3) a "pure" nerve such as a digital nerve. A sec-ondary suture is indicated in 1 to 5 weeks in (1) an "untidy" wound, (2) a proximal lesion, and (3) a "mixed" nerve such as the median nerve.

NERVE GRAFTS

The first documented nerve graft was performed by J. J. Philipeaux and A. Vulpian in

1870.[13] The lingual nerve was utilized as a donor to bridge a gap in the hypoglossal nerve.[27] A nerve graft provides a scaffold that assists the regenerating axons to find their way into the distal nerve stump and restore the original pattern of innervation. Nerve grafts are often utilized under less than optimal clinical conditions such as inadequate circulation, potential or previous infection, and a long time period after the initial nerve injury. The selected nerve graft must be acceptable to the host tissues without producing an inflammatory response or constrictive fibrosis; it should be small enough in diameter to readily vascularize; and it should have a funicular (fascicular) pattern similar to selected funiculi in the proximal and distal suture lines.

Following World War I, British surgeons concluded that autogenous nerve grafting was a failure. However, the technique utiilized was neither a cable nor full-thickness graft; instead a single nerve strand was encased in a tube of fascia or a vein.[20,27]

Grafting would perhaps have been abandoned after the dismal results of World War I except for the reports of Bunnell indicating successful grafting of digital nerves.[6]

The early attempts at nerve grafting during World War II involved use of eight fresh homografts obtained from patients who had undergone amputation. None of these grafts showed clinical regeneration, and on histological study, it was found that the best regeneration had never proceeded more than 20 mm into the proximal end of the graft.[30]

The consistent failure of fresh homogenous nerve grafts led to a trial of frozen dried homografts. Forty-six frozen dried homografts were performed at Walter Reed General Hospital and Cushing General Hospital in 1944 and 1945. Only two grafts demonstrated clinical recovery, a distal 3 cm defect of a median nerve and a facial nerve cable graft approximated by a plasma glue technique.[30,36]

There were 3415 definitive operations recorded in the Veterans Administration monograph concerning peripheral nerve injuries during World War II,[38] but only 30

Table 30-8. Results of nerve grafting (Seddon complete series)*

	Result		
	Bad	Fair	Good
Donor nerves (cutaneous nerves)			
Digital			
In palm	2	5	1
In digits	6	2	10
Other single strands	3	1	3
Cable	9	4	9
Inlay	1	4	6
Main nerve trunks			
Upper limb			
Free	6	2	17
Pedicle	0	5	8
Lower limb—free	4	5	0
(all common peroneal to tibial)			
TOTAL (113)	31	28	54

*From Seddon, H. J.: Surgical disorders of the peripheral nerves, ed. 2, Edinburgh, 1975, Churchill Livingstone.

nerve grafts were performed in that series. Barnes Woodhall commented: "With the exception of the successful autografting of small nerves, such as the facial and digital nerves, and an occasional impressive instance of regeneration in frozen dried homografts, the record of nerve grafting in man was a practically unbroken record of failures in World War II, as it had been in World War I."[38] These were full-thickness grafts.

In contrast, Seddon recorded a significant success rate for the autogenous nerve grafts performed in adults at the Oxford Center during World War II.[24,26,27] Seddon's total experience, until 1975, is recorded in Table 30-8[27] and includes 22 cable grafts.

Definition of successful result

One of the difficulties in evaluating nerve grafts, as with nerve sutures, is the definition of a successful clinical result. Seddon, who has recorded the most successful nerve graft series, states that he utilizes the grading system introduced by the Nerve Injuries Committee of the British Medical Research

Council in 1954. Seddon also states that a "successful" nerve graft should be as good as the best result observed after direct suture of the nerve. However, motor function is usually improved to a greater degree than sensation.[35]

Sanders[23] and Brooks[3] also recorded approximately 50% useful recovery in autogenous grafts in 143 documented cases.[9]

From this experience, it was possible to define some of the factors in a successful autogenous nerve graft: (1) The length of the graft (nerve gap) should be 6 cm or less in length.[9] Nicholson and Seddon reported 70% useful recovery in median nerve lesions under favorable conditions if the defect was less than 2.5 cm. If the defects ranged between 2.6 and 5 cm, the percentage of useful results dropped to 50%. Defects greater than 5.1 cm were regarded as "prejudicial" to a useful reinnervation.[16] In Europe a nerve gap of 2.5 cm is grafted routinely, while the gap is usually 5 to 7 cm before grafting is utilized in the United States. The graft should be 10% to 20% longer than the nerve gap.[9,27] (2) A cable graft is preferable to a full-thickness main nerve trunk graft. The full-thickness graft is in jeopardy of inadequate revascularization with central necrosis. The selected cutaneous nerve should contain large funiculi in order to reduce the interfunicular spaces that are responsible for the wasteful dispersal of regenerating axons.[9] The preferable cutaneous nerves for use as cable grafts include the sural and the medial cutaneous nerve of the forearm.[9] (3) The nerve graft should be done as soon as possible following the nerve injury, and it should occupy a well-nourished soft tissue bed. (4) A surgical "team" with experience will obtain better results than the "occasional surgeon."

Only a limited number of nerve grafts were performed at the Brooke Army Medical Center during the Vietnam War. Almost all were free cable grafts without consideration for precise longitudinal alignment of the funiculi. No information is retrievable concerning the nerve gap that was closed or the longitudinal tension on the nerve graft. All were delayed procedures, more than 3 months after injury. Only 5 of 34 grafts (15%) demonstrated clinical return (Table 30-9).

The nerve pedicle graft was introduced during World War II in an attempt to maintain adequate circulation in a full-thickness graft. The first procedure involved the median and ulnar nerves in the forearm, with the ulnar nerve filling a gap in the median nerve.[31] This was followed by other reports for the upper extremity[28] and lower extremity.[11] This technique was successful in three of five cases during the Vietnam War (Table 30-9).

No major series of nerve grafts has been reported in the United States that has utilized civilian injuries. Since the military experience in World War II and the Vietnam War, techniques have changed to include magnification of the operation site. In addition, the cable graft has changed to a bundle of interfascicular grafts. The opportunity for early grafting is common in "civilian" injuries as compared to "military" injuries but has not been utilized until recently.

Only nine autogenous nerve grafts were placed in eight patients at the University of New Mexico from 1971 through 1976. Only two of the eight grafts with follow-up had fair or good results (Table 30-10).

At the University of New Mexico the current method for nerve grafting involves a microsurgical anastomosis with several cables matched to funicular groups in the proximal and distal portions of the nerve. The pattern of funiculi in the proximal and distal ends are

Table 30-9. Major nerves—Vietnam war (autogenous grafts)*

Type of graft	No return	Clinical return
Upper limb		
Cable	20	2
Pedicle	2	1
Lower limb		
Cable	7	0
Pedicle	0	2
TOTAL (34)	29	5

*Brooke Army Medical Center, Fort Sam Houston, Texas.

Table 30-10. Autogenous nerve grafts (University of New Mexico—1971-1976)

Nerve and patient	Age at surgery	Graft type* (length)	Injury-graft time	Follow-up time	Result	Remarks
Median 16233	4	*Pedicle* from ulnar 13.5 cm forearm (L)	12 mo	61 mo	M4 S3+	Two-point discrimination: 8-10 mm APB-M4
Median 22-82-66	22	Double *cable* 6.5 cm at wrist (R)	9 mo	40 mo	M1 S1	Failed primary repair, Tinel sign 3 cm proximal to carpal crease
Common digital, index-long, long-ring 25-85-14	18	*Full-thickness* sural (2 grafts): 5 cm in palm and 4.7 cm in palm (R) (2 grafts)	10 mo	22 mo	M− not rated S1	Two-point discrimination: >20 mm No sudomotor Severe associated injuries
Median 28-04-30	13	Double cable *interfascicular* 2 cm in carpal tunnel proximal to thenar branch (L)	5 mo	14 mo	M3 S3+ Good tactile gnosis	Two-point discrimination: >12 mm middle; 5 mm thumb, index, APB-M3
Median 18-78-69	12	Double cable *interfascicular* 6.5 cm elbow level (L) plus tendon transfers	33 mo	13 mo	M1 S3+	Two-point discrimination: >12 mm index; 5 mm thumb, middle Pickup test: (R) 10 sec (L) 32 sec
Ulnar 27-56-90	20	Double cable *interfascicular* 3.5 cm at wrist (L)	23 mo	10 mo	M1 S2	No intrinsics; two-point discrimination: > 20 mm; Tinel's fixed; no sudomotor
Median 19258	17	Double cable *interfascicular* 12.5 cm forearm (L)	13 mo	13 mo	M1 S2	Two-point discrimination: 10 thumb, 18 index, long Tinel at wrist
Median 28-60-11	22	Triple cable *interfascicular* 4.5 cm at wrist (L)	18 mo	Lost to follow-up		Severe associated injuries

carefully evaluated for precise longitudinal alignment of the funiculi through the cable graft (interfascicular or interfunicular graft).

REFERENCES

1. Bora, F. W., Pleasure, D. E., and Didizian, N. A.: A study of nerve regeneration and neuroma formation after nerve suture by various techniques, J. Hand Surg. **1**:138, 1976.
2. Boswick, J. A. Jr., Schneewind, J., and Stromberg, W., Jr.: Evaluation of peripheral nerve repairs below elbow, Arch. Surg. **90**:50, 1965.
3. Brooks, D.: The place of nerve-grafting in orthopaedic surgery, J. Bone Joint Surg. **37A**:299, 1955.
4. Brown, P. W.: The time factor in surgery of upper extremity peripheral nerve injury, Clin. Orthop. **68**:14, 1970.
5. Buncke, H. J., Jr.: Digital nerve repairs, Surg. Clin. North Am. **52**:1267, 1972.
6. Bunnell, S., and Boyes, J. H.: Nerve grafts, Am. J. Surg. **44**:64, 1939.
7. Edshage, S.: Peripheral nerve suture, a technique for improved intraneural topography, evaluation of some suture materials, Acta Chir. Scand. **331**:(Suppl.)1, 1964.
8. Flynn, W. F.: Peripheral nerve injuries in the hand. In Flynn, J. E., ed.: Hand surgery, Baltimore, 1966, The Williams & Wilkins Co., p. 415.
9. Hakstian, R. W.: Microsurgery, its role in surgery of the hand, Clin. Orthop. **104**:149, 1974.
10. Highet, W. B., and Sanders, F. K.: The effects of stretching nerves after suture, Br. J. Surg. **30**:355, 1943.
11. MacCarty, C. S.: Two-stage autograft for repair of extensive damage to sciatic nerve, J. Neurosurg. **8**:319, 1951.
12. McEwan, L. E.: Median and ulnar nerve injuries, Aust. N.Z. J. Surg. **32**:89, 1962.
13. McFarlane, R. M., and Mayer, J. R.: Digital nerve grafts with the lateral antebrachial cutaneous nerve, J. Hand Surg. **1**:169, 1976.
14. Michon, J.: Nerve suture today. In Michon, J., and Moberg, E., eds.: Traumatic nerve lesions of the upper limb, Edinburgh, 1975, Churchill Livingstone, p. 69.
15. Moberb, E.: Surgical treatment for absent single-hand grip and elbow extension in quadriplegia, principles and preliminary experience, J. Bone Joint Surg. **57A**:196, 1975.
16. Nicholson, O. R., and Seddon, H. J.: Nerve repair in civil practice. Results of treatment of median and ulnar nerve lesions, Br. Med. J. **2**:1065, 1957.
17. Omer, G. E., Jr.: Injuries to nerves of the upper extremity, J. Bone Joint Surg. **56A**:1615, 1974.
18. Omer, G. E. Jr., and Spinner, M.: Peripheral nerve testing and suture techniques. In American Academy of Orthopaedic Surgeons: Instructional course lectures, vol. 24, St. Louis, 1975, The C. V. Mosby Co., p. 122.
19. Onnë, L.: Recovery of sensibility and sudomotor activity in the hand after nerve suture, Acta Chir. Scand. **330**:(Suppl.):1, 1962.
20. Platt, H.: On the results of bridging gaps in injured nerve trunks by autogenous fascial tubulization and autogenous nerve grafts, Br. J. Surg. **7**:384, 1920.
21. Rank, B. K., Wakefield, A. R., and Hueston, J. T.: Surgery of repair as applied to hand injuries, ed. 4, Edinburgh, 1973, Churchill Livingstone.
22. Sakellarides, H.: A follow-up study of 172 peripheral nerve injuries in the upper extremity in civilians, J. Bone Joint Surg. **44A**:140, 1962.
23. Sanders, F. K. The repair of large gaps in the peripheral nerves, Brain **65**:281, 1942.
24. Seddon, H. J.: The use of autogenous grafts for the repair of large gaps in peripheral nerves, Br. J. Surg. **35**:151, 1947.
25. Seddon, H. J., ed.: Peripheral nerve injuries, Medical Research Council special report series 282, London, 1954, Her Majesty's Stationery Office.
26. Seddon, H. J.: Nerve grafting, J. Bone Joint Surg. **45B**:447, 1963.
27. Seddon, H. J.: Surgical disorders of the peripheral nerves, ed. 2, Edinburgh, 1975, Churchill Livingstone.
28. Shelden, H., Pudenz, R. H., and MacCarty, C. S.: Two-stage autograft for repair of extensive median and ulnar nerve defects, J. Neurosurg. **4**:492, 1947.
29. Smith, J. W.: Factors influencing nerve repair, Arch. Surg. **93**:335, 433, 1966.
30. Spurling, R. G., and Woodhall, B., eds.: Neurosurgery, Medical department, U.S. Army, surgery in World War II, Washington, D. C., 1959, U.S. Government Printing Office (Chapter XX), Vol. 2.
31. Strange, F. G. St. C.: An operation for nerve pedicle grafting, Br. J. Surg. **34**:423, 1947.
32. Stromberg, W. B., Jr., et al.: Injury of the median and ulnar nerves, J. Bone Joint Surg. **43A**:717, 1961.
33. Sunderland, S.: Observations on the course of recovery and late end results in a series of cases of peripheral nerve suture, Aust. N.Z. J. Surg. **18**:264, 1949.
34. Sunderland, S.: Funicular suture and funicular exclusion in the repair of severed nerves, Br. J. Surg. **40**:580, 1953.
35. Sunderland, S.: Nerves and nerve injuries, London, 1972, Churchill Livingstone, p. 697.
36. Tarlov, I. M.: Plasma clot suture of nerve, Surgery **15**:257, 1944.
37. Thorburn, W.: Injuries to the peripheral nerves, Official History of the Great War, vol. 2, London, 1922, Her Majesty's Stationery Office.
38. Woodhall, B., and Beebe, G. W., eds.: Peripheral nerve regeneration, Veterans Administration Medical Monograph, Washington, D.C., 1956, U.S. Government Printing Office.

31

Clinical evaluation of epineurial suture of digital nerves

Norman K. Poppen

A group of 49 patients with 74 injured digital nerves and 14 patients with median or ulnar nerve injuries was studied more than 5 years following epineurial nerve suture.[1] The quality of return of sensibility was tested within the autonomous zone for the nerve using von Frey plastic filaments, a modified Weber two-point discrimination device, and a dynamic testing device—the plastic ridge (see Chapter 28).

On the basis of the von Frey test, we were not able to distinguish the injured digits from the normal digits with heavy callosities. This test was not useful in determining the end result sensibility after nerve suture.

Of the factors studied, the age of the patient at the time of suture was by far the most important determinant of the sensibility regained. For patients over 20 years of age at the time of suture, two-point discrimination was less than 10 mm in only 4 of 48 digital nerves. Normal ridge values (less than 2 cm) were found only in patients less than 20 years of age at the time of suture. In general, those patients over the age of 30 years at the time of nerve suture could not feel the ridge.

When compared with a group of median and ulnar nerve injuries at the level of the wrist, digital nerve injuries were found to have better return of sensibility by two-point discrimination and ridge criteria.

In patients with injury to a common digital nerve, the sensibility regained in the juxtaposed surfaces of the adjacent affected fingers was compared. The sensibility on the two digits tended to be equal or nearly equal.

Repairs performed within 24 hours of injury produced sensibility equal to that resulting from nerve sutures performed 3 to 6 months after injury. The few repairs performed after an interval of 6 months gave inferior results.

Neither the dominance of the affected hand nor the occupation of the individual affected the end result sensibility when compared on the basis of age at the time of nerve suture.

Few of our patients had persistent subjective complaints. Only two reported hyperesthesia that was functionally limiting; 63 of 74 nerve repairs had a mild Tinel's sign elicited after careful examination or none at all.

With injury to either index finger digital nerve on the dominant hand, three fourths of the patients continued to use the long finger for fine pinch. This was true even when the ulnar digital nerve was injured. Those who continued to use the index finger for fine pinch either had a distal lesion with a very small area of deficit or were less than 15 years of age at the time of suture. We felt that patients with index finger digital nerve injuries do well because most have one intact digital nerve and the long finger is easily accessible for fine pinch.

The sensibility regained after digital nerve suture is strongly dependent on the age of the patient at the time of suture. Few adults regain any tactile gnosis as determined by a dynamic test device. Functional limitation in these patients is minimal because the remaining intact nerves provide for easy adaptation to the area of deficit.

REFERENCE

1. Poppen, N. K. et al. Recovery of sensibility after suture of digital nerves, J. Hand Surg. 4:212, 1979.

32

Epineurial sutures of peripheral nerves

Svante Edshage

As long as repair of divided peripheral nerves has been performed by surgeons, the epineurial suture has been the method of choice. With minor changes in the technique, epineurial suture was the standard method until the technique of free nerve grafts performed under the operating microscope was introduced. When the microscope became more generally used, refined techniques for suturing peripheral nerves, for example, bundle sutures and single-fascicle sutures, were tried. Even if these techniques under certain circumstances have advantages over the epineurial nerve suture, the latter still has its place in the therapeutic arsenal of the surgeon. One may then ask, when, where, and how should an epineurial suture of a divided peripheral nerve be made.

WHEN
Primary treatment

As in many fields of reconstructive surgery the golden moment for repair of a peripheral nerve is immediately after the injury. Any clean nerve laceration, whether transverse or oblique, where the nerve ends do not require any resection, including replantation, is suitable for a primary epineurial nerve suture. This includes, for instance, suicide attempts where the median nerve is cut with a razor blade. It also includes glass injuries in which the nerve is similarly cut clean through. When resection of damaged parts of the nerve is necessary, it is very questionable if an epineurial suture should be tried. Some-

times it may be possible but generally not. Complicating injuries, for instance, flexor tendon severance at the wrist, were earlier regarded as a contraindication to peripheral nerve suture. In my opinion it is not necessary to postpone the peripheral nerve surgery; the repair of the flexor tendons and the epineurial repair of the peripheral nerve can be performed at the same time. Finger flexion can be started 3 weeks after the suture without jeopardizing the result of the epineurial suture providing the wrist is held in a straight position so as not to put tension on the suture line in the nerve. Extension of the fingers to the neutral position does not cause enough tension to make the result of the peripheral nerve suture questionable. The same thing holds for digital nerve injuries combined with flexor tendon injuries.

Secondary treatment

Epineurial sutures in secondary cases are possible when the nerve ends, after resection, can be joined without tension. This must not be accomplished by extreme flexion of surrounding joints. In the case of the wrist joint this means that the flexion must not exceed 10 to 20 degrees of volar flexion. If more volar flexion of the wrist is necessary, an epineurial suture should not be tried, rather a nerve grafting procedure should be the method of choice. An extensive mobilization of the peripheral nerve to lessen the tension at the suture line should be avoided as this may jeopardize the blood supply to the nerve and thus interfere with the regrowth of axons

279

across the suture line. Flexion of the joints to enable secondary epineurial suture repairs in children does not seem to be as dangerous as in adults. Here one can accept much more acute flexion of surrounding joints in order to be able to make an epineurial suture after some resection. Even in children extreme flexion positions must be avoided, and extensive mobilization is to be avoided. In these cases free nerve grafts are preferred.

WHERE

As a general rule, all peripheral nerves should be sutured by epineurial sutures if this is technically possible. There are some exceptions to this rule: Epineurial sutures of brachial plexus lesions should not be tried. This has been tried in the past, but the results have not been rewarding. Free nerve grafting is the only way to bridge the defect in this region.

Some nerves do not lend themselves to repair, especially in adults. In the tibial nerve the only result to be achieved may be a severe paresthetic sole of the foot and no real useful sensory function. I have not seen any tropic ulcers on the sole of the foot, even after resection of the tibial nerve, in cases where these difficult paresthesias have developed. In my opinion it is, therefore, dubious whether a tibial nerve at the ankle joint should be sutured in an adult. In the child, however, suture is indicated, as the results are superior to those in adults.

Another example where the nerve should not be sutured may be the purely sensory nerve supplying a field of minor importance to the function of the hand, for instance the superficial branch of the radial nerve in the lower arm. Here the only result may be a painful, irritating paresthetic field, and the sensation will only cause trouble to the patient. The result of not suturing the nerve will generally be quite acceptable to the patient. Furthermore, the neuromas in that nerve, if located in scar tissue, may sometimes necessitate resection of the neuroma and a part of the nerve in order to locate the neuroma in a non-skin–fixed, scar-free position in the forearm.

HOW
Anesthesia

The anesthesia may either be general or local. If local anesthesia is chosen, a high local block permitting a bloodless field for sufficent time should be used. New local anesthetic drugs, which are long acting, have been introduced and are excellent for this purpose. In my experience no damage to the nerve of any magnitude that is recognizable in the end results is caused by brachial plexus or axillary blocks.

Bloodless field

If at all possible, a bloodless field should always be used when making a peripheral nerve suture. If one cannot see exactly what one is trying to do, the result in peripheral nerve surgery is certain to be inferior. The gentle handling of tissues is also essential, and a bleeding field will not permit optimal, atraumatic surgery to be performed.

Exploration

The exploration of the nerve injury should always be large enough to permit good exposure of the nerve. The surgeon performing the peripheral nerve surgery must be used to handling the skin in the injured area in order to place his accessory incisions correctly and to avoid later scar contractures.

The dissection should start in undamaged tissue and proceed toward the injury. This is necessary not only in secondary procedures but also in primary procedures. This implies that the diagnosis of a peripheral nerve injury should be made before surgery is started and not during surgery. The nerve ends should be freed for a limited distance and then checked to determine whether they are of acceptable quality for an epineurial suture. The surgeon should also determine whether it is possible to join the nerve ends without flexing the surrounding joints excessively.

Magnification

In most cases of epineurial nerve suture, it is advisable to use some kind of magnification. It is usually not necessary to use an operating microscope in order to make a good epineurial nerve suture. A good magnifying glass may be quite sufficient. The operating microscope helps the surgeon considerably in evaluating the nerve ends and the amount of trauma to which they may have been submitted.

Resection of nerve ends

Resection of the nerve ends (Figs. 32-1 and 32-2) prior to epineurial nerve suture should only be necessary in secondary cases, where after resection they can be joined without tension. There are many helpful devices constructed for a good resection of a peripheral nerve. The only really necessary thing is to stabilize the nerve with some kind of plastic wrap. The nerve is then cut through this plastic wrap with a razor blade. In that way thin slices of the nerve can be cut away, and resection surfaces, which are perpendicular to the long axis of the nerve, can be achieved. Free resection should not be tried. When

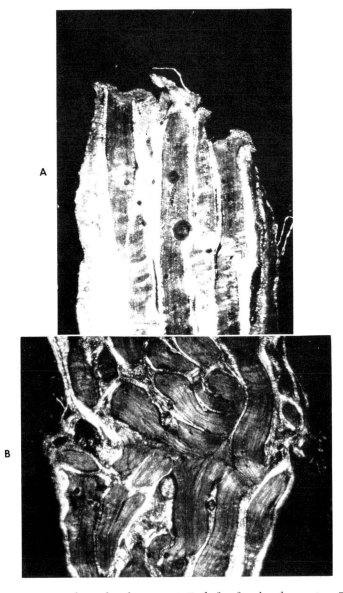

Fig. 32-1. Frozen sections of peripheral nerves. **A,** End after free-hand resection. **B,** Epineurial suture of two free-hand resected nerve ends.

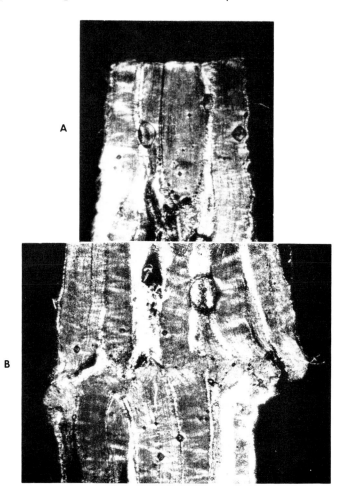

Fig. 32-2. Frozen section of peripheral nerves. **A,** Cut end after resection with the nerve wrapped in plastic and using a special holder. **B,** Epineurial suture of two "holder resected" ends. **A,** Severe inflammatory reaction around plain catgut thread implanted 3 weeks earlier. Note absence of reaction in perineurium in lower part of picture. **B,** Injured perineurium pulled into endoneurium. Very little reaction in perineurium.

scar-free tissue has been reached on both sides of the lesion, the nerve ends are handled in the same way as in primary nerve sutures. Only with perpendicular, evenly resected surfaces can good fascicular opposition be expected after the nerve suture.

Suture material

Any suture material but catgut may be used. It should be of a size from 8-0 to 10-0. A heavier suture material should not be necessary to keep the nerve ends together. If heavier suture is necessary, it is probably better to make a free nerve graft instead of an end-to-end suture.

Suturing

The sutures should be placed in the epineurium. In multifascicular nerves one or two sutures can be placed in the epineurium between the bundles of fascicles, but most of the time this necessitates an operating microscope. The sutures must not pass the epineurium. The use of stay-sutures should be employed.

Rotational displacement must be avoided by careful examination of the cut surfaces. The pattern of fascicles should match as very limited or no resection has been performed. Of course other landmarks such as longitudinal vessels should not be forgotten.

Surrounding tissue

The tissue surrounding the nerve suture should be as free from scar as possible. This means that the carpal ligament is better divided in order to give the median nerve less chance to be compressed both by the surrounding tissue and the ligament. Similarly, it is better to excise superficialis tendons that are cut at the same level as the nerve than to suture these and cause scar tissue to develop surrounding the nerve suture.

Immobilization

Immobilization of the injured extremity should be maintained for 4 to 5 weeks. It should not be necessary to change the immobilzation during this time as extreme flexion of any immobilized joints should be avoided.

Partial lesion

The best treatment for a partial nerve lesion is primary suture. In these cases bundle suture is carried out with the same technique as described for primary epineurial suture. The only difference is that under the micro-scope the injured bundle of fascicles should be dissected free from the intact part of the nerve. An exact match of the fascicles is usually possible. The bundles are joined by a couple of fine stitches in the epineurium that is always carried with the bundle. In these cases it is generally not necessary to flex the joints as the tension is relieved by the remaining, uninjured parts of the nerve.

Secondary sutures of partial nerve lesions should not be tried with the techniques of epineurial or perineurial nerve suture. In these cases free nerve grafts should be used. The earlier described method of looping the intact part of the nerve to make it possible to make an epineurial suture is not recommended.

CONCLUSION

Epineurial nerve suture without any wrapping is still a good method for repair of injured peripheral nerves including replantation. This is particularly true for nerve injuries in children, primary treatment of partial nerve injuries, and primary treatment of complete injuries of multifascicular nerves without any loss of tissue and with no contamination or laceration of the nerve ends. It is our general treatment for digital nerve injuries, and we rarely find it necessary to use free nerve grafts there.

In secondary procedures an epineurial suture should be performed when the resection surfaces can be joined without severely flexing the surrounding joints or mobilizing the nerve ends extensively to overcome tension at the suture line. If this is not possible, free nerve grafts should be inserted.

33

Materials and methods of microsurgical repair*

Harry J. Buncke and Harold D. McDonald

The development of microsurgical techniques and instrumentation has made it possible to align the structures involved in small vessel and nerve repair more accurately and thereby to improve the results of such repairs.[10,13] We will discuss the materials and methods of microsurgery and present some clinical cases for illustration.

MATERIALS
Loupes

Magnifying loupes have become readily available in recent years and are constantly being improved. They are generally available in powers of $\times 2$, $\times 2^1/_2$, $\times 3^1/_2$, $\times 4$, $\times 4^1/_2$ and $\times 6$. Some models provide a choice of two powers and have a variable interpupillary distance. The most useful loupes are those that are fitted to a single individual with the interpupillary distance fixed for best vision. We find magnifying loupes in either $\times 4^1/_2$ or $\times 6$ powers to be very useful in initial dissection and identification of severed vessels and nerves, particularly in the digits. One has more freedom of movement when using magnifying loupes to do the preliminary dissection and to identify structures. The operating microscope is reserved for the final repair.

*This work supported in part by funds from the Microsurgical Transplant Research Foundation, the Microsurgical Fund of the Ralph K. Davies Medical Center, and the Office of Naval Research, Grant No. NR 105-851.

Microscopes

Several companies presently make microscopes that are readily available. It is important to have a diploscope or a microscope that enables both the surgeon and the assistant to see the same field so that they will be better able to work together.

The magnification powers generally available on operating microscopes are $\times 6$, $\times 10$, $\times 16$, $\times 25$, and $\times 40$. In repairing larger structures, $\times 6$ and $\times 10$ are useful. However, for smaller structures such as digital nerves and vessels, $\times 16$ and $\times 25$ are needed.

The use of the monopolar-type cautery is not recommended for microsurgery because it is likely to cause heat damage to the surrounding tissue and initiate thrombosis of vessels. A bipolar-type electrocautery is recommended, since it will work under fluid and does not significantly damage surrounding structures. There are several available that work satisfactorily.

Forceps

Jewelers' forceps can be refined for use in microsurgery as forceps, pickups, and vessel spreaders. In some cases, the heavier jewelers' forceps can be used as needle holders. We use No. 1, No. 2, and No. 5 jewelers' forceps. The tips are finely ground and polished and the opening tension is properly adjusted. We also have the handles rounded with silicone rubber (Fig. 33-1, A). The rounded

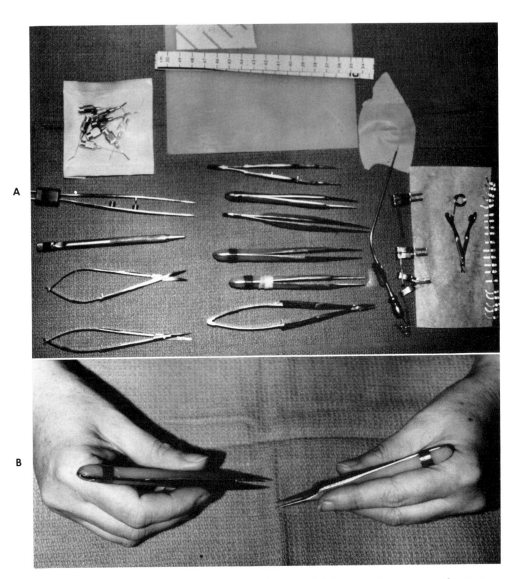

Fig. 33-1. A, Microsurigcal instruments. First column on left from top down: group of irrigating tips; bipolar coagulator tip; blade breaker; curved microscissors; straight microscissors. Center column from top down: plastic block to lay sutures on; centimeter tape; one flat-handled forcep; four jewelers' forceps with rounded handles; needle holder with rounded handle. Right column from top down: piece of rubber balloon for background material; suction tip; group of microclamps with applier; and to left of card, three sets of clamps mounted on bar used to approximate vessels. **B,** Jewelers' forceps with rounded handles showing ease of grip, rotation, and control. (Designed by Zoltan Szabo, Microsurgical Laboratory, R. K. Davies Medical Center, San Francisco, California.)

handles enable one to rotate the instrument in the thumb, index, and long fingers for better control of the instrument with stability and mobility improved over the flattened sides of the jewelers' forceps as they come from the manufacturer (Fig. 33-1, *B*). More expensive forceps are available from the various surgical supply houses.

Needle holders

A round-handled needle holder is preferred to the flat-handled instrument because of the ease of control between the fingertips. The needle holder should be the type that does not have a latch on it, as opening the latch under a microscope results in unnecessary, distracting motion and trauma. Some surgeons prefer a straight tip, and some prefer a slightly angled tip. Each surgeon should select the one he feels works best for him. We have a straight-tipped, modified Barraquer round-handled needle holder with small cups at the tip that hold the needle more securely at various angles (Fig. 33-1, *A*). The short and medium length handles seem to function well in peripheral microsurgery. For deeper work in a less accessible location, such as intercranially, the longer handled instruments may be preferable.

Clamps

Several different types of microsurgical clamps are available commercially. These include the Acland clamp and modified Heifitz clamp or Kleinert clamp. It is useful to have single clamps that can be used on individual structures and also clamps that are mounted on a sliding bar, which can be used to approximate the two ends of a vessel to simplify suturing (Fig. 33-1, *A*). Microvascular clamps should exert a pressure less than 30 gm/mm² so as not to damage the endothelial lining.[12] Clamps with a higher closing pressure than this should be discarded as they can result in a failure at the anastomosis secondary to thrombosis. There are special clamps for use in microapproximation of the vas deferens and fallopian tubes and for holding nerves in close proximity for ease of repair. These clamps used for the nerves, vas, and fallopian tubes usually have an extended circumferential opening at the tips to aid in atraumatic application.

Suture

One of the more significant advances in materials design that has done much to further microsurgery is the development of strong, fine microneedles and microsutures. A small German company, Springler and Trill, developed a steel microneedle that is strong, small, and sharp and can be swaged onto 9-0, 10-0, and 11-0 sutures. Soon after, the Japanese and Australians developed microneedles and microsutures that have proven useful in microsurgery. This development has overcome one of the major blocks to the advance of microsurgical technique, greatly simplifying the passing of the suture through structures at the microsurgical level. These needles are available now with nylon that ranges in size from 18 to 30 μ. We use 11-0 nylon swaged on a 70 μ needle for most vascular procedures, and we prefer the 70 to 100 μ needle on 9-0 or 10-0 nylon for microneurosurgical use.

Background material

A very inexpensive, useful material in microsurgery is a piece of brightly colored rubber balloon that can be cut into various sizes and placed behind the structures being worked upon (Fig. 33-1, *A*). The background material gives a good color contrast in the microsurgical field. Either a yellow or light blue seems to work the best for us. The rubber material also provides a surface from which sutures can be picked up with ease for tying, cutting, and so forth.

Blade breaker

A blade breaker is a useful instrument when doing endomicroneurosurgery (Fig. 33-1, *A*). It allows one to break small chips of razor blade and hold them firmly for use in splitting fascicles and fascicular bundles in an atraumatic fashion (Fig. 33-2). A large segment of blade held in the blade breaker can also be used to cut the ends of a fascicle or small nerve squarely in a guillotine fashion

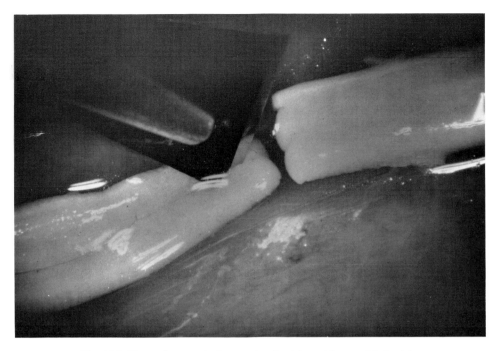

Fig. 33-2. Fascicular repair. Separating fascicles with razor blade chip.

(Fig. 33-3), thereby making it possible to carry out an accurate square-end approximation of the structures in the nerve.

METHODS
Microvascular

It is possible to anastomose a 1 mm vessel with microsurgical techniques with a high degree of success.[2] This technique has been carried from the laboratory into the clinical setting and is now used extensively in instances of replantation of severed parts[8] and transfers of vascularized tissue such as flaps of skin and subcutaneous tissue,[4] bone,[9] muscle,[6] and nerve.[11] We presently use the laboratory rat as a model for teaching and research in microvascular surgery.[3] The basic techniques and manipulations of surgery under the operating microscope are assimilated while learning to perform a successful repair of the rat femoral artery. After one has mastered the arterial anastomosis, it is possible to advance to the more difficult venous anastomosis. The next step is to more complex procedures such as anastomosis of the

rat femoral artery to the femoral vein or to place a segment of vein into an artery simulating an interposition graft in which one must do two anastomoses. End-to-side repairs are also important clinically and must be perfected in the laboratory.

Microneurosurgical

Microneurosurgical repairs of severed nerves have been done by three different methods. The first and, historically, the oldest method is by aligning the nerve according to the surface anatomy such as by identifying and aligning a large vessel. The nerve is then held together by sutures in the epineurium. It is important that this be done under the microscope with good, careful, atraumatic surgical technique (Fig. 33-3). The second method is by carefully separating out the individual fascicle bundles, mapping the pattern of like-appearing fascicle bundles, and suturing each bundle to its distal mate (Fig. 33-4).[1,5] The third method of repair is by the interfascicular bundle graft technique (Figs. 33-5 and 33-6). This last technique was

Text continued on p. 295.

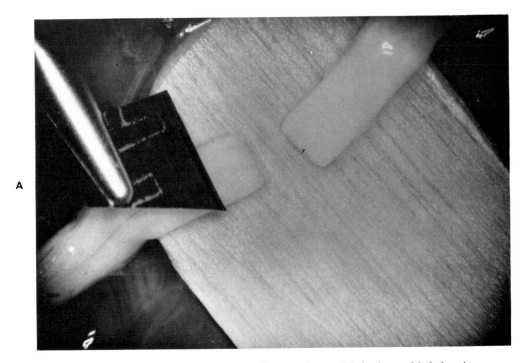

Fig. 33-3. Epineurial repair. **A,** Nerve ends cut with razor blade chip on blade breaker.

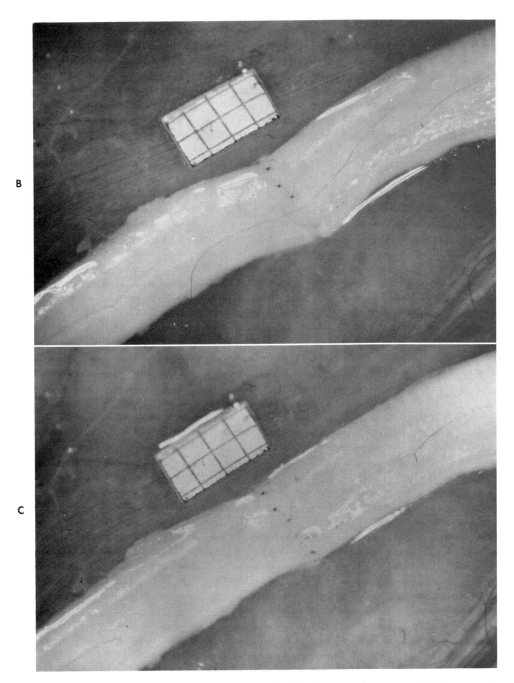

Fig. 33-3, cont'd. B, Nerve repair partially completed with 10-0 nylon suture. **C,** Nerve repair completed.

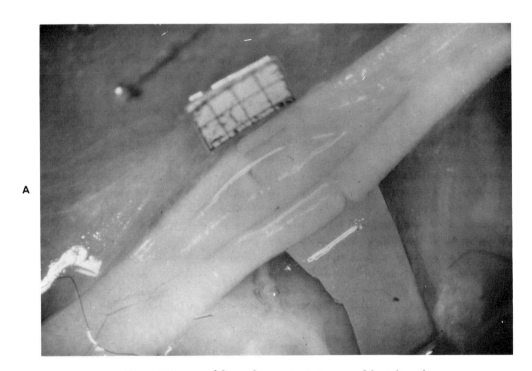

Fig. 33-4. Staggered fascicular repair. **A,** Staggered fascicle ends.

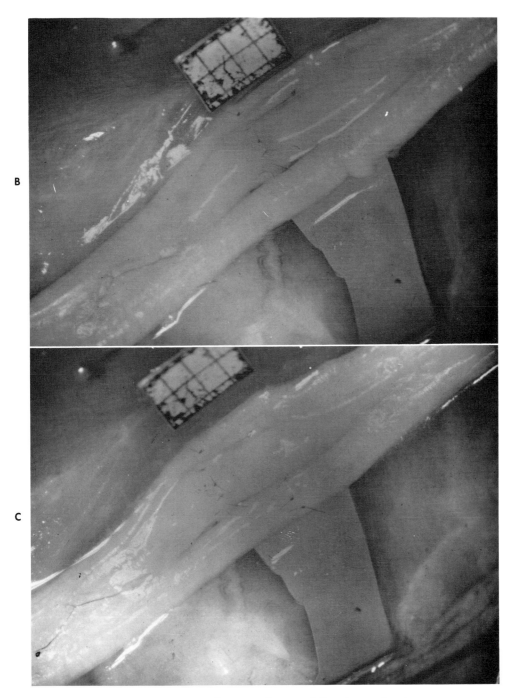

Fig. 33-4, cont'd. B, Repair underway. **C,** Repair completed.

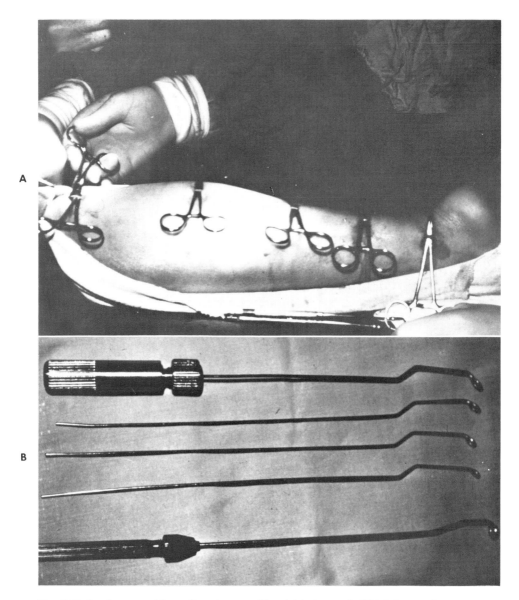

Fig. 33-5. Sural nerve cable grafts to lacerated brachial plexus. **A,** Obtaining sural nerve, step-ladder incisions. **B,** Nerve strippers.

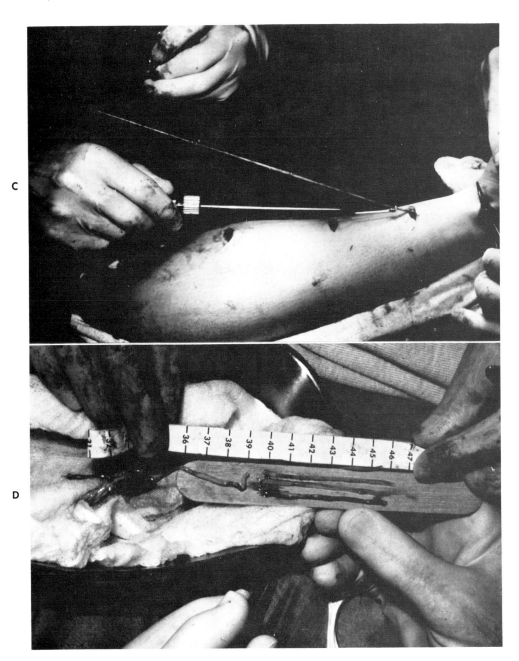

Fig. 33-5, cont'd. C, Nerve graft is mobilized by passing nerve stripper between incisions.
D, Cables for repair.

Continued.

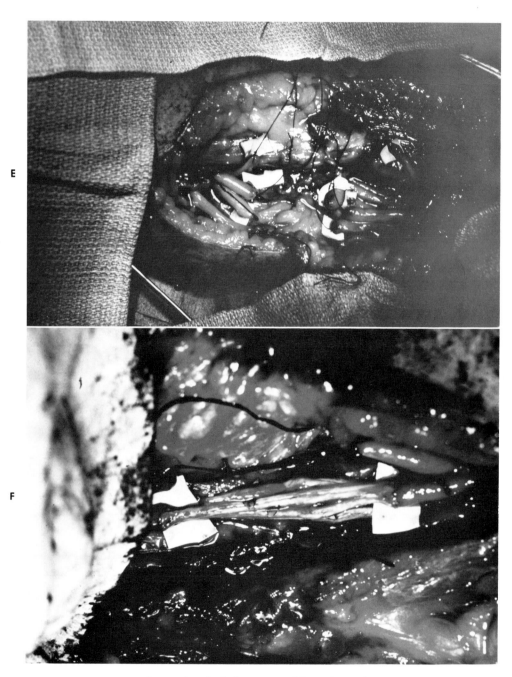

Fig. 33-5, cont'd. E, Defects in brachial plexus. **F,** Cable grafts in place. (Nerve strippers designed by Hans Andrel, Insbrook, Austria.)

devised to bridge defects and permit nerve repairs without tension. In the interfascicular bundle graft technique, the ends of the nerve are dissected from normal to abnormal or scarred tissue. The abnormal-appearing nerve is then excised, cutting the bundles of fascicles at different levels, and removing a small band of epineurium to a level just beyond the area where the fascicles appear normal. An interposition graft (usually from the sural nerve) is then interposed between the fascicular bundles and held in place with one or two sutures. Within a very short period of time, fibrin clotting stabilizes the repair. This technique has been shown to yield good results in situations where there is likely to be tension at the site of nerve repair.[7]

The instruments presently available for use in microsurgery are continually improving. With improving technology, the bulky microscopes we use today could be replaced with a three-dimensional televised image, picked up from the operative field and reconstituted holographically over the field magnified 10 to 20 powers. The excessive manipulations necessary in microsuturing will surely be replaced in the future by simplified mechanical vessel and nerve approximators or quick-setting biological adhesive substances specific for vessel or nerve tissue.

Illustrative cases
Case No. 1

M. R. is a 49-year-old female who was injured 2 months prior to her admission when she was struck in the right axilla by a piece of flying glass, which resulted in a laceration of her axillary artery, vein, and all cords of the brachial plexus (Fig. 33-5, *E*). She was treated on an emergency basis by repair of the axillary artery and vein and was referred for treatment of her brachial plexus laceration. On examination of the right upper extremity, the deltoid muscle was found to have some action, but the remainder of the muscles in the extremity distal to that point were denervated as was the sensory component of the right upper extremity.

Treatment for the brachial plexus injury consisted of sural nerve grafts that were taken from both lower extremities and used as interfascicular grafts (Fig. 33-5, *F*). The sural nerve grafts were obtained by turning the patient prone and making a transverse incision just behind the lateral malleolus where the sural nerve was picked up. It was gently tugged on, and stepladder type incisions were made proximally up the lateral and posterior aspect of the lower legs up to the level of the popliteal fossa. When the highest point on the popliteal fossa was reached, the nerve was transected and a nerve stripper was used to deliver the sural nerve retrograde between the stepladder transverse incisions (Fig. 33-5, *A* to *C*); 38 cm of sural nerve was obtained from each leg. The patient was then turned supine and the brachial plexus explored. The axillary nerve was found to be intact. The radial, ulnar, median, musculocutaneous, medial brachiocutaneous, and antebrachiocutaneous nerves were all found to be cut (Fig. 33-5, *E*). The sural nerve grafts were cut to bridge the gaps produced after excision of the neuromas and gliomas (Fig. 33-5, *D*) and sutured in an interfascicular fashion to repair the radial and median nerves. The medial antebrachiocutaneous nerve was used as a graft for the musculocutaneous nerve, and the medial brachiocutaneous nerve was used as grafts to repair the ulnar nerve (Fig. 33-5, *F*).

Case No. 2

J. F. is an 18-year-old male who, 7 months prior to his admission, suffered an avulsion of his left hand, which had been drawn into a hydraulic packaging machine. The hand was successfully replanted at our hospital immediately after the avulsion (Fig. 33-6, *A*). Seven months following the replantation, the patient was readmitted for repair of the median and ulnar nerves, which had been avulsed at the time of the amputation of the hand. On exploration of the right upper extremity, the distal neuroma of the median nerve was found in the proximal third of the forearm (Fig. 33-6, *C*) and the neuroma of the ulnar nerve was found just distal to the elbow joint.

Sural nerve cable grafts were obtained in a

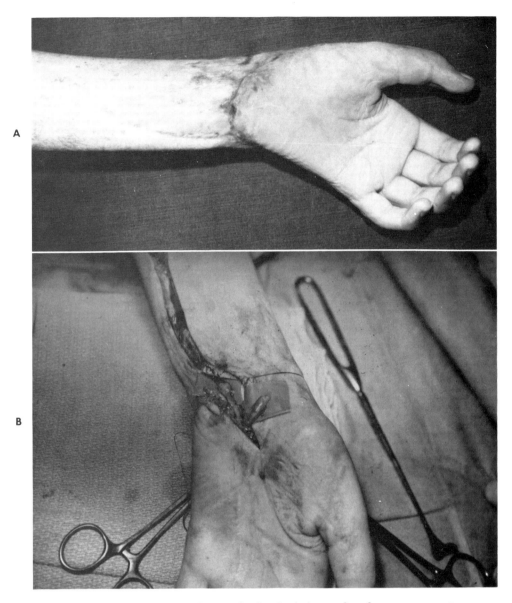

Fig. 33-6. A, Replanted hand. **B,** Ends of avulsed ulnar and median nerves at wrist.

manner similar to that described for Case No. 1 using stepladder incisions over each calf. At the level of the popliteal fossa, a Z-type incision was made and the nerve was split off the common peroneal nerve in the distal posterior thigh. At this point, the nerve was transected and a stripper, was used to free the nerve from the level of the distal thigh down through the stepladder incisions; 55 cm of sural nerve were harvested from each leg.

The median and ulnar nerve neuromas and gliomas were resected. Two 20 cm interfascicular grafts of sural nerve were placed in the median nerve passing the nerve grafts beneath a tunnel of skin graft to a level just proximal to the carpal tunnel. The ulnar

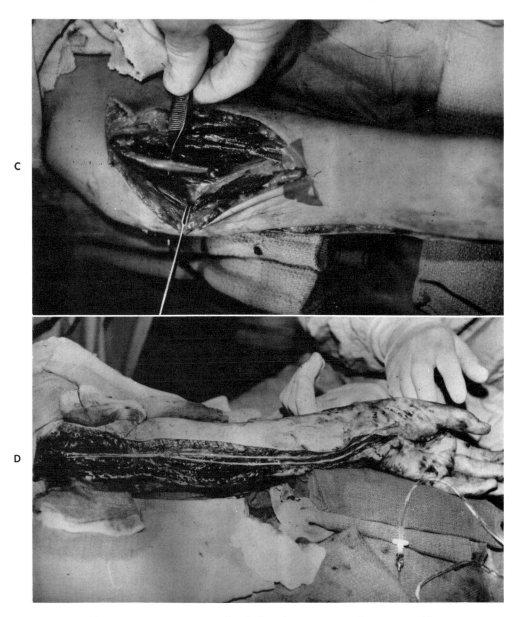

Fig. 33-6, cont'd. C, Proximal end of median nerve. **D,** Ulnar nerve cables.

nerve was reconstructed with two 30 cm grafts from the proximal ulnar nerve to the ulnar nerve sensory fascicles at the level of Guyon's canal (Fig. 33-6, *D*). A medial bundle of ulnar nerve fascicles was sutured with a third graft to the proximal motor branch to the flexor carpi ulnaris muscle. All the interfascicular grafts were approximated with interrupted 9-0 nylon sutures.

SUMMARY

The future of microsurgery holds many possibilities for helping mankind in a variety of ways. One of these is the increased use of free muscle transplants innervated by long nerve grafts. Such transplants could be used to repopulate paralyzed limbs with expendable muscles from elsewhere in the body, innervating these new muscles with nerve grafts to ipsilateral and contralateral proximal expendable motor roots. Direct cortical stimulation with implanted electrodes has been used to give the blind a visual stimulus. The thousands of pacemakers attest to the fact that muscle will respond to external stimuli for an indefinite period of time. With the use of ultrarefined microelectric circuitry borrowed directly from the "space program," it may be possible to pick up impulses from the motor cortex and transmit them to specific muscles by microtelemetry, thus bypassing the cerebrospinal neuroconductive link.

CONCLUSION

We have presented the materials of microsurgery including loupes, microscopes, electrocauteries, round-handled instruments, clamps, sutures, background material, and blade breakers. A method of microsurgery training using the rat as a laboratory model is recommended. Epineurial, perineurial, and interfascicular cable grafts have been illustrated. Two cases are presented to demonstrate the materials and methods of microsurgery. Future use of microneurosurgery is discussed.

REFERENCES

1. Bora, F. W.: Peripheral nerve repair in cats, the fascicular stitch, J. Bone Joint Surg. **49A:**659, 1967.
2. Buncke, H. J., and Shutlz, W. P.: Total ear replantation in the rabbit utilising microminiature vascular anastomosis, Br. J. Plast. Surg. **19:**15, 1966.
3. Buncke, H. J., Chater, N. J., and Szabo, A.: Manual of microvascular surgery from Ralph K. Davies Medical Center, Microsurgical Unit, San Francisco, 1975, Printed and distributed by Davis & Geck Co.
4. Daniel, R. K., and Taylor, G. I.: Distant transfer of island flap by microvascular anastomosis, Plast. Reconstr. Surg. **52:**111, 1973
5. Grabb, W. C., et al.: Comparison of methods of peripheral nerve suturing in monkeys, Plast. Reconstr. Surg. **46:**31, 1970.
6. Harii, K., Ohmari, K., and Torii, S.: Free gracilis muscle transplantation with microneurovascular anastomoses for treatment of facial paralysis, Plast. Reconstr. Surg. **57:**133, 1976.
7. Millesi, H., Meissl, G., and Berger, A.: The interfascicular nerve-grafting of the median and ulnar nerve, J. Bone Joint Surg. **54A:**727, 1972.
8. O'Brien, B. M., and Miller, G.: Digital re-attachment and revascularization, J. Bone Joint Surg. **55A:**714, 1973.
9. Ostrup, L. T., and Fredrickson, J. M.: Distant transfer of free living bone graft by microvascular anastomosis, Plast. Reconstr. Surg. **54:**274, 1974.
10. Smith J. W.: Microsurgery of peripheral nerves, Plast. Reconstr. Surg. **33:**317, 1964.
11. Taylor, G. I., and Ham, E. J.: The free vascularized nerve graft, Plast. Reconstr. Surg. **57:**413, 1976.
12. Thurston, J. B. et al.: A scanning electron microscopy study of micro-arterial damage and repair, Plast. Reconstr. Surg. **57:**197, 1976.
13. Wise, A. J., and Camalottin, I. A.: Comparative analysis of macro and microsurgical neurorrhaphy techniques, Am. J. Surg. **117:**566, 1969.

34

Interfascicular nerve repair and secondary repair with nerve grafts

Hanno Millesi

In the early 1870's Hueter[16] introduced the technique of epineurial nerve repair. This technique represented a great advance in the surgery of peripheral nerves; it provides a good coaptation of the stumps of a peripheral nerve without traumatizing the nerve tissue. One must not forget that before this technique was accepted generally surgeons hesitated to touch a nerve stump and attempted to achieve an approximation of the nerve stumps by uniting other structures like muscles in the neighborhood (nerve repair "cum carne"). For nearly one century the epineurial nerve repair was the standard technique, and it was applied to all nerves regardless of their internal structure. The disadvantage of epineurial nerve repair was recognized soon. In many instances suturing the circumferential epineurium does not provide an optimal alignment of the individual fascicles within the nerve stumps. Attempts to improve this situation by coaptation of the individual fascicles, using perineurial stitches,[18] failed because they were connected with increased surgical trauma.

During the past 15 years microsurgical techniques, combined with improved atraumatic technique, have been developed that exploit the magnification of the microscope. Microsurgery makes it possible to extend surgical activities into delicate tissue layers without causing a punishing tissue reaction. This gives the surgeon the possibility to adapt his technique to the structure of the involved nerve segment. Interfascicular nerve repair is one of these adapted techniques that applies to nerve segments consisting of many fascicles of different sizes arranged in fascicle groups. It happens that such arrangement is present in the majority of the common sites of nerve injuries. Different structural arrangements of the involved nerve segment need different techniques.

The concept of interfascicular nerve repair proved extremely useful if nerve grafting was necessary because it solved the problem of the discrepancy between the stumps of a severed nerve trunk and the segments of skin nerves available for nerve grafting. Instead of combining several skin nerve segments to produce a cable of the same size as the nerve to be repaired,[33] the nerve stumps are prepared by interfascicular dissection, separating the individual fascicle groups. Nerve grafts have been used since long ago and considerable successes have been reported.* Still, confidence in the results of nerve grafts was not too great, and grafts were not considered as an alternative to end-to-end nerve repair but rather as a technique of second choice if end-to-end nerve repair was completely impossible. The developments of the past 15 years changed this attitude very much in favor of nerve grafting. The development is perhaps best expressed by remembering that Smith,[39] who became famous because of the development of cross-face nerve grafting,

---

*See references 2, 5, 7, 8, and 33 to 35.

299

stated in 1966 that "nerve grafts have not proved very satisfactory."[36,37]

PRIMARY VS. SECONDARY NERVE REPAIR

The terms of primary and secondary nerve repair are not always used in the same way. There is an overlapping in the use of the terms "delayed primary" and "early secondary" repair. It therefore seems necessary to give a definition of these terms as used by the author.

Primary nerve repair

The two nerve stumps of a severed peripheral nerve are united at the time when wound closure is achieved. This can be done immediately when the patient comes in or as a delayed procedure after 24 or 48 hours, if one follows the "opération avec une chance urgence différée"—according to Iselin.[17] The main point is that the nerve repair is done at the same time when a final wound closure is achieved, and by performing the delayed nerve repair no opening of the wound is necessary.

Early secondary nerve repair

In early secondary nerve repair the nerve repair is not performed with the original wound closure, but it is delayed to a second operation that might be performed a few days, a week, or several weeks after the original injury. The wound is closed at the time of injury and has to be opened again to perform the nerve repair.

Late secondary nerve repair

If for one reason or another the optimal time for nerve repair has passed and the nerve repair has to be performed more than 6 months later than the original injury, a late secondary nerve repair is performed. Consequently, one performs a late secondary nerve repair if primary nerve repair has failed and a second attempt is to be made.

It is obvious that nerve repairs, performed as late secondary repairs, have a much poorer prognosis than primary or early secondary repairs.

There would be no discussion at all if primary nerve repair would offer an advantage as far as nerve regeneration is concerned. In the past some surgeons hoped that, according to Schife,[32] the degeneration of the nerve fibers in the peripheral stump could be avoided by immediate nerve repair; this could not be proved. Holmes and Young[15] demonstrated that the proliferation of Schwann cells reaches its peak 3 weeks after the injury. The metabolism of the ganglion cells after nerve lesions has its maximum in the third week.[11,12] McQuarrie, Graftsein, and Gershon[20] observed an increased axon sprouting after a second injury to a nerve stump.

Therefore from a theoretical point of view, early secondary nerve repair offers better chances. On the other hand, primary nerve repair has its merits: Only one operation is necessary, and the anatomical situation is much clearer, usually. The nerve stumps might have retracted because of elastic forces, but this can be overcome easily because no fibrosis has occurred yet. On the other hand, the estimation of the amount of tissue damage is difficult, even by the use of the microscope. It might happen that two damaged stumps are coaptated, and the axon sprouting does not commence immediately above the level of transection of the proximal stump but far more proximal. Then the axons have to grow quite a bit along a fibrotic proximal stump until they reach the level of coaptation. There is a potential danger of contamination of the wound and this is increased if the operative field has to be extended in order to look for retracted nerve stumps. Other injuries, like skin loss, bone fracture, and so forth, may create a complicated situation. The conditions, as far as personnel, equipment, and timing are concerned, are not always ideal.

If early secondary repair is selected, several advantages can be exploited. Complicating injuries have been controlled. The general state of the patient has improved. Asepsis is secured, and the operation can be performed as an elective procedure under optimal personnel, technical, and time conditions. The surgical approach can be selected as necessary. The disadvantages are that a second operation has to be performed and time has been lost. The retraction of the stumps might be fixed already, and end-to-end coaptation is more difficult to achieve. A neuroma has formed at the proximal stump and a glioma at the distal stump. They have to be resected, including fibrotic tissue, at the two stumps. Therefore usually a larger defect is created as compared with primary nerve repair. But this, in fact, is not a real disadvantage, because it is secured that normal nerve tissue is present in the cross section before coaptation is performed. Anyway, direct end-to-end coaptation can be more difficult to achieve, and, therefore, the tension at the suture site is increased. This disadvantage can be avoided by the wider use of the nerve grafts in early secondary repairs.

To achieve a direct end-to-end coaptation is even more difficult in late secondary repairs, and, therefore, under these circumstances, nerve grafting is indicated in many cases.

The decision whether primary or early secondary nerve repair should be performed is an individual decision, depending on the patient and on the surgeons' experience and temperament. His decision will be a correct one as long as he remembers the following points:

- The main concern is to do no harm to the patient.
- If primary repair is forced under unfavorable conditions when a nerve defect is present and other injuries complicate the situation, this may cause additional damage to the nerve.
- The nerve stumps may suffer a traction lesion if a direct coaptation is forced in a case of a nerve defect beyond a certain limit.
- It is also harmful for the patient if the failure of a primary nerve repair is not recognized early enough and precious time is lost to make a second attempt.

GENERAL CONSIDERATIONS— ANATOMICAL ASPECTS

The macroscopical unit of a peripheral nerve is the fascicle, which contains a number of nerve fibers (axons, Schwann cells, and myelin sheath), the endoneurial framework, and the endoneurial capillary plexus and is surrounded by the perineurium. The term "funicle" (funiculus) is synonymously used. The term "fascicle" (fasciculus) is preferred because the meaning of the Latin word, *fasces*, defines a collection of homologous longitudinal structures kept together by circular structures. Funiculus is also used in the anatomical terminology in another sense, for example, funiculus spermaticus, a formation that contains several different structures.

The fascicles of a peripheral nerve are embedded in, and surrounded by, the epineurium. The epineurium contains the intraneural vessels, which show many anastomoses with each other and with the vascular plexus in the perineurium and the endoneurium.[19] By careful surgical dissection it is possible to elevate and resect the superficial layer of the epineurium, which surrounds all the fascicles in a circumferential way. As seen by the surgeon, it is on top of the fascicles and it could be referred to as the "epifascicular part" of the epineurium, in contrast to the remaining epineurial tissue, which remains between the fascicles after such a dissection. The latter part of the epineurium can be referred to as the "interfascicular" epineurium. Within the interfascicular epineurium two parts can be differentiated: the lose interfascicular tissue, which just fills the spaces between the fascicles and contains the vessels, and the more tense structures, which surround several fascicles, uniting them into a group of fascicles within the cross section.

Generally speaking the cross section of a peripheral nerve can be divided into a fascicular and a nonfascicular part. According to Sunderland[41] the percentage of nonfascicular area in the cross section of the median nerve varies between 30% and 75% with an average of a little more than 50%. For this reason there is a rather high risk that—in case of stump-to-stump coaptation—the cross section of a certain fascicle meets a nonfascicular area.

The fascicular pattern of a peripheral nerve changes along its course.[40,41] In certain levels

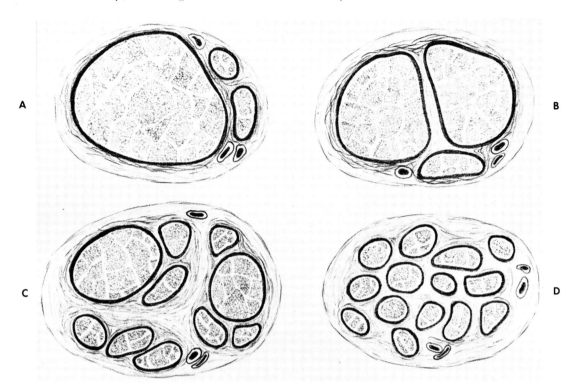

Fig. 34-1. Four basic patterns of fascicular structure. **A,** Monofascicular pattern. **B,** Oligofascicular pattern. **C,** Polyfascicular pattern with grouping. **D,** Polyfascicular pattern without grouping.

a plexiform arrangement of the fascicles could be demonstrated.

Four basic patterns can be distinguished (Fig. 34-1).

Monofascicular pattern (Fig. 34-2, A)

In a monofascicular pattern a cross section contains one big fascicle. There might be some small fascicles in the periphery that can be neglected. In this case the relation of fascicular to nonfascicular tissue is much in favor of the fascicular tissue.

Oligofascicular pattern (Fig. 34-2, B)

In an oligofascicular pattern the cross section contains several large fascicles. If there are two large fascicles, the relation of fascicular to nonfascicular area is still much in favor of the fascicular area. But with an increasing number of fascicles, the relation changes in favor of the nonfascicular area.

Polyfascicular pattern without grouping (Fig. 34-2, D)

In a polyfascicular pattern without grouping the cross section consists of many small fascicles that are diffusely distributed over the cross section.

Polyfascicular pattern with grouping (Fig. 34-2, C)

In polyfascicular pattern with grouping the cross section consists of many fascicles of different sizes. The fascicles are arranged in several groups that can be separated easily by interfascicular dissection. Great efforts have been made to study the intraneural topography of the nerve fibers of certain qualities.[40,41] In distal levels the nerve fibers supplying the same end-organ are arranged in certain fascicles and fascicle groups, respectively. In proximal levels there is a rather diffuse distribution of the nerve fibers,

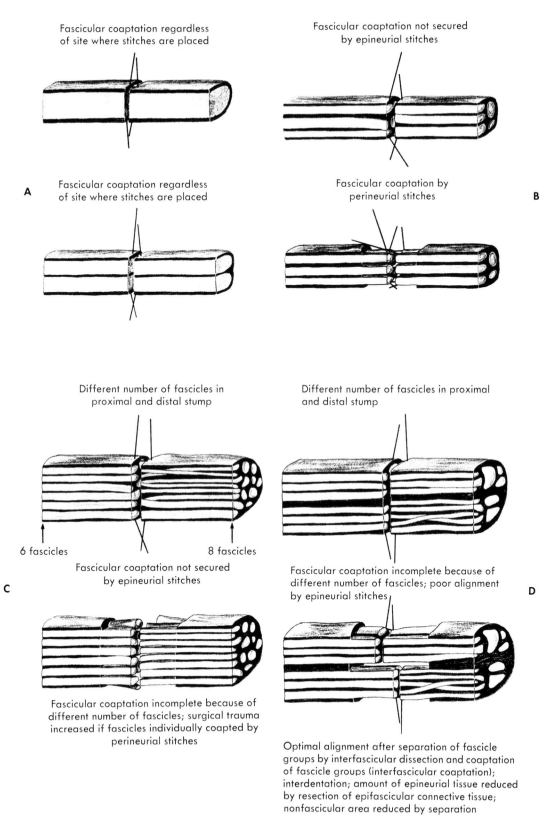

Fascicular coaptation regardless of site where stitches are placed

Fascicular coaptation not secured by epineurial stitches

A

Fascicular coaptation regardless of site where stitches are placed

Fascicular coaptation by perineurial stitches

B

Different number of fascicles in proximal and distal stump

Different number of fascicles in proximal and distal stump

6 fascicles   8 fascicles

Fascicular coaptation not secured by epineurial stitches

Fascicular coaptation incomplete because of different number of fascicles; poor alignment by epineurial stitches

C

D

Fascicular coaptation incomplete because of different number of fascicles; surgical trauma increased if fascicles individually coapted by perineurial stitches

Optimal alignment after separation of fascicle groups by interfascicular dissection and coaptation of fascicle groups (interfascicular coaptation); interdentation; amount of epineurial tissue reduced by resection of epifascicular connective tissue; nonfascicular area reduced by separation

Fig. 34-2. A, Monofascicular pattern and oligofascicular pattern. **B,** Oligofascicular pattern. **C,** Polyfascicular pattern without group arrangement. **D,** Polyfascicular pattern with arrangement in two groups.

supplying a certain end-organ over the cross section. In spite of this diffuse distribution, in many instances nerve fibers of the same function are represented in higher numbers in certain sectors of the nerve. A few millimeters outside the stylomastoid foramen the facial nerve usually consists of one large fascicle with a few small satellites. Missl[22,23] demonstrated by cadaver dissection and serial sections that nerve fibers supplying different muscle groups are cumulated in certain sectors. From Sunderland's tables[41] it seems that in proximal levels of the radial nerve, motor fibers going to the posterior interosseous nerve are represented in a higher frequency in the dorsal quadrant of the nerve.

GENERAL CONSIDERATIONS— TECHNIQUE

The aim of all surgical efforts to repair a transected peripheral nerve is to achieve a most exact and accurate coaptation of the fascicles to offer an optimal chance to the axon sprouts to grow into corresponding peripheral fascicles. This aim should be achieved by the use of a minimum of surgical trauma and a minimum of disturbing factors like buried foreign material, tension, and so forth, to avoid everything that might impede the axons from crossing the suture line. In addition, everything has to be avoided that might exert any deteriorating influence, like compression, traction, and so on. It could be demonstrated[29] that axon sprouts, having already crossed the suture line, may be damaged by compression owing to shrinkage of scar tissue or by stretching of scar tissue.

During the past years the problem of epineurial versus perineurial nerve repair was studied again. The experimental results of Bora[3] and Grabb and co-workers[14] favored the perineurial repair. In contrast to early work Bora and co-workers[4] published experimental results that were interpreted as showing epineurial repair to be superior. Cabaud and co-workers[10] did not see much difference in experiments with the ulnar nerve of the cat.

The results of such experiments can be interpreted with extreme caution only: it is not only the fact that results of animal experiments cannot be applied to human patients, but also the structural differences between different nerve segments may lead to wrong conclusions.

In a nerve segment with monofascicular pattern the relation of fascicular to nonfascicular tissue is very much in favor of the fascicular tissue; the danger of malalignment is nil. In such a case epineurial nerve repair must yield better results. Resection of epineurial tissue would not provide any benefit. The stumps of the large fascicle are in such a broad area of contact that connective tissue proliferation deriving from the epineurium cannot interfere with the coaptation.

The same is true if one has to deal with an oligofascicular nerve with a few large fascicles. Again it will be easy to achieve exact fascicular coaptation just by epineurial repair.

With an increasing number of fascicles it becomes more and more difficult to achieve fascicular coaptation just by epineurial stitches. The relation of fascicular to nonfascicular tissue changes in favor of the nonfascicular tissue, and the danger of malalignment increases. The fast proliferation of connective tissue, deriving from the epineurium, may interfere with the coaptation before a firm union is achieved. In this case resection of the epifascicular epineurium may reduce the amount of epineurial proliferation at the site of coaptation. Coaptation of the individual larger fascicles by perineurial stitches helps to secure fascicular coaptation.

In nerves with a polyfascicular pattern this consideration becomes more important. It seems logical that, even in such a nerve segment consisting of many small fascicles an individual fascicular repair as suggested by Tupper[42] may increase the chances. But there is a certain limit beyond which an exact alignment in a nerve with many small fascicles needs so much manipulation and surgical trauma that the gain of exactness does not repay. One must not forget that the trauma caused by one stitch becomes relatively more important the smaller the involved fascicles are. In addition, in cases of even small defects, owing to the rapid change in the number of fascicles the two stumps contain a different number of fascicles, which makes complete fascicular coaptation impossible.

In nerves with polyfascicular pattern without grouping it might be the better solution to perform a truncular coaptation, attempting to achieve a maximum of exactness by the use of guide sutures.[24,38] In case of nerve grafting, the grafts are coapted with the fascicles of certain sectors of a nerve (sectoral nerve grafting) exploiting all the knowledge about intraneural topography.

The interfascicular coaptation represents a compromise between truncular coaptation and fascicular coaptation especially designed for nerve segments with a polyfascicular pattern and grouping of the fascicles. Resection of the epineurium reduces the source of proliferative connective tissue at the site of coaptation. By interfascicular dissection the preformed groups of fascicles within the cross sections are separated. The corresponding groups are identified, which is much easier than the identification of individual fascicles. It does not matter if there is a different number of fascicles present in the two stumps, provided that the number of groups is identical. Optimal alignment can be achieved between the fascicle groups or between fascicle group and graft in the case of interfascicular nerve grafting. Stepwise transection with interdentation after coaptation increases the lateral stability.

In conclusion

The procedure of restoration of continuity of a transected peripheral nerve is defined by description of the way good coaptation is achieved and not by determining the site where the stitches are placed. In all the above-mentioned types of coaptation stitches could be placed in the perineurium or the epineurium. Stitches in the epineurium can be placed in the circumferential epifascicular epineurium (epineurial stitch *sensu strictorii*) or in the interfascicular epineurium (interfascicular stitch). All types of stitches might be used in the same surgical procedure. Therefore the terms "epineurial" or "perineurial"

nerve repair do not really describe what was done.

Besides the coaptation there are three more essential steps during nerve repair that can be performed in different ways and have to be defined to describe the whole procedure.

Preparation of stumps

Especially in secondary nerve repairs the two stumps have to be prepared. The preparation can be performed by resection of small sections until normal nerve tissue is present in the whole cross section. This can be done by the use of a razor blade or a diamond knife, and different technical devices have been designed to make the resection easier. This way of preparation is applied in nerves with a monofascicular pattern, an oligofascicular pattern with very few fascicles, or a polyfascicular pattern without grouping. The other way of preparing the stumps is to incise the epineurium proximal and distal to the lesion and to perform an interfascicular dissection to separate individual fascicles or groups of fascicles. This way of preparation is extremely useful in oligofascicular nerves with more fascicles and in polyfascicular nerve segments with grouping of the fascicles. It is also applied in lesions in-continuity and in reoperation after failure of a previous nerve repair. Its advantage is that the group arrangement can be recognized. Near the division of a nerve the fascicle groups can be defined according to their function in a distal stump by extending the exposure to the division and following the fascicle groups in retrograde direction to the level of transection. It usually is not very difficult then to make a good guess as to which one corresponds to which by comparing the fascicle groups of the two cross sections.

Approximation

The next step is the *approximation* of the two stumps. This can be done by grasping the nerve tissue with an instrument or by the use of a stay-stitch. If there is no tension in a longitudinal direction, a single stitch would be sufficient to provide a good area of contact. If there is tension, contact will be established only at the point of the stitch. The remaining area of the two cross sections will tend to spread apart, and more stitches will be necessary to achieve good contact. At this point the surgeon has to decide how much tension he is ready to accept. The selection of further technical steps will depend very much on this decision. Truncular coaptation, with stitches in the epifascicular epineurium, will provide rather good tensile strength but at the expense of exactness. Fascicular or interfascicular coaptation fulfills the requirements of exactness much better but cannot be used if there is tension at the site of coaptation. In this case too many stitches have to be used and the surgical trauma is very much increased. If one wants to use these techniques and a given defect cannot be overcome by tranposition and limited mobilization, one should use a nerve graft. Flexion of the adjacent joints to ease tension does not solve the problem. The site of coaptation will be stretched gradually when mobilization is commenced, and this may have a deleterious influence on the regenerating axons.

Maintaining the coaptation

Finally, the achieved coaptation, which has been discussed previously, has to be maintained. It can be easy or difficult, according to the tension that is present at the time of surgery or might be expected during mobilization if the approximation has been achieved by flexing the adjacent joints.

If tension is avoided completely, one stitch per fascicle with fascicular coaptation and per fascicle group with interfascicular coaptation very often is sufficient to maintain the coaptation until fibrin clotting provides additional tensile strength. As this tensile strength is minimal, the tension has to be really zero. Extreme care is necessary to avoid shearing forces during wound closure and during the first postoperative days. After 8 to 10 days the tensile strength is sufficient to commence mobilization. Only exceptionally a second or a third stitch may be necessary.

The tensile strength at the site of coaptation can be increased by application of an allogenic fibrinogin concentrate along with thrombin factor XIII and calcium ions according to the suggestion of Matras and co-workers[21] and Duspiva and co-workers.[13] Extreme care is necessary to avoid touching the nerve cross section with this solution. If tension is really zero, such additional measures are not necessary.

If a surgeon is ready to accept some tension immediately or later on, in order to be able to overcome larger defects by direct coaptation, he has to use more stitches, and the amount of surgical trauma increases. This may be acceptable if truncular coaptation and stitches in the epifascicular epineurium are used. There will be a limit, different in different individuals, beyond which the consequences of tension at the sutures will be more important than the disadvantage of using a nerve graft with its two sites of coaptation.

At the present time all surgeons agree on the fact that in a clean cut a direct end-to-end coaptation is the treatment of choice, and, in the case of a defect beyond 4 cm, grafting is the better solution. Between these extremes there is an area of disagreement. Surgeons with vast experience with nerve grafts, like Brunelli,[9] Samii,[31] Buck-Gramcko,[6] and myself,[27] use a nerve graft in small defects that are managed by direct coaptation by other surgeons.

TECHNIQUE OF INTERFASCICULAR NERVE GRAFTING

The technique of interfascicular nerve grafting is especially designed for polyfascicular nerves with group arrangement. It combines a minimum of surgical trauma with a maximum of accuracy. It is used in early or late secondary repairs. If the fact of complete transection and the exact site of the lesion is known from the primary treatment of the injury, the proximal and distal stump can be exposed using a minimal incision, and the grafts can be introduced across the tunnel. Otherwise the whole length of the involved nerve has to be explored. The proximal and distal nerve stumps are exposed in normal tissue proximal and distal to the lesion (Fig. 34-3, *A*). Therefore marking stitches at the time of primary surgery is not useful.

After exposure of the two stumps the

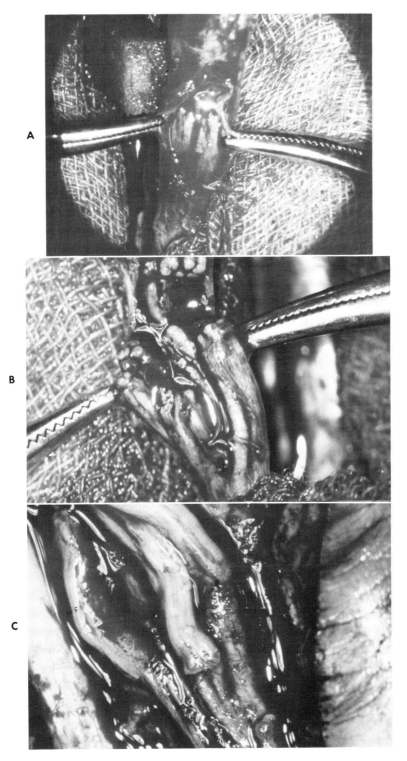

Fig. 34-3. Median nerve. **A,** Epifascicular epineurium was incised. Two fascicle groups are exposed. (×6.) **B,** After interfascicular dissection, five fascicle groups have been isolated and transected proximal to neuroma. (×10.) **C,** Five nerve grafts have been approximated and coapted to fascicle groups. One 10-0 nylon stitch has been used for each graft end.

epineurium is incised proximal to the lesion and elevated. A strip of epineurium approximately 1 cm in length is resected. After resection of the epifascicular epineurium, one enters the space between two fascicle groups by careful microsurgical dissection. The preformed fascicle groups are separated. The dissection continues toward the neuroma in the proximal stump and the glioma in the distal stump. For each fascicle group the level where the neuroma or the glioma commences is defined, and at this level the fascicle group is transected by the use of a special scissors with undulated blades (Fig. 34-3, *B*).

After this interfascicular dissection the nerve stump consists of several protruding fascicle groups of different lengths. The exposure is extended distally to the division of the involved nerve. There the individual branches can be identified. By following these fascicle groups in a retrograde direction, it can be recognized which fascicle group contains nerve fibers of a certain function. It is especially important with the median and ulnar nerves to recognize the fascicle groups containing the motor fibers. A sketch is made of the fascicular pattern of the proximal and distal stumps. Comparing the fascicle groups, a guess is made as to which fascicle group contains the corresponding fibers in the proximal stump. The distance between the two stumps is measured. Up to this moment the operation is performed under tourniquet, if possible. Now the tourniquet is released and the wound is compressed for hemostasis. During this period of time the nerve grafts are provided. The first choice is the sural nerve, which can be easily excised if the patient is in a side position, that is, one leg is on top of the other. The sural nerve is identified behind the lateral ankle (Fig. 34-4, *A*) using a small transverse incision. By a gentle pull the course of the nerve can be palpated. A second incision is made 4 to 5 cm proximal to the lateral ankle on the dorsal aspect of the calf. The nerve is identified here; it usually is found dorsal and medial to the small saphenous vein. Now the sural nerve is transected at the level of the

distal incision. By a gentle pull on the nerve at the proximal incision, other smaller branches of the nerve are identified and transected at the level of the distal incision. After transection of these additional branches, the whole nerve can be extracted from the proximal incision. Again a gentle pull is exerted on the nerve, and the course palpated in a proximal direction. Using another small incision at the midcalf and a fourth incision just beneath the popliteal fossa, the nerve is identified, transected at the proximal level, and extracted. Sometimes the nerve receives a second source at the level of the midcalf. This can be recognized by palpation. Both parts are excised. This possibility is the reason why the use of a stripper is not recommended. It would not be possible to recognize this variation, and a part of the nerve would be destroyed. By excision of the sural nerve a segment of 35 to 45 cm can be gained.

In its proximal part the sural nerve consists of one or a few large fascicles. In its distal part there are many small fascicles. As mentioned above, at a distal level, the sural nerve is already branching. Following these branches in a proximal direction, the nerve can be divided into smaller subunits, each of them consisting of several fascicles. Proper segments can be selected according to the fascicular pattern of the nerve at different levels. If one sural nerve is not sufficient, the second sural nerve can be used as a graft. If one knows that a lot of nerve grafts will be needed, the two sural nerves can be excised as a first step with the patient prone. Up to this date there have been no problems as far as painful neuromas of the sural nerve are concerned. It has to be stated that in all cases the sural nerve was transected at a level where the proximal stump is buried underneath the fascia and not exposed to irritation in the subcutaneous tissue. The whole sural nerve should be excised even if only a small piece is needed.

Another suitable nerve graft is the cutaneous femoris lateralis nerve. This nerve can be identified easily, just beneath and medial to the spina iliaca ventralis, where it emerges

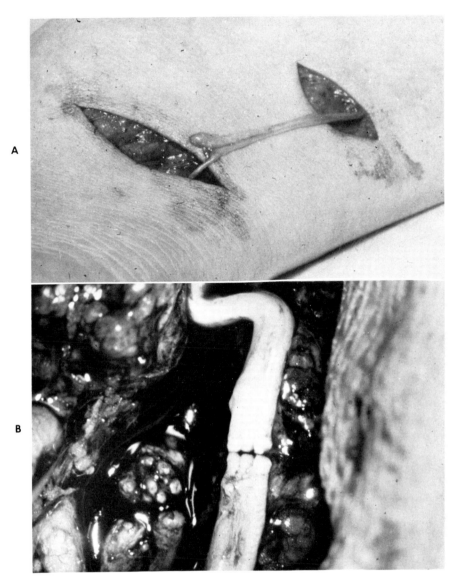

Fig. 34-4. A, Exposure of sural nerve behind lateral ankle of left leg. Nerve is already divided. After transection of main trunk, small branch is identified by pull at more proximal incision. **B,** Transection of sural nerve in segments of proper length. Epifascicular epineurium has to be pushed back gently to expose fascicles.

from the abdominal wall and runs in a caudal-lateral direction in the subcutaneous tissue of the thigh. It divides into several branches. By selecting the common nerve or one of the branches, a proper graft can be provided. The nerve can be followed into the pelvis if a longer segment is needed. Transec-

tion within the pelvis would have the advantage that the neuroma at the site of transection is buried in the depths of the pelvis. A segment about 20 cm in length can be removed.

The third choice is the cutaneous antebrachii medialis nerve. This nerve is found at the border between the axilla and upper arm by a small transverse incision. It is in close relation to the brachial vein. A piece of about 25 cm can be obtained by two additional transverse incisions in the midarm and at the level of the elbow joint. At the distal level the nerve is already divided into two or three branches. This nerve is not used as a graft if a lesion of the ulnar nerve of the same extremity is present.

Further donor nerves would be the cutaneous antebrachii dorsalis nerve, the intercostal nerves, and the saphenous nerve. The saphenous nerve and the sural nerve of the same extremity are not excised to avoid a major sensory loss of the foot. The ramus superficialis of the radial nerve is not used as a donor because of its known tendency to develop painful neuromas. We have used it only in cases of brachial plexus lesions, when the nerve was functionless anyway.

After removing the grafts, proper segments are prepared a little bit longer than the defect, measured in neutral position of the limb. Transection of the grafts is performed by scissors with undulated blades. The transection is done by several partial bites, and after each bite the epineurial tissue of the graft ends is pushed back to avoid capping of the cross section by epineurial tissue (Fig. 34-4, *B*). The epineurial tissue of the grafts is not resected routinely. Because these are free grafts and tissue proliferation commences with a certain delay after circulation is reestablished, there is no danger that connective tissue proliferation from the epineurium of the graft will interfere with the site of coaptation. The graft segments that fit best to the individual fascicle groups are selected. Using one 10-0 nylon stitch, which is anchored in the epineurium or the interfascicular tissue of the graft on the one side and the interfascicular tissue of the fascicle group on the other side, a gentle approximation is achieved (Fig. 34-3, *C*). As there is usually no tension this stitch is sufficient to provide good end-to-end contact. Rarely, for instance if gravity is involved, a second stitch might be necessary to achieve good contact. After the graft has been in contact with the

cross section of the fascicle group for a while, fibrin clotting will provide a sufficiently strong coaptation. Nothing else is done to maintain the coaptation. As the fascicle groups have been cut at different levels, an indentation is achieved between each graft and other neighboring fascicle groups. This side-to-side contact increases the surface of contact and adds to the lateral stability. After all grafts have been placed, the wound is closed with extreme care to avoid shearing forces and dislocation of the grafts. After skin closure a plaster cast is applied to immobilize the extremity in exactly the position it had during operation. This immobilization is continued for 8 to 10 days. Thereafter no further immobilization is necessary.

For a successful grafting a proper recipient site is essential. The grafts do not survive as well in bad scar tissue. In such a case a proper recipient site should be prepared by a previous plastic surgical procedure. Circumscribed areas of scar tissue can be bypassed. It does not influence the result in such a case if the graft is a little bit longer. The quality of the result is dependent on the length of the defect rather than on the length of the graft. The more nerve tissue has been lost, the more different are the fascicular patterns. As the fascicle groups are constant over a longer distance, the recognition of crresponding fascicle groups is possible even in cases of defects of a few centimeters.

In longer defects the problem of identifying corresponding fascicle groups becomes more difficult. In long defects one can be forced to face the fact that in the distal stump there is a polyfascicular pattern with group arrangement, but in the proximal stump a different type of fascicular pattern is present. In this case the proximal ends of the grafts are united with sectors of the cross section that provide—according to the general knowledge of intraneural topography—a good chance of containing a number of fibers of the desired quality. In very proximal levels, we have to reckon with a diffuse distribution of fibers over the entire cross section. But even with this diffuse distribution, there is still a chance that at least some of the fibers will grow into the correct pathway. Obviously the result will be worse in these cases than in patients with shorter defects.

RESULTS

Between 1964 and the end of 1970, 98 patients with traumatic lesions of the median, radial, and ulnar nerves have been operated on using the interfascicular grafting technique. Ninety patients could be followed and evaluated with a sufficiently long follow-up period. The evaluation was performed using the scheme of Highet, as used by Nicholson and Seddon[30] for the median and the ulnar nerve, respectively. The M0 to M5 scale was used for evaluation of the radial nerve.

Radial nerve

Thirteen of sixteen patients operated on because of defects of the radial nerves could be evaluated. Five of thirteen could be graded M5 (average age 24 years [8 to 42 years], average length of defect 5.7 cm [3 to 10 cm]). Five cases were listed as M4 (average age 32 years [22 to 53 years], average length of defect 7.6 cm [4 to 12 cm]. There were two patients listed M3 (average age 25 years [8 to 42 years], average length defect 10.5 cm). One patient did not achieve a useful recovery (M2 only): his age was 62, and there was a defect of 10 cm to be bridged (see Table 34-1).

Median nerve

Thirty-eight patients with lesions of the median nerve could be evaluated. Eleven of them had only a partial loss of thenar muscle function owing to partial innervation of these muscles by the ulnar nerve. These cases could not be used for motor evaluation. From the remaining 27 patients suitable for motor function evaluation, 16 achieved a motor recovery of M4 or M5 (average age 27.7 years [9 to 64 years], average length of defect 6.3 cm [2 to 16 cm]). Six cases achieved a motor recovery of M3 (average age 38.6 years [15 to 55 years], average length of the defect 9.6 cm [4.5 to 20 cm]). There were two cases with recovery of M2 (average age 58 years [47 to 69 years], average length of defect 6 cm [5.7

Table 34-1. Thirteen cases of radial nerve repair by the interfascicular grafting technique

M5 n = 5/13(38.5%)			M4 n = 5/13(38.5%)			M3 n = 2/13(15.4%)			M2 n = 1/13(7.6%)			M1	M0
Current number	Age	Defect (cm)	Current number	Age	Defect (cm)	Current number	Age	Defect (cm)	Current number	Age	Defect (cm)		
9	21	10.0	11	34	12.0	12	8	12.5	7	62	10.0		
1	8	8.5	8	25	8.0	16	42	9.0					
2	19	4.0	15	26	8.0								
3	30	3.0	5	22	6.0								
10	42	3.0	6	53	4.0								

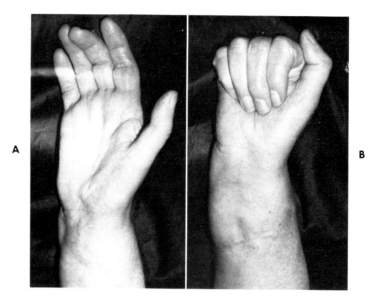

Fig. 34-5. Female patient: 51 years of age. Transection of median and ulnar nerve and all flexor tendons in distal forearm. Tendon repair by suture, nerve repair by nerve grafts (four sural nerve segments of 2 cm length for each of nerves). **A** and **B,** Short time after repair.

cm]). Three patients had only M1 motor recovery (average age 20.6 years [12 to 38 years], average length of defect 12.5 cm). These three patients had suffered extremely severe injuries. Two nerves (cases 38 and 39) belong to the two extremities of a 12-year-old boy who had sustained a severe electrical burn. The major part of the muscle was damaged directly by the electric burn, and motor recovery could not be expected. But there was return of protective sensibility (S3). The third failure was a median nerve of a 38-year-old man in whom a postoperative infection, after primary repair, had resulted in prolonged suppuration. The scar tissue did not provide a satisfactory bed for the nerve grafts. A pedicle flap to restore soft tissue prior to nerve grafting might have improved the result.

As far as sensibility was concerned all 38 cases could be evaluated. There were two cases listed as S4 (average age 14 years [10 to 18 years], average length of the defect 6 cm [5 to 7 cm]). Thirteen patients achieved the result of S3$^+$ (22 years [9 to 46 years], average

length of the defect 7 cm [2 to 20 cm]). Protective sensibility was achieved in 22 cases (average age 37.7 years [12 to 69 years], average length of defect 6.6 cm [2 to 19 cm]) (Fig. 34-5). There was one failure, a 47-year-old patient with a defect of 7 cm. The repair was performed 13 months after the original injury (see Table 34-2).

All but one nerve were repaired as secondary repairs, the majority of them as late secondary repairs. There were five patients with high median nerve lesions included.

Ulnar nerve

Thirty-nine patients could be evaluated. Nineteen of them achieved a motor recovery of M4 to M5 (average age 29.2 years [7 to 67 years], average length of the defect 4.7 cm [2 to 12 cm]). Twelve patients achieved a recovery of M3 (average age 43 years [13 to 69 years], average length of the defect 6.4 cm [2 to 20 cm]). In three nerves there was a recovery of M2$^+$ (average age 37 years [15 to 58 years], average length of the defect 12.6 cm [6 to 20 cm]). Two patients had a recovery of

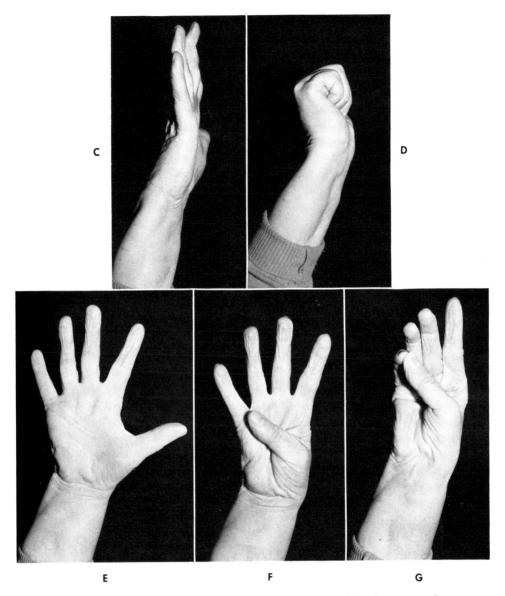

Fig. 34-5, cont'd. C to **G,** Two years after repair. Protective sensibility has returned. No two-point discrimination.

M2 (ages 17 and 31 years) and the length of the defects were 6 and 20 cm. Three patients had a recovery of only M1 (average age 41.3 years [33 to 53 years], average length of defect 9.3 cm [4 to 19 cm]). Ten patients achieved a recovery of S3$^+$ or better (average age 15.8 years [7 to 28 years], and 23 patients reached protective sensibility (S3) (average age 41.6 years [13 to 69 years], average length of defect 6 cm [2 to 20 cm]). Six patients did not achieve a useful degree of sensibility (average age 40.5 years [17 to 62 years], average length of defect 10.3 cm [5 to 20 cm]) (see Table 34-3).

Table 34-2. Thirty-eight cases of median nerve repair by the interfascicular grafting technique

n	Patient n	Partial loss 11/38(28.9%)			M4-5 16/27(59.26%)			M3 6/27(22.22%)			M2 2/27(7.41%)			M1 3/27(11.11%)		
		Current number	Age	Defect (cm)	Current number	Age	Defect (cm)	Current number	Age	Defect (cm)	Current number	Age	Defect (cm)	Current number	Age	Defect (cm)
S4	2/38 (5.26%)				20	18	7.0	5	15	20.0						
					14	10	5.0									
S3+	13/38 (34.21%)	23	46	4.5	2	10	16.0									
		21	24	4.0	4	39	13.0									
		29	27	4.0	13	21	6.0									
		30	25	3.5	9	9	5.0									
		17	20	2.0	36	20	5.0									
					40	13	5.0									
					12	19	2.5									
S3	22/38 (57.90%)	22	52	8.0	8	44	12.0	10	55	16.0	43	69	5.0	38	12	19.0
		27	21	6.0	16	22	10.0	3	48	7.0				39	12	12.0
		24	24	5.0	37	19	5.0	15	25	5.0				41	38	6.5
		25	21	3.4	1	64	3.0	36	43	5.0						
		28	34	4.0	18	50	3.0	7	46	4.5						
		26	46	2.0	6	51	2.0									
					11	35	2.0									
S2	1/38 (2.63%)										19	47	7.0			

Table 34-3. Thirty-nine cases of ulnar nerve lesions repaired by the interfascicular grafting technique

n	Patient n	Partial loss			M4-5 19/39(48.72%)			M3 12/39(30.77%)			M2+ 3/39(7.69%)			M2 2/39(5.13%)			M1 3/39(7.69%)		
		Current number	Age	Defect (cm)	Current number	Age	Defect (cm)	Current number	Age	Defect (cm)	Current number	Age	Defect (cm)	Current number	Age	Defect (cm)	Current number	Age	Defect (cm)
S4	1/39 (2.56%)				28	7	4.5												
S3+	9/39 (23.08%)				36	12	10.0												
					9	20	7.0												
					29	17	7.0												
					2	10	6.0												
					11	11	6.0												
					10	23	5.0												
					37	19	5.0												
					16	28	3.0												
					18	11	3.0												
S3	23/39 (58.98%)				13	67	7.0	23	34	20.0	8	15	20.0				41	8	4.0
					40	13	5.0	5	39	10.0	6	39	12.0						
					14	46	4.0	44	48	6.0	19	58	6.0						
					3	63	3.0	43	69	5.5									
					4	12	3.0	12	13	5.0									
					31	25	3.0	24	45	4.5									
					7	51	2.0	34	34	4.5									
					17	55	2.0	15	55	4.0									
					26	64	2.0	27	54	3.0									
								25	18	2.0									
S2+	1/39 (2.56%)													33	31	20.0			
S2	3/39 (7.69%)							1	62	7.0				38	17	5.0			
								30	47	5.0									
S1	2/39 (5.13%)																22	33	19.0
																	20	53	5.0

SENSIBILITY TESTING AND TRAINING

To improve the results of sensibility, different training techniques have been developed. At our department we use a method that was developed on the basis of the Braille's system.[26] Small plates made of aluminum foil with standardized prominences are provided. The prominences in one of the plates are arranged in two converging lines; this gives the opportunity to test two-point discrimination (Fig. 34-6, *A*). The distance between the pair of prominences must be an irregular one; otherwise the patient knows that there have to be two points and he believes

he feels them. In other plates the prominences are arranged as a straight or a curved line or as a circle, a quadrangle, or a triangle (Fig. 34-6, *B*).

Rinderer[28] studied the range of normal values by testing 80 patients with normal sensibility. The average value for the two-point discrimination test was 2.85 mm, with a range between 1.5 and 6 mm (see Fig. 34-7, *A*).

The geometrical figure test was classified into six levels:

- Level 5 means the test person could identify the line of prominences immedi-

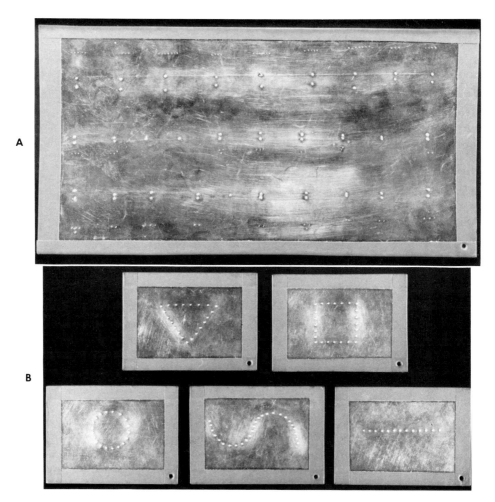

Fig. 34-6. Small plates of aluminum foil with standardized prominences are used for testing two-point discrimination, **A,** and ability to distinguish geometrical figures, **B.**

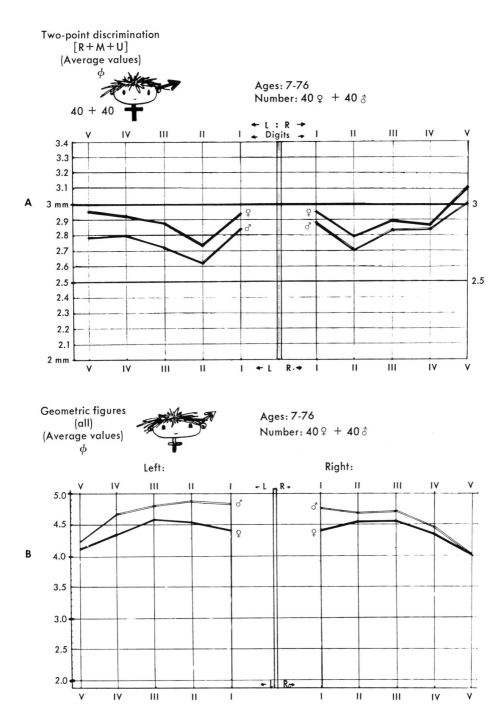

Fig. 34-7. Normal values for all digits of right and left hands using aluminum plate devices. **A,** Two-point discrimination. **B,** Geometrical pattern recognition.

ately and follow it very securely without losing it, not even once. The test person could recognize the figure at once.

- Level 4 means that the patient or the test person follows the line just a bit insecurely, losing it up to two times. They could identify the figure but not as quickly as in level 5.
- Level 3 means that the test person recognized the line but followed the line of an expected or imagined figure, and, therefore, gave an instant answer but a wrong one.
- Level 2 means the test person could follow the line with great difficulty only. The line was lost up to five times, and the figures were recognized with great difficulty.
- Level 1 means the test person was almost unable to follow the line, lost the line five times, and had great difficulty locating it again. The test person was incapable of recognizing the figure.
- Level 0 means the test person was incapable of following the line at all. The prominences were not recognized.

Of the normal test persons 80% reached level 5, 10% reached level 4, and the remaining 10% were under level 4 (see Fig. 34-7, *B*). As expected, the results were much better in the younger age group than in the older test persons. It is a great advantage of the test that each finger can be tested independently on three aspects (radial, palmar, and ulnar). The results with the index finger were far better than the results with the little finger. The test is useful in determining whether the test person belongs within the normal range or not. If the test person is outside the normal range, improvement can be followed as the results gradually approach the normal range.

For training purposes the patient is first tested and his level determined. Needless to say, the test is performed with the patient blindfolded. The patient is then encouraged to repeat the palpation of the plates with open eyes and blindfolded—in alternation. Although he will obtain less sensory information on which to base a decision than a nor-

mal individual, with training he should learn to come to correct conclusions on the basis of this diminished sensory input. Many different plates with different figures can be used to avoid guessing. From time to time standard tests are performed to see if the patient has already climbed to a higher level.

REFERENCES

1. Albert, E.: Einige Operationen am Nerven, Wr. Med. Presse. **26**:1285, 1885.
2. Ballance, C., and Duel, A. B.: Operative treatment of facial palsy by the introduction of nerve grafts into fallopian canal and by other intratemporal methods, Arch. Otol. **15**:1, 1932.
3. Bora, W.: Peripheral nerve repairs in cats, J. Bone Joint Surg. **49A**:659, 1967.
4. Bora, F. W., Pleasure, D. E., and Didzian, N. A.: A study of nerve regeneration and neuroma formation after nerve suture by various techniques, J. Hand Surg. **1**(2):138, 1976.
5. Brooks, D.: The place of nerve grafting in orthopaedic surgery, J. Bone Joint Surg. **37A**:299, 1955.
6. Buck-Gramcko, D.: Discussion at Symposium on Hand Surgery, Vienna, May 21-23, 1977. In print.
7. Bunnell, S.: Surgery of the nerves of the hand, Surg. Gynecol. Obstet. **44**:145, 1927.
8. Bunnell, S., and Boyes, H. J.: Nerve grafts, Am. J. Surg. **45**:64, 1939.
9. Brunnelli, G.: Discussion at Symposium on Hand Surgery, Vienna, May 21-23, 1977. In print.
10. Cabaud, H. E., et al.: Epineural and perineural fascicular nerve repair: a critical comparison, J. Hand Surg. **1**(2):110, 1976.
11. Ducker, T. B., and Kauffman, F. C.: Metabolic factors in surgery of peripheral nerves, Clin. Neurosurg. **24**:406, 1977.
12. Ducker, T. B., Kempe, L. G., and Hayes, G. J.: The metabolic background for peripheral nerve surgery. J. Neurosurg. **30**:270, 1969.
13. Duspiva, W., et al.: Eine neue Methode der Anastomisierung durchtrennter peripherer Nerven, Chir. Forum p. 100, 1977.
14. Grabb, W. C., et al.: Comparison of methods of peripheral nerve suturing in monkeys, Plast. Reconstr. Surg. **46**(1):31, 1970.
15. Holmes, W., and Young, J. Z.: Nerve regeneration after immediate and delayed suture, J. Anat. **77**:63, 1942.
16. Hueter, K.: Die allgemeine Chirurgie, Leipzig, 1883, Vogel Verlag.
17. Iselin, M.: Urgence avec opération différée, Mém. Acad. Chir. **83**:232, 1957.
18. Langley, J. N., and Hashimoto, M.: On the suture of separate nerve bundles in a nerve trunk and on internal nerve plexus, J. Physiol. Lond. **51**:318, 1917.
19. Lundborg, G.: Structure and function of the in-

traneural microvessels as related to trauma, edema formation, and nerve function, J. Bone Joint Surg. **57A:**938, 1975.

20. McQuarrie, I. G., Graftsein, B., and Gershon, M. D.: Axosprossung bei Zweitwunden, Brain Res. **132:**443, 1977.

21. Matras, H., et al.: Zur nahtlosen interfaszikulären Nerventransplantation im Tierexperiment, Wien. Med. Wschr. 122 Jhrg. **37:**1517, 1972.

22. Meissl, G.: Intraneural topography of the extracranial facial nerve. In Fisch U., ed.: Facial nerve surgery, Birmingham, Ala., 1977, Kugler Medical Publications.

23. Meissl, G.: Die intraneurale Topographie des extrakraniellen N. facialis, Acta Chir. Aust. In press.

24. Michon, J.: Die Nervennaht unter dem Mikroskop. Paper read at eighth symposium d. Deutschsprachigen Arbeitsgemeinschaft für Handchirurgie, Vienna, May 28-30, 1967.

25. Michon, J.: Etat actuel des techniques de réparation des nerfs peripheriques, Orthop. Traumatol. p. 273, 1970.

26. Millesi, H.: Fortschritte in der Behandlung peripherer Nervenläsionen, Krankengymnast **23:** 138, 1971.

27. Millesi, H.: Discussion at Symposium on Hand Surgery, Vienna, May 21-23, 1977. In print.

28. Millesi, H., and Rinderer, D.: A method for training and testing sensibility of the finger-tips. Abstracts of the Seventh International Congress of the World Federation of Occupational Therapists, Jerusalem, March 12-17, 1978, p. 98

29. Millesi, H., Berger, A., and Meissl, G.: Experimentelle Untersuchungen zur Heilung durchtrennter peripherer Nerven, Chir. Plast. **I:**174, 1972.

30. Nicholson, O. R., and Seddon, H. J.: Nerve repair in civil practice. Results of the treatment of median and ulnar nerve lesions, Br. Med. J. **2:**1065, 1957.

31. Samii, M: Discussion at Symposium on Hand Surgery, Vienna, May 21-23, 1977. In print.

32. Schiff, H.: Sur le réunion des nerfs moteurs d'origine et de fonctions différents, Arch. Sci. Physiol. Nature **3:**13, 1885.

33. Seddon, H. J.: The use of autogenous grafts for the repair of large gaps in peripheral nerves, Br. Hand Surg. **35:**151, 1947.

34. Seddon, H. J.: Nerve grafting, J. Bone Joint Surg. **45B:**447, 1963.

35. Seddon, H. J.: Surgical disorders of the peripheral nerves, Edinburgh, 1972, Churchill Livingstone.

36. Smith, J. W.: Factors influencing nerve repair: I. Blood supply of peripheral nerves, Arch. Surg. **93:**433, 1966.

37. Smith, J. W.: Factors influencing nerve repair: II. Collateral circulation of peripheral nerves, Arch. Surg. **93:**433, 1966.

38. Smith, J. W.: In Grabb, W. G., and Smith, J. W., eds.: Plastic surgery, Boston, 1968, Little Brown & Co.

39. Smith, J. W.: A new technique of facial animation, Transactions of the Fifth International Congress of Plastic Surgery, Australia, 1971, Butterworth & Co., p. 83.

40. Sunderland, S.: The intraneural topography of the radial, median and ulnar nerves, Brain, **68:**243, 1945.

41. Sunderland, S.: Nerve and nerve injuries, Baltimore, 1968, The Williams & Wilkins Co.

42. Tupper, J.: Discussion at Symposium on Hand Surgery. Vienna, May 21-23, 1977. In print.

35

Fascicular nerve repair

Jack W. Tupper

Within a peripheral nerve, the nerve fiber (axon and its sheath) is the smallest functional unit. Bundles of these fibers contained by a specialized tubular membrane, the perineurium, form the smallest surgical unit, the fasciculus. This may vary from less than 0.1 mm to several millimeters in diameter. The fascicular contents are under axoplasmic pressure and, therefore, are always round in cross section (Fig. 35-1). In contradistinction to the epineurium, the perineurium forms not only a physical but also a physiological barrier as well, allowing preferential passage of some materials. Capillaries form the only true intrafascicular vessels.

Fasciculi may pass singly along the nerve or may be arranged in groups (Fig. 35-2). Surrounding fasciculi and fascicular groups, binding them all together, is a loose areolar tissue, the intraneural epineurium. In this tissue are the blood and lymph vessels. Surrounding all of this to form the outer layer of the peripheral nerve is a more or less tubular membrane, the circumferential epineurium (Fig. 35-3).

From an anatomical standpoint, nerve repairs may be of several types:

1. Epineurial—sutures through the circumferential epineurium only
2. Epineurial plus a few sutures in corresponding bundles (in large nerves)
3. Large bundle repair—removal of circumferential epineurium and suturing of large bundles (in large nerves)
4. Perineurial (fascicular)—both circumferential and intraneural epineurium are discarded at the repair site. Fasciculi are repaired with sutures in the

perineurium only. Even in this type, bundles of very small fasciculi (less than 0.2 mm) are usually sutured as a unit.

There are approximately 25 fasciculi in the median nerve at the wrist (Fig. 35-4) and four or five (Fig. 35-8) in a proper digital nerve.

If an epineurial repair is done, there is gross orientation of the nerve ends but poor fascicular coaptation. A tight closure inhibits escape of budding axons but may make intraneural hematoma more likely. Since a peripheral nerve is often 50% interfascicular tissue, it would follow that regenerating axons would have approximately that percentage chance of growing down a distal perineurial tube rather than into the tissue between. A specific fascicular juncture, if motor and sensory can be sorted, theoretically would give a better percentage.

Accurate fascicular matching can be done only in primary repair of sharply divided nerves. At the wrist level, the motor fascicle of the median nerve is separate and can usually be identified, but proximally fascicles will be mixed in their motor-sensory content.

If a graft is to be used, the repair may be either epineurial or perineurial. The sural nerve is the usual donor nerve. If a fascicular graft is to be carried out, the epineurium must be removed and the fasciculi dissected into lengths determined initially by the distance between branches so that the length of fascicular graft is essentially one fairly homogeneous strand. Not all fascicular material within a nerve is useful; many are too small in size. These grafts may then be sutured to bridge the gap between proximal and distal fasciculi in the injured nerve.

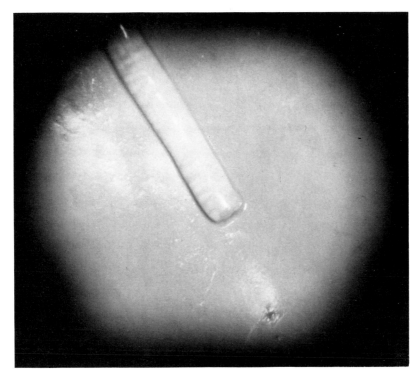

Fig. 35-1. Single fascicle. Cross section is always round. Cross-striations in perineurium are bands of Fontana.

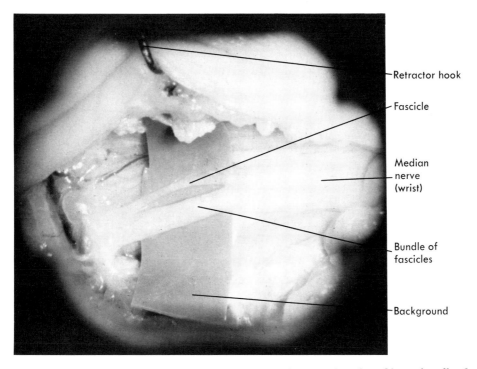

Retractor hook

Fascicle

Median nerve (wrist)

Bundle of fascicles

Background

Fig. 35-2. Median nerve at wrist has been divided into single upper fascicle and lower bundle of fascicles.

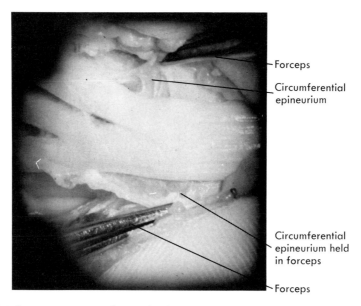

Fig. 35-3. Median nerve in carpal tunnel. Three major branches are to left. Circumferential epineurium has been divided longitudinally and reflected to sides where it is held in forceps.

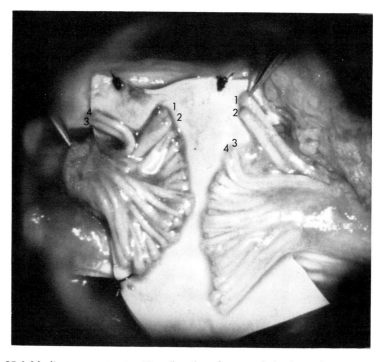

Fig. 35-4. Median nerve at wrist. First four fascicles on radial side are being matched.

TECHNIQUE OF FASCICULAR REPAIR

A piece of light blue ordinary latex balloon serves nicely as a background. It is readily available, inexpensive, and does not give a light reflection. Frequent flushing using a plastic BSS bottle* with a blunt needle allows easier identification of tissues to be discarded. The irrigant solution is heparinized saline, which keeps the fine suture materials from sticking to the wound surface. My preference in suture material is the S & T 50 μ (5-v) *short* (3 mm) straight needle swaged onto 18 μ nylon.† It is difficult to carry out accurate perineurial sutures with larger needles.

1. Dissect away the circumferential epineurium from the end of the nerve for a distance approximately equal to the diameter of the nerve.

2. If dealing with a large nerve, identify fascicular bundles and dissect them initially as bundle units, proximally and distally. Match them with what appear to be corresponding units and temporarily loosely suture them together. Then, one bundle at a time, dissect all fasciculi from each other removing all the intraneural epineurium. Frequent flooding of the field will aid in cleanly preparing the fasciculi. Each fasciculus shows a spiral pattern in the perineurium (bands of Fontana) (Fig. 35-1). These are pleats that disappear on axial stretch and reappear when tension is relaxed. The fascicles from the two paired bundles are arranged in a fan-shaped pattern on a flat surface facing each other (Fig. 35-4). These are then matched one to another by size. Protruding from the perineurial cuff are the gelatinous intrafascicular contents (Fig. 35-5). This is trimmed flush with the perineurium, and two sutures are then placed at 180 degrees from each other. Axoplasmic leak will then usually cease. If only one suture is used, there is a possibility of torsion of the fasciculus with loss of contact (Fig. 35-10). The rest of the fascicles in the bundle are then matched and sutured in like manner. Then the next bundle is dealt with in similar fashion until repair is complete (Figs. 35-6 and 35-7).

In smaller nerves such as the digital nerve,

---

*Alcon Co., P.O. Box 2664, Fort Worth, Texas 76101.
†S & T, Chirurgische Nadeln, 7893 Jestetten FRG, West Germany.

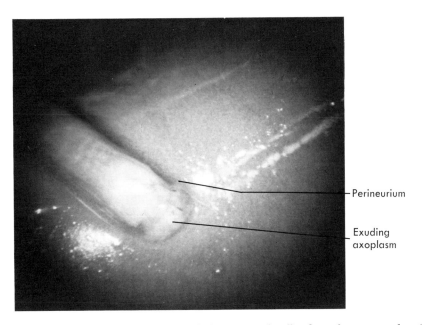

Perineurium

Exuding
axoplasm

Fig. 35-5. Single divided fascicle showing end of perineurial cuff and axoplasm protruding from cut end.

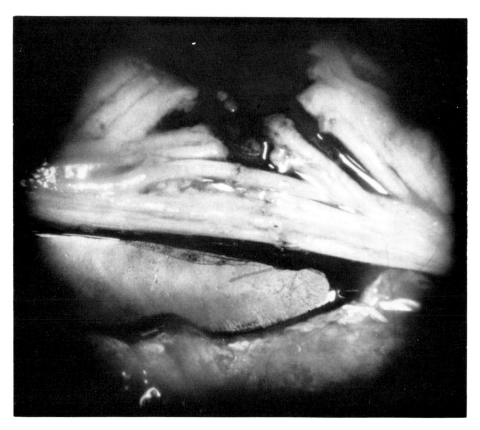

Fig. 35-6. Partially completed fascicular repair of median nerve.

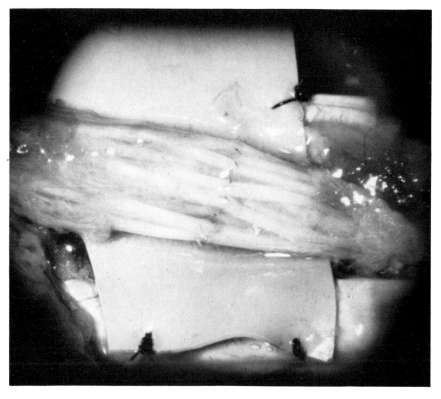

Fig. 35-7. Completed fascicular repair of median nerve at wrist.

the fascicles number three to five and are not formed into bundles but pass singly through the nerve (Figs. 35-8 and 35-9).

A delay of only a few days will result in shrinking of the distal perineurial tubes and make repair slightly more difficult.

A secondary repair after scar and neuroma formation have occurred requires a resection of the scar regardless of whether the repair is to be perineurial or epineurial. If a fascicular juncture is to be used, then the multiple new fascicular sprouts must be removed until a

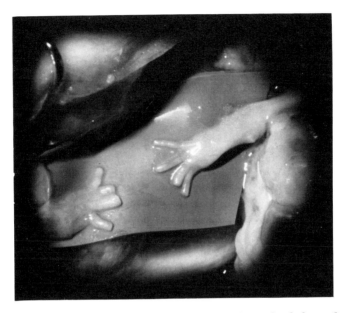

Fig. 35-8. Digital nerve fascicular repair. Nerve ends have been divided into four individual fascicles and ends trimmed.

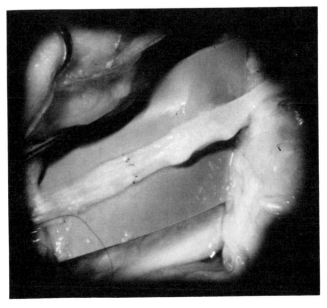

Fig. 35-9. Digital nerve fascicular repair has been completed using two sutures for each of four fascicles.

normal anatomy is reached. This may leave a sufficient gap so that a graft is required.

FASCICULAR GRAFT TECHNIQUE

The sural nerve is the best donor nerve. It may be removed while the patient is supine, but this is carried out more easily in the prone position, particularly if both sural nerves are to be removed. Frequently, the grafts are removed and prepared the day prior to insertion if the necessity for grafting is known. These may then be stored at 4° C overnight. Blood storage refrigerators are kept at this temperature.

Working on a moist plastic surface, each fascicle is dissected free from the others. The fascicle is kept as a unit until branching occurs where it is transected. Usually the larger fasciculi in the nerve are the ones most suitable. These fascicular lengths are then stored in a sealed jar with a slightly moist sponge overnight. Then, after preparation of the proximal and distal nerve stumps in the manner described above, these fascicles are trimmed to the necessary length, and suturing is carried out (Fig. 35-10). The original proximal-distal orientation of the graft fascicles is not thought to be important, but no facts are available. The proximal nerve stump will usually have more fascicles than the distal; therefore all distal junctures are made first. These are then covered with a piece of plastic to prevent sticking to gloves, gowns, and so forth, and then the proximal junctures are carried out. An attempt is made to place grafted material in a vascular bed of muscle, fat, or areolar tissue.

It is not yet possible to define the usefulness of fascicular repair because insufficient nerves have been repaired and followed at the present time. Preliminary results are as follows: In digital nerve repairs on a fascicular basis, there were 14 cases over age 21 followed for 1 year or more. All cases with vas-

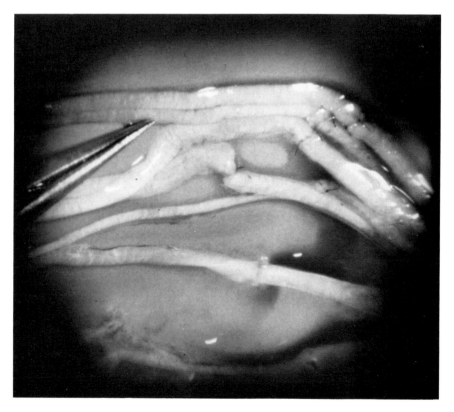

Fig. 35-10. Fascicular grafts obtained from sural nerve have been sutured at one end. Note central fascicle that has twisted because only one suture was used.

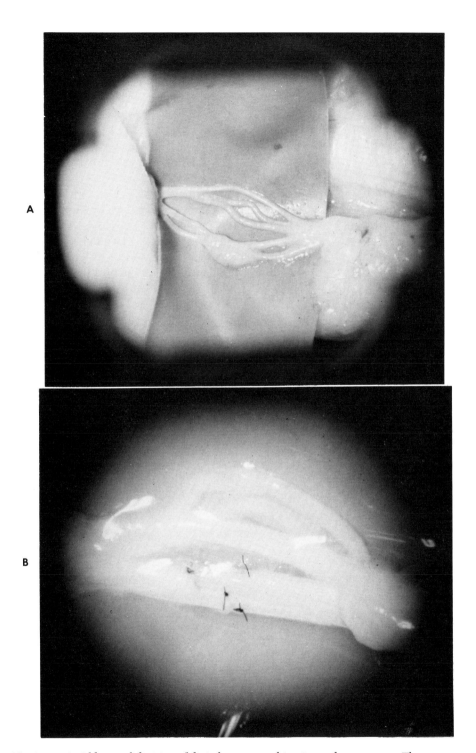

Fig. 35-11. A, Old partial division of digital nerve resulting in tender neuroma. There was partial loss of sensation. Fascicles involved in neuroma have been separated from normal fascicles. **B,** Neuroma has been resected and individual fascicles repaired. Uninjured fascicles remain intact and unimpaired.

cular damage, crush, or skin loss were deleted from the series. In these cases, the von Frey tests were 2.48 compared with a normal 1.65. Two-point discrimination was 10.1 if all patients with no two-point discrimination at all were measured as 15 for purposes of obtaining an average.

There were 27 patients with epineurial repairs with the same qualifications—all done in the same time period as the fascicular repairs so as to minimize differences in technique. The microscope was used in all cases. In these, von Frey tests equalled 2.55 and two-point discrimination was 7.63. This indicates little difference.

In nerve grafts with the same qualifications, there were two cases that had epineurial grafts and these both had a von Frey test result of 1.65 and two-point discrimination of 15 (no two-point discrimination at all).

There were six fascicular nerve grafts done on digital nerves. These had a von Frey test result of 1.9 and two-point discrimination of 9.5.

There have been insufficient numbers of median and ulnar nerves above the wrist to draw general conclusions. Individual cases would indicate that dissecting the fascicles from a sural nerve does not do any particular harm. In general, one may say that for repair or for grafting completely severed nerves, there is no indication at the moment that fascicular repair is either better or worse than epineurial repair.

It would seem that the ideal indication for fascicular dissection and repair or grafting would be in the partially divided nerve, for the uninjured fascicles could be dissected free from the severed fascicles and a specific repair could be carried out (Fig. 35-11). This would prevent additional surgical damage to the uninjured fasciculi, reduce the chance of neuromatous pain, and encourage restoration of some sensation.

REFERENCES

1. Bora, F. W.: Peripheral nerve repair in cats: the fascicular stitch, J. Bone Joint Surg. **49A:**659, 1967.
2. Sunderland, S.: Nerves and nerve injury, Philadelphia, 1968, The Williams & Wilkins Co., Chaps. 7, 8, 29, 30, and 45.

36

Overview of surgical technique and clinical results

At the Bunnell symposium, the topics of surgical techniques and the results of clinical application of those techniques were discussed separately. The following discussion includes material related to both topics.

DISCUSSION

Gary Frykman (Loma Linda): I have a question I'd like to direct to both Dr. Millesi and Dr. Sunderland. We've talked about groups of fasciculi and that this is perhaps a satisfactory way to repair nerves. I would like to have their comments as to how constant these groups are from one patient to the next at the different levels of the nerve.

Millesi: There is a full fascicular pattern with group arrangement in peripheral nerves distal to the upper arm. More proximally, there is less group arrangement. The pattern may differ from patient to patient requiring an individual dissection for each patient. One thing I can state from several hundred cases operated by this technique is that the group structure remains more constant than the fascicular pattern. A lot of the changes in the fascicular pattern occur within a group. The group pattern, therefore, remains more constant over a longer distance.

Sunderland: I think in certain regions the anatomical arrangement in terms of fiber localization is very constant. For example, at the wrist there is a constant internal structure for the median nerve, likewise

for the ulnar nerve at the wrist and for the disposition of the dorsal cutaneous nerve of the hand bundles in the ulnar nerve. More proximally in the arm, the localization that is going to be of any value is lost. In the case of the median and ulnar nerves above the elbow, this presents no problem because you know that just about every funiculus contains fibers from every peripheral branch. So localization doesn't become a factor of any significance. The radial nerve is a little different because it terminates in the supracondylar region to divide into superficial radial and posterior interosseous divisions. These groups of fibers are well localized, and the relationships are quite constant up to the level of the spiral groove. In these regions we can be absolutely certain about the distribution of the various groups of funicular structures in terms of their fiber representation.

There are at present three methods a surgeon can use to identify funicular groups. One is the anatomical method. This is a fairly rough way, but within the limits of the regions I've indicated, it is accurate, and I think it's the best. The second is an electrophysiological technique that is being used particularly in nerve lesions at and just above the wrist. With this technique, identification depends on stimulation of the proximal and distal stumps. The distal stump, however, must be stimulated within 72 hours, because

329

beyond that time the axons will have degenerated. Within about 72 hours, stimulation of the funiculi in the distal stump will produce a motor response. Some have stimulated digital nerve sensory endings to see if they can pick up potentials at the distal stump. That is a little more difficult but would allow separation of motor-bearing funiculi from sensory-bearing funiculi. The problem is, of course, that within a short distance sensory and motor fibers mix, and the fact that you get a motor response does not mean that you have no sensory fibers in the funiculus. So, there are problems.

To identify sensory funiculi in the proximal stump, you must have a conscious patient. The proximal stump funiculi are then stimulated to see whether or not there is a sensory response. Theoretically, this allows identification of sensory funiculi, but, again, there is the problem that at a certain level there will be mixed funiculi. I think that the electrophysiological method of identifying funiculi is still an open-ended issue, but at the moment it looks as if it is not attracting a great deal of attention.

The third identification method is a little more complicated. It is based on the histochemical finding that acetylcholinesterase stains differently in motor and sensory fibers. The procedure is to take biopsy specimens at an initial operation within 72 hours of the injury. These are stained for acetylcholinesterase, a procedure that requires about 38 hours of incubation time. This results in a cross section of the nerve with the motor funiculi only stained a deep brown. That allows you to identify motor and sensory funiculi. The problem is again mixed funiculi.

The published illustrations of sections that have been prepared in this manner are a beautiful confirmation of our findings based on anatomical and histological analyses. I think that at present there are insuperable difficulties with electrophysiological and histochemical identification of funiculi. We are better off, at the moment, relying on good, old-fashioned anatomy.

Niebauer: Sir Sydney, I think the real problem is that when they put Adam together, they didn't color-code him. It seems almost insurmountable to achieve what we would like to, because there are patients who have Martin-Gruber anastomoses. I have had patients with their median nerves cut at the wrist who immediately, in fact before I sutured them, could use their thenar muscles. When you add this fact to the problem of identifying funiculi far distances apart, it seems it is pretty much a hit-and-miss situation if the lesion is one of any distance. I wonder whether that's true or not.

Sunderland: I think that is correct. With increasing loss of nerve, you do reach a situation where the gap is so great that it's not possible to get any correspondence between the proximal and distal stumps. You then use your best judgment with a funicular cable graft to provide the nerve replacement that is going to guide regenerating axons into the distal stump. Particularly when you're dealing with nerves that are very mixed, where the percentage of sensory fibers is about the same as the percentage of motor fibers and they're battling it out for endoneurial tubes, the situation is not good. When dealing with the median nerve in the distal fourth of the forearm, where motor and sensory fibers have blended together in funiculi, you put your money on sensory regenerating processes because they represent 94% of the cross-sectional area of the nerve. The motor fibers then represent only 6% of the area. There are, of course, bound to be some variations. If you have an all median hand in which the median nerve is providing the entire motor innervation to the hand, then that percentage would increase, but the percentage of motor fibers in the ulnar nerve would decrease. So there is at the wrist an interplay between median and ulnar nerve innervation that can be very significant.

Dr. Niebauer has mentioned the importance of the Martin-Gruber anastomosis. I have a patient who had his median nerve torn out between the axilla and the elbow. Now that median nerve is gone, but he has almost perfect function in his hand. He has an almost all-ulnar hand. The only deficit he has is in pronation, flexion of the terminal phalanx of the thumb, and a slight disability in flexion of the index finger. Sensation is within normal limits. Obviously he has a Martin-Gruber anastomosis that is doing this, and if you block the ulnar nerve at the appropriate level, you eliminate the function. All of these factors must be taken into consideration when you evaluate a case and, very importantly, when you evaluate the end result.

Omer: When the mix is 50-50, Sir Sydney, when it's 50% motor and 50% sensory, is there a gap distance that makes it probably a good idea to side with Dr. Tupper and take out the sural nerve graft and do a biopsy of the cut nerve ends at a first operation? Then, at a second operation in 3 days, you can utilize the histochemical findings to guide placement of the grafts. Is there a point at which that becomes the preferred method rather than sheer anatomy?

Sunderland: I think that is a very difficult question to answer. I would point out that in the proximal stump the funiculi would all be mixed, each funiculus probably containing motor and sensory fibers in about the same proportions. Under those circumstances, the graft receives a random distribution of fibers that proceed from proximal stump through the graft into the distal stump. This, of course, is where the results can vary a great deal. You may be extremely fortunate and pick up an element of localization that just happens to be there in that particular patient. That is why results vary so much when you perform the same technique at the same level with the same gap distance. The results can be very different.

Omer: Dr. Millesi, your colleague in Vienna, who does histochemical staining, does he have a gap distance for us?

Millesi: The staining technique has two disadvantages. One disadvantage is that it takes 2 or 3 days until you get the result. The second disadvantage is that you cannot use it at the distal stump after 48 hours, because when wallerian degeneration has commenced, the stain does not.work. It is, however, still possible to stain the proximal stump. A third point is that the technique works well at peripheral levels, but there anatomical facts alone already provide satisfactory results. At more proximal levels there is the problem of the mixed fascicles that this technique does not solve. So, I think it's a good technique for study and for research but, unless the incubation time can be shortened, a doubtful technique for clinical application.

When we hear that the motor fibers in the median nerves constitute only 6% of the area and that the chance to get them to regenerate is a very poor one, the situation sounds quite desperate. The clinical results, though, tell us that this is not so and that in spite of these problems useful motor recovery can be achieved in a high percentage of cases. This excludes cases of mixed innervation. Because of this very important point, if you do research work in this field, you should use cases where the median and ulnar nerves are both repaired. Then you are certain that the recovery is because of your repair.

R. T. Dauphine (Monterey): I have a question for Dr. Tupper who has mentioned the ooze from the cut fascicles. If wonder if this is not just apparent and may be due to retraction of the perineurium from the end of the fascicle with drying and so on with time.

Tupper: No, if you cut it off, it comes back, and if you cut it off again, it comes back. You're cutting off no perineurium each time, you're just cutting off ooze and it keeps coming back. It's not apparent, it's very real.

Sunderland: I think that this is a reflection of the intrafunicular pressure that is maintained by the perineurium. If you just nick the perineurium, if you breach it, you immediately get a herniation of the contents of the bundle out through that opening.

It's just like a little hernia. If the fibers have been damaged, they will begin to yield axoplasm.

This was one of the early observations that led people to think that there was an intrafunicular pressure that was of some significance. I think J. Z. Young was one of the first to direct attention to it. There's other evidence, of course, that there is a normal intrafunicular pressure. It takes a long time to dissipate that pressure along the length of the funiculi. They just go on slowly oozing like sap coming out and collecting at the cut. The same process also occurs initially at the distal stump but it's soon lost because the axons and myelin begin to degenerate. The accompanying loss of funicular contents reduces the intrafunicular pressure. I think that this is the probable explanation.

Tupper: I think further evidence of the intrafunicular pressure is the fact that all funiculi are round and this is because they're under pressure.

B. O'Brien (Melbourne): Surgery should really be an aid to healing, and I think it can be done a little too enthusiastically. There are dangers in doing a lot of interfascicular dissection. Excessive handling can damage the nerve fibers and interfere with the blood supply. I think some of the funicular repairs we have been shown fit into that pattern. I, personally, just peel back the epineurium and do a group interfascicular suture anatomically aligned as Sir Sydney advocated. I cut the nerves with a very fine pair of sharp scissors, which has a guillotine effect. At one stage we had electrically operated nerve cutters, but they did no better than straight scissors used only for that purpose.

We have been involved in comparing suture techniques in experimental animals for some years. We repaired the common peroneal nerve in 60 dogs using epineurial repair, funicular repair with the epineurium cut back, and combined epineurial and funicular repair.* We studied the end

result using histology, nerve conduction studies, electromyography of muscles just beyond the union and the small muscles in the paw, and we estimated the area below the action potential. We found no difference between the different techniques nor could we confirm Sir Sydney's observation of excessive fibrosis around 10-0 sutures. We repeated the study in monkeys, using the peroneal and anterior tibial nerves at the midleg level. There were 60 sutured nerves in the same three groups, and they were studied in the same way. We have not completed the histochemical material for this study, but, so far, we have been unable to show any difference between the three groups. In this model, which was one of nontension or normal tension, we were unable to demonstrate that the epineurium was a proliferative structure that interfered with neural regeneration. So Dr. Edshage may be correct in saying that a clean laceration at the wrist without loss of nerve tissue can be sutured in an epineurial fashion. The results from this experimental model, which was as good as we could get and as near as possible to what Sir Sydney and Professor Millesi asked for, perhaps cannot be extrapolated with absolute accuracy to the human situation. I think that the only way that we'll resolve this matter is to do a carefully controlled, prospective study in humans involving suture of many nerves in many patients. I think such a study is essential for future progress.

Niebauer: I would like clarification of a particular point. I would like to know whether most surgeons do a bundle repair and talk of it as a funicular repair, or do most do a funicular repair like those described by Dr. Tupper. Do you approximate four or five bundles of funiculi, or do you individually suture 10 to 30 funiculi? I think this is an important point.

Omer: Dr. Kutz, would you like to answer that? What do you do at home, Joe? Do you suture each funiculus or do you do an interfascicular bundle repair? Incidentally, I think Gary Mulberg is right, we really

---

*Burke, P. F., and O'Brien, B. McC.: A comparison of three techniques of micro nerve repairs in dogs, The Hand. To be published.

mean suture, don't we? We're not repairing a nerve, we're suturing it.

J. Kutz (Louisville): We're just approximating it. Most of our cases are done as described by Dr. Millesi, It's an interfascicular bundle group. In most cases we don't go to the extreme of doing model sutures, we do the minimum number of sutures to achieve close approximation under the microscope.

Tupper: I just don't want to leave the impression that I do this every time. I do it sometimes, a few times, attempting to analyze it and see what happens. I'm not a proponent of the method yet.

J. Terzis (Montreal): I would like to point out that what Dr. Sunderland and the rest of us have so far called pure motor fascicles also contain sensory fibers. We have completed a study* on the deep motor branch of the ulnar nerve of the monkey, a large primate. We found that over 60% of that motor nerve was composed of sensory fibers. So, it's amazing that the results of nerve suture are so good considering that even with a very distal repair we are still dealing with a mixed fascicle.

Omer: Is the problem that none of these repair techniques do well simply because we align a lot of axons with tissue that doesn't have neural elements in it? Is the debate about whether it's motor or sensory not nearly as important as whether we just sort of put things end-on-end? Is that what we're getting around to saying? You're telling me you're not sure about sensory, you're not sure about motor, you can't identify them on either side, and you show me a lot of pictures of tubes that really just don't match. Are we ending up saying we ought to make sure that the little tubes inside the tubes sort of match each other, and the imperfect regeneration is because they don't meet each other exactly? Is that a fair statement?

McCarroll: Referring back to Dr. Horch's

*Terzis, J. K., and Dykes, R. W.: Clin. Orthop. Rel. Res. **128:**167, 1977.

and Dr. Bunge's presentations, I think that what they and others were saying is that the nerve elements have something that helps them grow back together. Thus the surgeon does the patient a great service if he stays out of the way as much as possible and approximates the nerve ends using the simplest applicable technique. I think that if a nerve knows how to grow back to one of twelve sensory endings in cat hairy skin, it is already way ahead of where surgery is going to be in the next 100 years. To match that surgically, you don't want to be suturing 30 fascicles in the median nerve at the wrist, you want to be suturing 15,000 axons; that's only about 30,000 sutures for one nerve. Then, you could align something and try and get things straight. This applies to clean, simple lacerations. It's the type of injury used in all the animal experiments. If you add complicating problems such as scar tissue, lost segments of nerve, the things that you face every day when you suture a human nerve injury, there are good reasons for wanting to use more complicated techniques than the simple, epineurial approximating suture that stays out of the way.

Sunderland: Well, if there's one thing I've learned here, it's what spaghetti really is. You know, in Australia, we have a saying "horses for courses." I'm sure there are situations where the only way to repair a divided nerve is by a conventional epineurial suture, getting the best possible match in terms of orientation of the nerve ends. Where the bundles are large, where there is very little epineurial connective tissue, where there is a reasonable correspondence of funicular pattern, and where there is no fiber localization that you can take advantage of, then quite clearly an end-to-end union is preferred. There are, however, two situations to be considered: one, a very clean transection, and two, where there is loss of nerve tissue resulting in a gap.

The problems are very different in the two cases. With a clean transection, even at the wrist with an absolutely clean transection, I think a straight epineurial conventional repair, maintaining appropriate axial alignment, will do the job. But I'm sure there are locations, and I've already illustrated the classical one of the ulnar nerve in the distal fourth of the forearm, where if you miss the internal anatomy of the nerve trunk, you are going to approximate dorsal cutaneous nerves of the hand bundles to motor funiculi in the distal stump, and that's the one thing you don't want to do. So, the point I would make is that there is no one single solution. You look at a particular situation and then decide what type of repair is justified in that particular case. I do believe that this is very important. The second point I would like to emphasize is that there are regions where failure to recognize the internal anatomy of nerve trunks can get you into very big trouble indeed. Now, regarding the others, the mixed motor and sensory fascicles, you just use the best human judgment.

There's no doubt whatsoever in my own mind that there could be chemotrophic influences. But I think that these relate only to attracting regenerating axons to funiculi. I don't think there's any chemotrophic influence that attracts axon *A* back to endoneurial tube *A*, it's just not on.

Now it is a common experience that distal repairs do better than proximal repairs. If you're looking at recovery in the hand, the results after repair of the median nerve at the wrist are better than after repair at a high level just distal to the axilla. And the reason is because everything is mixed up in the proximal part of the limb. You will take advantage of what fiber localization there is whether you do a straight epineurial repair or whether you do a group funicular repair.

Another factor I do think you must keep in mind is this cross-sectional area of the nerve that is devoted to epineurial tissue on the one hand and funicular tissue on the other. If you're not careful, when you approximate the nerve ends by a straight epineurial repair, you will produce a considerable degree of overlap with funiculi

opposed to interfunicular tissue. All of you must have experienced those unfortunate cases in which you finish up with a very large painful neuroma of the median nerve at the wrist after a repair, and the reason for that is that there's been nonfunicular alignment. With the changing funicular pattern and the large area devoted to epineurial tissue, the repair has encouraged regenerating axons to grow into interfunicular spaces. They'll do this; they'll whirl around, and they are responsible for the formation of the large painful neuromas that occur in this situation.

So, I think that this is not an open-ended issue. It's not an either/or situation in the sense that one method should always be used in preference to the other. You can't go away and say every repair must be an epineurial repair or every repair must be a group funicular repair. It's not as simple as that. You must look at each case and analyze it in terms of the various factors that comprise the nature of the lesion. I would like to suggest that you take a very careful look at biopsy specimens of the proximal and distal stumps to see, if only as a matter of record, whether or not you've got a reasonable correspondence of proximal funiculi to distal funiculi or whether, when you put the ends together, most of your regenerating axons are not going to get into funiculi in the distal stump, let alone get into corresponding or functionally related endoneurial tubes.

A. Daniller (New York): Can Professor Milesi give us an indication as to the time element involved in cases where he would not go back to do a nerve repair because the muscle is irrevocably damaged? He mentioned one case, for example, of 1½ years, but it was my impression that there had been some function prior to inserting the grafts.

Millesi: The time interval is a very important factor. We should do these late secondary repairs, if necessary, as early as possible, hopefully within 6 months time. But if this 6 months time has elapsed, there is no reason not to try a repair after a longer time interval. We have cases of 1½ years or even more with useful recoveries, but, of course, the recovery would have been better if the patient had been operated on within a shorter time interval. It also depends on which nerve is involved. In a case of a median nerve laceration, I would do such a later secondary repair even after 3, 4, or 5 years, because I would expect at least protective sensibility to return. I wouldn't expect very much motor function after such a long period but some sensibility. Then I could do a tendon transfer to provide opposition. In these cases there is actually no time limit.

Niebauer: One certainly must congratulate Dr. Millesi, and we can't argue with success. I also admit that we have a big microscope mounted on a computer, and we use it, and put in nerve grafts, and do all these things. But I must think back to the days of watching Dr. Bunnell take hold of a nerve and pull on it, and I would sort of close my eyes as he did. I learned to do the same thing, and we overcame up to 2, 3, or 4 cm of discrepancy in the defect. These nerves were sutured, and the arm was put up in flexion, and the wrist was put up in flexion, and the arm and wrist finally were gradually straightened out. Some of these nerves did remarkably well. Now, I'm not saying that we should all go back and do that again, but as orthopaedists many of you know that patients can have severe flexion contractures of their knees, and if you straighten them out slowly you will not get a peroneal nerve palsy, whereas, if you do it abruptly, you certainly will. So, we must think of these things, although I certainly do not advocate them.

Anonymous: Dr. Millesi, I'd like for you to comment on how you localize the motor and sensory branches in the proximal and distal ends in order to put your cable grafts in.

Millesi: It all depends on the level of the repair. When suturing the median nerve in the forearm, it's not so far to its division. What we do is to dissect the stumps in the way described and make a sketch of the fascicular pattern of the proximal and distal stumps. Then we proceed distally until the nerve divides. At that level we can define the thenar motor branch very well and follow it back proximally to the repair site. Then we know for sure which bundle at the lesion contains the motor fibers. Now we have to match the two cross sections using our best judgment. We try to define which proximal bundle will match with this motor branch in the distal stump. This of course is a guess, but the results show that the guess was correct in the majority of the cases. If you have to deal with a large gap, things are a little bit worse, because the fascicular pattern changes very much. There is an advantage, though, and this advantage is that the more proximal the lesion, the more the fibers are distributed on the whole cross section. Using our knowledge of internal topography, we know that in certain sectors there is a predominance of certain fibers. We then use the fasicle groups of these sectors to unite with identified bundles in the distal stump. Evidently, with the length of the defect, a lot of fibers are lost, and this is the reason why the results become worse if the defects are longer. This is not so much due to the length of the graft itself as to the length of the defect and the changing fascicular pattern. But still you can have good results.

Niebauer: Are there any other questions?

L. Milford, (Memphis): I don't wish to ask a question but rather to make an observation and philosophical statement. For 2½ days we have concerned ourselves with the question of the proper pathway. We have asked, "How do we get there from here?" We have discussed the minutiae of where we're going as if we were checking a road map. A number of beautiful experiments and microdissections have been presented, but they were all based on the assumption that this part must go to that part by a connection. There has been allusion made to some humoral element, to the possibility of a factor we have no concept of.

For example, Dr. Tupper presented the case of the child who had no anatomical connection of the nerve but obtained a result that is much more impressive than what we usually obtain by reestablishing the anatomical connections in older age groups. We have raised the possibility that there is something else there yet to be discovered. So, I'm asking the experimentalists and philosophers about this. Is it possible to think in terms of flying when we're trying to figure out how to get from this town to that town instead of by road? When Kanavel was trying to figure out appropriate hand incisions to drain abscesses without destroying the nerves, what would he have thought if someone had asked, "Well, what about antibiotics?" Is there anything to this magnetic field in the salamander that Dr. Diamond suggested would do certain things to these specialized cells? What is it that directs the nerve to these? The salamander and starfish can regenerate an entire extremity but we know little about that.

I simply suggest that maybe there is another tack or solution to the severed nerve other than suturing it. I hope that someone can see over the horizon and envision a new approach other than establishing the old pathway that we have so long attempted and so long been disappointed and frustrated with the results.

37

Clinical and experimental approaches to nerve repair, in perspective

Sir Sydney Sunderland

The extent to which interest in nerve injury, nerve regeneration, and nerve repair has blossomed in recent years is really astonishing. The results of nerve suture and nerve grafting in two world wars and the years between left a legacy of disappointment and discouragement. Today the situation is very different. Effective means of controlling wound infection, the fabrication of finer suture materials, improvements in microsurgical techniques, and, importantly, a better understanding of factors influencing the quality of recovery after nerve repair have combined to convert a generally discouraging outlook into one of guarded optimism—some would say unqualified optimism. However, many mischievous biological barriers remain to bedevil the surgeon, and it is important not to underestimate the limitations that these continue to impose on the surgeon's attempts to achieve an acceptable degree of useful functional recovery following nerve repair.

Today many investigators working in diverse fields are attacking the problems of nerve regeneration and nerve repair with unrelenting vigor and with a variety of new experimental techniques and new technical weapons. The result of this phenomenal activity has been a growing mass of data that experimentalists pour daily in a continuous stream into the scientific literature. However, despite the massive accumulation of information in recent years, there are areas where uncertainty and controversy persist, and many questions to which we have yet to find acceptable answers.

The pressure of expanding knowledge and the vast literature that has grown up about it makes it difficult to integrate information in a meaningful way so that the threads of our understanding are becoming tangled and disconnected, perspective is becoming blurred, and inquiries come to lack design and purpose. If new information is to be fully effective, some synthesis, however imperfect, of all of the work done and currently in progress must be attempted from time to time in order to see where we stand and to establish a vantage point from which we may be able to see new and possibly more rewarding lines of investigation. Finally, it is of value periodically to reexamine practices established by long usage and enforced by authority with the object of determining what should be retained and what should be amended or discarded.

There are, however, obstacles to following such a progressive approach to the elucidation of unsolved problems of nerve injury and nerve repair. In the first place the experimentalist seeking to satisfy only his curiosity, in itself a highly commendable pursuit, proceeds in one direction and all too often is oblivious to the pressing practical realities of the clinical situation, while the clinician, laboring to satisfy not only his curiosity but also to meet a clinical need, moves at a much slower pace and often in a different direction. This inevitably results in a widening of the gap between experimental and clinical attitudes and between what is professed and what is practiced. To complicate the situation still further, the emergence of a variety of clinical subspecialties in recent years has meant that patients with a peripheral nerve lesion are now so scattered throughout the various specialities that any one consultant rarely accumulates a series that is sufficiently large to excite his investigational instincts.

Unfortunately, meaningful dialogue between the different groups concerned is uncommon, although clearly some pooling of experience and ideas is not only desirable but essential if we are to resolve those issues and differences that are the subject of continuing disagreement and controversy. The day should be over when experimentalist talks only to experimentalist and clinician only to clinician. This volume on nerve repair has been a splendid example of how the barriers between different disciplines can be broken down and how investigators working in different fields, but with a common objective, either overt or covert, can be brought into productive and harmonious conjunction. While it has not been possible to settle all differences of opinion or to provide acceptable answers to all questions, each is at least aware of, understands, and has a clearer appreciation of the other's point of view. The importance of maintaining a continuing communication between all interested parties cannot be overemphasised.

Finally, in the search for improvements in nerve repair, the central objective of the exercise should be kept constantly in mind. For most tissues and structures, once mechanical repair has been effected, the natural processes of healing attend to the return of function. The surgeon can expect no such reward after nerve repair because factors far more complex than the simple restoration of nerve trunk continuity and axon regeneration are involved. These factors, and the manner in which they aid or impair regeneration, must be recognized and clearly understood because this information provides the clue to the steps to be taken during nerve repair to assist orderly regeneration

with the object of ensuring that the restored pattern of innervation approximates as closely as possible to the original. The ideal, of course, would be to devise measures to restore the original pattern of innervation in every respect, but this is currently beyond our technical expertise. Nevertheless there is still room for improvement and in our search for perfection we now have a wide range of new and greatly improved experimental techniques to assist us, while at the laboratory level the study of axon transport mechanisms and the electron microscope are proving invaluable in filling in the gaps in our knowledge of the ultrastructural processes and changes involved in degeneration and regeneration.

EVALUATION OF NEW METHODS AND TECHNIQUES OF NERVE REPAIR

Any new method, procedure, technique, or management policy introduced with the object of improving the results of nerve repair should only survive if it can be conclusively demonstrated that it is responsible for giving superior results. The greatest obstacle to reaching finality in this matter is the absence of valid audits that can be used as a basis for comparing conflicting claims. End result evaluation, which is the basis of any comparative study, presents more difficulties than may at first appear, for more careful consideration reveals that it is complicated in two important ways. The first concerns the impossibility of isolating many of the variables influencing recovery so that each can be subjected to separate study and evaluation. The second relates to differing interpretations of what is meant by "recovery" and the frequent failure to measure and express it reliably and objectively.

It is now clear that many factors influence the outcome after nerve repair and that each of these is subject to a considerable range of variation. As we have seen, some are built into the anatomy of nerves, others are introduced by the injury and the accompanying degenerative and regenerative processes, while superimposed on these are those technical procedures associated with repair and treatment that require critical evaluation before their final acceptance.

Although we have some understanding of the manner in which each factor operates, we have not yet progressed beyond the stage of being able to express the degree to which it does so in any but the most general and relative terms. To add to our difficulties these factors are also interrelated in such an intricate manner that it is impossible to isolate any one factor for separate study and evaluation. A study of the relative merits of any new method or procedure would require standard conditions as these relate to the nerve injured; the nature, level, and severity of the injury; equivalent retrograde effects; identical conditions at the suture line; and so on. While this may be attainable in the experimental animal, it is certainly not possible in the clinical situation for in no two patients will the conditions established by the transection be identical in every respect.

Failure to recognize and appreciate these complexities of nerve repair means that, when the effectiveness of a particular procedure or technique is under investigation, it is usual to find it equated with the quality of the recovery without regard to the other variables contributing to the end result. The results of such an approach are capable of grave misinterpretation. One must, therefore, emphasize the need for exercising continuing caution in evaluation studies.

Before taking this subject further, it should be noted that recovery proceeds in three phases. The first involves axon regeneration and the reestablishment of axonal connections with the periphery. The second involves the return of function in its simplest form, as revealed by the reappearance of contractions in individual muscles in response to voluntary effort and the return of protective sensation to denervated skin. The third involves the return of complex movements requiring the coordinated activity of groups of muscles and the return of the more discriminative aspects of sensation.

The first two phases relate to axon regeneration and are completed well within 3 years. The last phase, which implies useful functional recovery, involves additional, more complicated, and time demanding processes and takes years longer to complete. Its assessment requires searching tests that provide a measure of the quality of the performance of a wide range of normal daily tasks.

Axon counts below the level of a nerve repair in the experimental situation are not a reliable guide to the final outcome as this is expressed in terms of functional recovery and for this reason should not be used in evaluation studies. Similarly the application of electrodiagnostic procedures to detect the presence of axon tips, to follow their advance distally, and to study the conduction properties of regenerated axons, provides information of very limited value in evaluation studies. Regarding the use of Hoffmann-Tinel's sign as a guide to prognosis, it should be noted that even when the test indicates that axons are regenerating down the nerve trunk, this information may be misleading. The sign gives no clue to the destination of regenerating sensory "axons," for the latter are not necessarily contained within endoneurial tubes that will lead them to the skin. Nor does the test provide any indication of the number of axons regenerating down the nerve so that the probable outcome of regeneration as regards the quality of sensory recovery remains uncertain. While, therefore, the sign is a useful indicator of regeneration, it is not a reliable measure of *useful* regeneration. Although this test should always be used, the results should be interpreted with caution.

Information on the second phase of recovery is obtained by the simple testing of individual movements and the response to pinprick, crude touch, and extremes of temperature, which combine to provide the elements of protective sensation. It should be noted, however, that expressing recovery in these terms relates only to the lowest level of motor and sensory function and no more than this should be inferred from an evaluation based on such limited testing.

It is the third and final phase of functional recovery that is the most difficult to evaluate and where reporting is most open to question. Examining and evaluating individual movements in terms of range and power tell us little about manipulative skills and more complex movements to express sensory function simply and solely in terms of graduated punctate stimuli is also misleading because such stimuli are not physiological in the sense that sensory receptors of diverse kinds are normally stimulated not singly but in varying numbers and combinations and at different intensities and intervals. This results in complex patterns of activity involving the interaction of many systems. Furthermore, although sensory units combine and summate to provide the basis for sensory perception, this does not occur in any simple fashion but involves processes of great complexity.

While it is true that testing for tactile localization, texture, and two-point and temperature discrimination provides information about the basic elements or precursors of discriminative sensation, it is equally true that sensory recovery expressed in such terms still gives an incomplete picture of the real functional value of that recovery to the patient. Consequently information restricted to such testing is inadequate for an end result evaluation. What is of greater importance to the patient is the extent to which a residual defect limits, for example, the practical use of the hand in the efficient performance of normal daily tasks. Here it is sufficient to say that sensory testing is not complete until it has included an examination and assessment of the quality of the sensory recovery in relation to its effect on the total function of the part. It is the totality of the sensory experience that is all important.

Clinical tests for integrated motor and sensory functions are limited only by the ingenuity of the clinician and the time at his disposal. How rapidly and efficiently can the patient pick up and handle dexterously a series of objects of varying size and shape, first under visual supervision and then blindfolded? How efficiently can he screw a nut on a bolt and how accurately can he recognize objects solely by feeling and handling them? Testing manipulative and discriminative skills in this way represents a step in the right direction, but these are still simple tests

that tell us little about the functional value of the recovery to the patient. What is required for an acceptable end result assessment of the quality and functional value of regeneration is information relating to the patient's ability to cope with a wide range of daily activities. Does the patient know whether or not he is holding an object when the act cannot be checked visually? Is he constantly dropping objects? Does the hand become useless in the dark or when he is unable to see what he is attempting to do with it? Are movements clumsily performed, because of a lack of sensory information and persisting muscle weakness and incoordination, when carrying out such daily tasks as writing, sewing, cooking, handling cutlery, tools and utensils, dressing and undressing? This list could easily be extended. Finally, and importantly, to what extent does the affected part suffer from repeated trauma and trophic changes, which are a measure of the loss or inefficiency of protective sensory mechanisms. Admittedly, it is often difficult to put a value, other than one expressed in subjective terms, on these refinements of functional recovery, but unless end result assessments include a reference to them, the evaluation will have a limited value as a basis for comparing the relative merits of different procedures and techniques.

That anatomical motor and sensory reinnervation does not necessarily ensure functional recovery is illustrated in those infants with brachial plexus birth palsies who despite good "clinical recovery" refuse to use the arm.[11,34] This is attributed to the lack of development of "functional cerebral motor patterns of coordination" and possibly the organization of the body image, owing to the isolation of the limb from the central nervous system at a critical period of development. This proposition had been tested experimentally by Zalis and his associates in 1965.[35] They found that sensorimotor deprivation during the immediate postnatal period produced a long-term impairment despite the development of essentially normal muscle reinnervation. Evidence that there is a limited critical period during which sensorimotor deprivation interferes with the development of motor programming and the body image was shown by the excellent recovery observed in rabbits when the injury was delayed for several months.

To recapitulate, the quality of useful motor and sensory recovery depends not only on the numbers of regenerating axons reinnervating skin and muscles and the degree to which their structural features are restored but also on the restoration of those patterns of innervation, involving motor and sensory fibers of diverse sizes and function, which are the basis of the coordinated activity of groups of muscles and sensory discrimination. Additionally, motor and sensory functions are interdependent. Thus much of a residual motor incoordination and clumsiness may be due to a sensory defect rather than muscle weakness. At the same time objects must be handled, as well as felt, in order to give full scope to sensory discrimination and object identification.

The question now arises as to whether the residual disability left in the wake of incomplete and imperfect axon regeneration can be improved by central readjustments to neural circuits through retraining directed to increasing the patient's ability to utilize, to the greatest advantage, new and modified patterns of motor and sensory innervation. Clinical evidence endorsing the notion of flexible neural circuits and the effectiveness of retraining techniques in improving function comes from several sources.

1. The substantial improvement that follows intensive motor and sensory retraining after nerve repair cannot be explained solely on peripheral adjustments but must involve, at least in part, the reorganization of central mechanisms to offset the anatomical alterations and deficiencies in patterns of motor and sensory innervation.

2. There is the known success of reeducational therapy after tendon transfers in which muscles normally producing one particular action are trained to perform others.

3. Nerve section and repair in the very young introduce the same hazards at the suture lines as are found in adults. Despite this, remarkable recoveries occur in children that are never seen in adults. These superior results are not due to the more effective regeneration of axons and their maturation but are best accounted for by the intervention of some central factor. Almquist and his associates[2] have concluded from their experimental studies on transected median and ulnar nerves of infant and adult Fascicularis monkeys that axon regeneration is comparable in the two age groups. The better functional outcome in infant animals was attributed to a much greater capacity for reeducation.

Although these clinical observations confirm the existence of some central factor participating in the recovery process, and one that is of greater potential in the young than in the adult, they throw no light on the mechanisms by which this might be effected other than to offer the oversimplified and obscure explanation that this is due to readjustments to central neural circuits.

However, they point to the importance of intensive remedial training program that should be directed to increasing the range and quality of more complex movements and to improving sensory discrimination and the stereognostic sense during which the patient learns to recognize and identify an altered profile of sensory impulses and to relate these new sensations to past experience.

This explains why the third phase of recovery is so protracted. It is, in fact, difficult to put a time limit on it, depending as it does on a further set of complicating factors such as the general attitude, intelligence, patience, perseverance, and motivation of the patient. It certainly extends into the fifth year, and, on the basis of my own observations, I am convinced that it can extend well beyond this time. While it is true that the effects of some innovations may be immediately apparent, it may not be possible to assess others until many years after the repair.

This third phase of recovery and the role of rehabilitatory measures in the restoration of function deserve far more attention than they have received to date.

This admonition cannot, of course, be divorced from the broader issue of how long costly and time-consuming forms of organized reeducational therapy should be continued and at what stage they should be regarded as an unnecessary luxury and the patient left to his own devices. It should be noted that persevering with the use of the affected parts in daily tasks is a significant factor in improving the quality of the recovery, the outcome being largely determined by the attitude of the patient. Here the motto is "practice makes perfect." With the passage of time the dedicated patient has a remarkable capacity for improving on the quality of the recovery and for adjusting to his residual disability.

Finally, there is abundant evidence that, when planning and conducting end-result assessments, more care should be exercised to exclude such variables as anomalous innervations and trick movements. All too often we hear too much of the unsubstantiated triumphs of techniques and procedures and too little of their failures—too much of rosy predictions and too little of the difficulties and complications to be overcome. This point is illustrated by directing attention to a recent inquiry into the merits of homografting in West Germany.

In the early 1970's some sensational claims in favor of homografting were made by Jacoby and his associates.[13-17] The homografts were disantigenized and disenzymatized, and Jacoby stressed the importance of shielding the suture lines with lyophilized dura. These impressive claims, which were in striking contrast to the experience of other surgeons, were criticized, particularly by Millesi, and were subsequently referred to the German Society of Neurosurgeons for an opinion on the merits of the method. The society, mindful of the necessity to investigate operative successes that differed so radically from those of other surgeons, set up a neutral commission consisting of three neurologists and three neurosurgeons to undertake a critical evaluation of Jacoby's results. Jacoby was requested to submit, for examination by the commission, what he regarded as his best eight patients operated on 12 to 18 months previously and this he willingly did. The

commission's inquiries revealed that the allegedly good results were not the result of axon regeneration and the return of function in the repaired nerves but were based on the misinterpretation of neurological findings, such as the failure to appreciate the significance of anomalous innervations, trick movements, and so on.[21]

This illustration will serve to stress the critical importance of end result evaluation in assessing the effectiveness of a particular method or procedure introduced to improve the quality of recovery.

Some of the more controversial issues and areas of uncertainty relating to nerve repair will now be considered, at all times, however, keeping in mind the importance of reliable recovery assessments as a basis for evaluating and comparing methods, procedures, and techniques.

CHEMOTROPIC INFLUENCE OF THE DISTAL STUMP ON REGENERATING AXONS

The generally accepted view is that the only factors influencing the direction taken by regenerating axons are physical and not chemical. There are, however, grounds for believing that the concept of a chemotropic effect should be subjected to further and more critical scrutiny. Should further investigation reveal that the distal stump does, in fact, attract regenerating axons then current views on many of the suture line phenomena associated with regeneration and nerve repair would require modification.

PROSPECTS OF ACCELERATING AXON REGENERATION

Reference has already been made to the great capacity of axons to regenerate and to the unsolved problem of devising ways to prevent this. However, the ability to accelerate axon regeneration would have the dual effect of shortening the time for which tissues remain denervated and hastening the onset of recovery. All attempts to achieve this have so far failed. A wide range of chemical agents (for example, thyroid extract, methylprednisolone acetate, dexamethasone, and dibutyl cyclic AMP) have been shown to be ineffective. However, recently Forman and Berenberg[12] have reported accelerated motor recovery after the administration of triiodothyronine, but this was attributed to an effect on the maturation of the regenerating axon rather than on axon growth.

Ducker and his associates[10] suggested that axon growth might proceed more rapidly after a second lesion, 2 to 3 weeks later, than after an original lesion. McQuarrie and his associates[22-24] tested this suggestion experimentally and reported that although the onset of regeneration was unchanged, the rate of axon growth was increased following the second lesion. They attributed this faster rate to a growth-enhancing effect introduced by the first or priming lesion. Some aspects of this study are questionable and further work on this interesting concept is required, particularly in view of their finding that the effect of a conditioning lesion was to retard the advance of regenerating noradrenergic axons.

In any experimental or clinical study directed to accelerating axon growth it should be remembered that regeneration rates vary from individual to individual and that in any one individual the rate will be faster in the proximal than in the distal part of the limb.

EFFECT OF OVERLOADING OF NEURONS ON NERVE CELL FUNCTION

During regeneration, neurons may become overloaded as the result of (1) axon sprouting, and (2) the entry, after high repairs, of what were originally short axons into long endoneurial tubes down which they grow to form axons much longer than those originally supported by the parent cell.

While there is evidence that neurons may hypertrophy under these conditions, the manner and extent to which nerve cell function is affected by these changes is unknown, although one suspects that they could affect the quality of the recovery.

CAPACITY OF NEURONS TO SPIN NEW AXONS AND TISSUE SURVIVAL AFTER DENERVATION

How long do neurons surviving amputation of the axon retain the capacity to spin a new axon to the periphery, and how long do tissues survive denervation and retain the capacity to function efficiently when reinnervated?

There is as yet no conclusive answer to either of these questions, although the time scale is certainly to be measured in years. Such information is necessary because it determines when considerations of nerve repair should be abandoned even when repair is technically possible.

As regards the survival of denervated tissues, comment will be confined to striated muscle although this is not to be interpreted as denying the importance of skin and joints. Data relating to the survival time of denervated muscles come from both experimental and clinical sources.

Using the Australian opossum, muscles have been maintained in a denervated state for periods extending to 485 days.[31] Histological examination of the denervated muscles revealed that muscle fibers, although grossly atrophied, retained those essential structural features on which their identification is based. The few small scattered foci of degeneration seen appeared to be vascular in origin.

Clinically, the survival of denervated muscle for long periods is evidenced by:

1. The examination of biopsy material from denervated muscles
2. The persistence of fibrillations for 11,[27] 18,[33] and 74 years[25]
3. The recovery occurring in muscles following reinnervation after prolonged denervation[28]

There is now good evidence that, providing denervated muscles are maintained in the best possible state by preventing venous and lymphatic stasis, prolonged exposure to cold, trauma, and overstretching, they not only survive prolonged denervation but also retain the capacity to function efficiently following satisfactory reinnervation. My own detailed records cover only periods of a little more than 12 months. Clearly more detailed data covering much longer periods are required.

OPTIMUM TIME FOR REPAIRING A SEVERED NERVE

What is the optimum time for repairing a severed nerve? The simple answer to this question is, of course, as soon as local conditions are favorable. Such an answer, although it emphasizes the urgency of nerve repair, evades the central issue of when conditions are to be judged favorable. At this point it is important to draw a distinction between complicated nerve severance in a lacerated wound with extensive destruction of tissue, and clean nerve severance in a tidy sharply incised wound where there is minimal loss of tissue. In the former there is general agreement that delayed repair is obligatory. In the case of the latter, however, some advocate primary repair of the nerve while others argue in favor of early secondary repair 2 to 3 weeks after the injury.

It will be difficult to resolve this particular issue because, in any comparative study, the time of the repair is not the only factor affecting the outcome, and, as has already been noted, it is impossible to isolate it for separate study and evaluation. It is important, therefore, to examine the clinical and experimental evidence on which the arguments in favor of each are based.

The short delay of 2 to 3 weeks is claimed to have the following advantages.

1. It permits injured tissues to return to a state that facilitates repair.
2. The relation of the nerve ends to the surrounding tissues can by then be clearly defined.
3. The limits of intraneural fibrosis and funicular damage at the nerve ends can then be determined more accurately and the unfavorable tissue safely trimmed away until a level is reached where the arrangement offers good prospects for a satisfactory repair.
4. The epineurium is then thicker and stronger. This facilitates suturing and gives a more secure union at the suture line than would the more delicate tissue normally comprising the nerve sheath.
5. After primary repair, the suture line must be left in the wound surrounded by healing tissues. As a result, the suture line ultimately becomes involved in adhesions that may pull on the nerve when movements are commenced. In early secondary suture this complica-

tion can be avoided by approaching the nerve clear of the primary scar.
6. The repair can be planned and carried out in an unhurried manner as an elective procedure.

At this juncture it is appropriate to discuss the experimental data that have been advanced in support of the claims for early secondary repair and to which some experimentalists and clinicians attach great importance. This is necessary because a critical examination of the experimental findings reveals that the confidence placed in them is ill-founded.

The biological arguments advanced in support of deferring repair to about the third week are based on claims that at this time Schwann cell activity and the condition of the endoneurial tubes in the distal stump and the parent neurons are all in an optimal state for regeneration.

1. In 1942, Abercrombie and Johnson[1] reported that Schwann cell activity at the nerve ends, which contributed to union and to the success of regeneration, was maximal between the nineteenth and twenty-fifth days after nerve section in the rabbit. This report greatly influenced British thinking at the time. However, our investigations, also at that time and using other experimental material, revealed intense Schwann cell activity much earlier and there is now considerable evidence confirming this. Furthermore, an examination of the course of regeneration and the quality of the recovery after nerve repair, performed at and outside the third week claimed for maximum Schwann cell activity, indicates that effective union occurs at the suture line regardless of when the nerve is repaired.

2. It was further claimed that the products of wallerian degeneration in the denervated endoneurial tubes would obstruct the advance of regenerating axons. This, it was believed, would apply in the case of primary suture, whereas a short delay before the nerve was repaired would allow time for the endoneurial tubes to be cleared of this obstructing debris. After second degree injuries regenerating axon tips descend along that section of the nerve below the lesion earlier and more rapidly than after a primary suture and

at a time when the affected portion of the endoneurial tubes is still occupied by the products of degeneration. Cravioto[8] has reported new axons enclosed in Schwann cells that still contained partly degenerated myelin. Despite the coexistence of regenerating axon tips and debris after a second degree injury, regeneration proceeds smoothly and rapidly to complete recovery. There is no evidence that, following primary nerve repair, the debris of wallerian degeneration or the reaction associated with its removal hinders the advance of regenerating axon tips.

3. The retrograde changes in the biochemistry and metabolism of the cell bodies following severance of a nerve have been subjected to intensive investigation in recent years. Out of this work has emerged the belief that the parent cell bodies are in an optimal state for regeneration about 2 to 3 weeks after nerve severance.[9,10] There are several reasons why this claim and its application to nerve repair should be questioned.

In the first place not all cell bodies react to axon severance in precisely the same way or to the same degree. Some cell bodies show surprisingly little change, while the retrograde reaction in others progresses steadily to the death of the cell. Likewise some neurons take longer to recover than others so that the onset of regeneration is delayed in some in comparison with others. These variations make it extremely difficult to decide, in any given case, precisely when conditions are optimal for regeneration. In any event, although primary nerve repair certainly antedates the onset of regeneration, this is not in itself a disadvantage.

It has also been established that successive transections of a nerve are, on each occasion, followed by a repetition of the retrograde neuronal response. This means that, even if it were confirmed that the parent neurons are in an optimal state for regeneration at the third week, there remains the obvious difficultly of again precipitating a retrograde neuronal reaction as the result of those further insults on the nerve occasioned by the preparation of the proximal stump for repair.

To date animal experimentation has been unable to produce any convincing evidence to support early secondary suture, and, in this respect, clinical experience must take priority over animal experimentation.

The disadvantages associated with early secondary repair should not be overlooked.

1. When a nerve is severed, the ends retract in the surrounding tissue and if left there they become fixed in the shortened position as healing proceeds and scar tissue forms; in addition, bulbs form at the nerve ends. Some preparatory resection and trimming of the proximal and distal stumps is then inevitable at the second operation in order to expose healthy bundles for end-to-end union. Sacrificing tissue when preparing the nerve ends for repair complicates repair in two ways:
   a. Widening the gap to be closed (This may then require mobilization and suture under tension. Although mobilization is, if skilfully executed, a harmless procedure, suture under tension is a common cause of failure.)
   b. Disturbing funicular relations at the nerve ends to a degree that adds to the loss of regenerating axons at the suture line
2. With delay, the nerve ends often become lost in scar tissue so that they become difficult to identify at a later date.
3. It involves a second operation.

Turning now to the case for primary suture.

1. Since the nerve has been cleanly severed, there is negligible tissue loss so that it is easier to align the nerve ends correctly when they are anastomosed.
   a. Little or no trimming of the nerve ends is required to prepare them for suture. At the same time it should be remembered that failure to determine the true limits of damage means anastomosing nerve ends that will heal with extensive fibrosis at the suture line.
   b. Minimal loss of nerve substance means that the funicular patterns at the nerve ends are more likely to correspond.
   c. Satisfactory suture can be performed without tension.

d. Mobilization is not necessary to effect end-to-end union of the nerve ends.

2. The looseness of the epineurium at this time could be an advantage rather than a disadvantage in that it would prevent too much tension at the suture line. When the epineurium is thick and strong, there is the temptation when sutures are holding well to finish with greater tension at the suture site than is desirable.

3. Repairing the nerve with the least possible delay reduces the time for which peripheral tissues are denervated and the period for which the patient is incapacitated.

4. The primary suture should obviate the need for any further surgery. Should resuture prove necessary, the second operation is made technically easier by the first suture, which prevents the retraction and shortening of the nerve ends and reduces the amount of tissue to be resected and, therefore, the gap to be closed.

Finally, the protagonists for early secondary, as opposed to primary, repair maintain that such a policy takes the surgical treatment of nerve injuries out of the hands of the inexperienced casualty surgeon and makes the repair an elective procedure performed by an experienced specialist. It is true that the quality of the end result is largely determined by the skill, experience, and judgment of the surgeon, and it is important that the repair of these injuries should not be left to the inexperienced. Primary suture should obviously be reserved for those cases where the conditions of wounding justify it and where capable and experienced staff are available. Such a policy is known to produce excellent results.

As things currently stand, the decision of whether to undertake a primary or an early secondary repair must be determined solely by the circumstances of the injury and the clinical findings. However, one final point can be made in defense of primary repair. Having inadvertently severed a nerve in the course of an operation, when should it be repaired? Is there a surgeon who would advocate a delay of 3 weeks?

EPINEURIAL VS. GROUP FUNICULAR REPAIR

The rationale of funicular nerve repair was outlined in Chapter 3, where it was demonstrated that because of differences in the funicular numbers at the nerve ends it was not possible to restore nerve trunk continuity on a funiculus-to-funiculus basis. A compromise was to so group the funiculi at the nerve ends that repair could be effected on a group-to-group basis. What we are discussing in this section then are the relative merits of conventional methods of epineurial repair on the one hand and group funicular repair on the other.

Studies comparing epineurial and group funicular suture as alternative methods of repair have been largely based on end result evaluations. This approach, as we have seen, can be misleading in that it inevitably disregards the participation of the many other variables contributing to the end result. Such comparative studies also miss the point that the two methods are not in fact competitive alternatives. On the contrary each has a clearly defined and specific place in nerve repair although to appreciate this requires an understanding of the criteria that determine when one method should be employed in preference to the other. Dispute over the relative merits of these two methods of repair will continue as long as there is a failure to recognize the rationale of group funicular repair, when the method should be used, and when its use can bring no advantage to the repair.

Indications for epineurial repair

1. The nerve has been cleanly severed so that the funicular patterns at the two nerve ends correspond in every respect, and correct axial alignment of the nerve ends can be preserved.

2. Despite discrepancies in the funicular patterns at the nerve ends, the funiculi are so closely packed that there is little intervening epineurial tissue into which regenerating axons may grow.

3. There is no worthwhile branch fiber

localization to be exploited by grouping the funiculi.

Indications for group funicular repair

1. There is an acceptable degree of branch fiber localization within specific funicular groups that can be safely identified at the nerve ends.

2. The funiculi are so arranged and so widely separated by epineurial tissue that simple end-to-end union of the nerve ends would result in large numbers of regenerating axons failing to enter the funiculi in the distal stump.

3. Conventional epineurial suture, despite correct axial alignment of the nerve ends, would aggravate the wasteful regeneration of axons into foreign and functionally unrelated endoneurial tubes. Lesions of the ulnar nerve in the distal forearm that leave the bundle group, representing the dorsal cutaneous nerve of the hand branch at the proximal nerve end but not at the distal end, are a case in point. Fig. 3-13 shows two sections from a serially sectioned specimen of an ulnar nerve 25 mm apart. Following the destruction of the blackened segment of the nerve, the proximal and distal stumps would present the funicular patterns illustrated; the funiculi for the dorsal cutaneous fibers would be present in the proximal stump but not in the distal stump. If the nerve were repaired by simple end-to-end union, or continuity restored by the insertion of a graft, these "cutaneous" funiculi would be opposed to those in the distal stump, which are destined for the deep terminal (muscular) branch. In such a situation the dorsal cutaneous bundle group should be isolated, mobilized, and transferred to supplement the reinnervation of sensory funiculi in the distal stump.

From this discussion it is clear that group funicular repair has a limited role in the end-to-end repair of nerves. In this respect it is important not to make demands on the method that it cannot possibly meet, and it is pointless to embark on a long and complicated group funicular repair when a simple epineurial repair would be just as effective. Furthermore, restoring nerve trunk con-

tinuity by the group funicular method is by no means trouble-free, as illustrated by the following enumeration.

1. In any form of funicular repair some sutures are buried and these are bound to promote some intraneural fibrosis. For this reason the number of bundle groups should be small and the number of buried sutures should be kept to a minimum.

2. In general, group funicular suture and tension at the site of repair are incompatible. That is why some prefer to close even small gaps by a nerve graft replacement, using group funicular repair at the nerve-graft junctions in order to avoid all tension at those sites.

3. The method involves time-consuming preparation of the nerve ends in order to free the funiculi from epineurial tissue so that they can be collected into groups for group funicular union. In doing this there is the risk of damaging fine nutrient vessels as well as funiculi, both of which could aggravate scarring at the suture site.

4. There is the additional time required to undertake the repair. Group funicular repair has the most to offer in the surgical repair of severed median and ulnar nerves in the lower forearm and at the wrist.

Although group funicular repair has only a limited application in the end-to-end repair of nerves, the method is obligatory for effecting nerve union in limb and digital replantation surgery and particularly for completing the union at nerve-graft junctions where it has been largely responsible for the greatly improved results that can now be expected from that method of repair.

POSSIBLE CENTRAL EFFECTS OCCASIONED BY THE NERVE REPAIR

The possibility of harmful effects on the parent neurons occasioned by the trauma caused during the preparation of the nerve ends for repair has assumed significance with the introduction of funicular nerve repair where mechanical, thermal, and chemical interference with the funiculi at the proximal nerve end may be unduly prolonged.

If adverse retrograde neuronal effects are confirmed, do these differ in any significant respect from those occasioned by the original injury? To what extent might they adversely affect regeneration and recovery and can they be minimized by:

1. Shortening the time of the operation
2. More careful and gentle handling of the nerve during the preparation of the proximal nerve end for repair
3. Blocking the nerve central to the level of the repair in the hope of preventing those peripheral effects generated at the nerve end from being transmitted centrally to reach and affect the neuron. Such a suggestion raises the fundamental question of the trigger, or signal, responsible for provoking the retrograde reaction and whether this is based on nerve impulse activity or on axon transport systems.

These suggestions are purely speculative but it seems reasonable to assume that repeated and prolonged trauma to the proximal nerve end would aggravate the retrograde neuronal reaction.

ENCLOSING THE REPAIR SITE WITH CUFFS OR WRAPPINGS OF FOREIGN MATERIAL

The site of nerve repair has been enclosed in cuffs or wrappings of foreign material in order to:

1. Effect sutureless end-to-end union, thereby eliminating the need for implanted sutures
2. Provide the suture line with a protective sheathing designed
   a. To protect this critical area from becoming involved in harmful scarring and adhesions
   b. To confine regenerating axons to the suture line
   c. To prevent the ingrowth of extraneural connective tissue between the nerve ends where it would hinder the advance of growing axon tips
   d. To encourage the longitudinal alignment of the components of the junctional tissue that would, in turn, facili-

tate the smooth passage of axons across the suture line
   e. To provide mechanical support for the suture line thereby minimizing torsion and displacement

Many have been so impressed with the arguments in favor of wrappings that they have adopted the use of shielding materials as a routine procedure during nerve repair, supplemented in many cases by fixing the cuffs with a tissue adhesive. Others, however, remain adamant that enclosing the site of the repair with any foreign material promotes harmful fibrosis and is associated with inferior results.

To date the ideal wrapping has been regarded as one that is effectively ignored by the body and yet meets the conditions outlined above. However, by virtue of their inertness, such materials remain permanently as a potential mechanical irritant unless removed at a second operation. In this respect inertness becomes a continuing liability. Tantalum, which had a vogue during World War II, was discarded in favor of Millipore, which in turn was discarded in favor of Silastic, which is now attracting its share of criticism. It is of interest that none of these materials, which were launched with such extravagant claims in their favor, has established a permanent place in peripheral nerve repair.

The use of protective cuffs can be challenged on the following grounds.

1. With the condition of the nerve ends fluctuating during healing from edema, cell proliferation, and revascularization, the cuff could be too tight at one moment and too loose at another. Its influence on the alignment of tissues at the junctional zone is questionable.

2. They carry the risk of impairing the blood supply at the suture line.

3. The inertness claimed for the material may in itself prove to be a disadvantage in that it persists as a foreign body to produce harmful effects by physical irritation. There is already discussion of removing such protective sheaths once nerve union has consolidated and this means a second operation.

4. The threat to the suture line in terms of

scarring does not come from extraneural elements but from the proliferating fibroblasts of the epineurium and this is occurring inside the cuff. The reason for this is clear when one considers the internal structure of nerve trunks. In human nerves, unlike in many animals used for experimental purposes, the monofunicular arrangement is uncommon. The usual arrangement is of a multifunicular nerve trunk with varying, but large, amounts of epineurial tissue separating the funiculi and enclosing the nerve trunk. It is this epineurial tissue that is the source of most of the harmful scarring at the suture line, and the protective wrapping does nothing to curtail this reactive fibrosis.

5. There is no conclusive proof that the use of protective cuffs improves the quality of the recovery.

The only advantage that can be claimed for isolating the suture line in this way is to prevent the formation of troublesome adhesions that might attach the nerve to its bed. However, more convincing arguments in their favor will need to be produced before the use of cuffs gains general acceptance.

What is required is a biologically degradable membrane that would be absorbed once its primary function of ensuring sound, effective, and uncomplicated union of the nerve ends has been fulfilled. This would make a second operation for its removal unnecessary. Kline and Hayes[19] have reported on collagen membrane wrapping for suture line protection. The membrane was prepared from irradiated bovine flexor-tendon collagen and had the advantage of being absorbed with an absorption time that could be controlled by varying the tanning process. However, the repetitive use of the collagen was associated with an increased cellular response that suggested the activation of an immune mechanism. They felt that the potential of collagen membrane as a protective wrapping required further study. Of the several nerve union techniques investigated by Braun,[5,6] sutureless tubulation using a collagen membrane fixed by stay-sutures some distance from the junctional zone was said to produce an excellent fiber pattern and the

best results. Berger and co-workers,[4] however, found collagen tubulation unsatisfactory. Metz and Seeger[26] refer to a new type of collagen membrane prepared from bovine submucosa, which is absorbable with an absorption time that can be modified by tanning with aldehyde. It has yet to be tested for the repair of nerves.

And so the search for a biologically ideal membrane for nerve repair continues and new and promising data have been reported in Chapter 25.

NERVE GRAFTING

The subject of nerve repair by replacement grafting offers unlimited opportunities for disputation. In fact it is probably fair to say that there are few facets of the subject where there is complete agreement. It is also true to say that disagreement flourishes where knowledge is incomplete.

Conflicting views on predegenerating the autograft

Predegenerating the autograft by nerve section in situ has been advocated with a view to improving the qualities of the graft as a medium for conducting regenerating axons across the gap to the distal segment of the severed nerve. The advantages claimed for grafts prepared in this way are based on the following considerations.

1. The predegenerated graft is firmer, which makes it easier to handle thereby facilitating union at the nerve-graft junctions.[3,7]

2. Predegenerated nerve is more likely to withstand the initial and temporary ischemia of transplantation because the increased metabolic activity associated with wallerian degeneration demands an increased blood supply, and this activity has subsided by the time the graft is transplanted.

3. Schwann cell proliferation and the outgrowth of Schwann cells from the cut ends of the nerve and graft have been claimed to be maximal 19 to 25 days after nerve section. This factor has been discussed in relation to nerve suture, where it was pointed out that the peak of Schwann cell activity varies con-

siderably and that healing at the suture site is just as effective immediately after nerve severance as it is some days or weeks later.

4. It has also been claimed that debris in the degenerating nerve fibers in the autograft presents an obstacle to the advance of axons and that, if sufficient time is allowed for the endoneurial tubes to be cleared of this material, regenerating axons will then advance along them more easily and rapidly. As previously noted, a histological and clinical study of the pattern of recovery following a second degree nerve injury demonstrates that there is no foundation for this claim.

There is, in fact, much experimental evidence to show that the rates of axon advance through predegenerated and fresh grafts are not significantly different. If the predegenerated graft has any advantage over the fresh graft, it is not based on a more rapid growth of axons into and through the graft.

From this it will be seen that the only advantage that could be claimed for the predegenerated autograft is the greater ease of handling during repair. It has the disadvantage, however, that it requires a two-stage operation. Experimental and clinical evidence offers no support for predegenerating the graft.

Conflicting views on the distal nerve-graft anastomosis

The graft is customarily attached proximally and distally at the same operation. However, there are those who claim that by the time regenerating axons traverse the graft and reach the distal suture line, particularly in the case of long grafts, scarring at that site will present an impenetrable obstacle to their further advance. On this premise there are now those who treat the distal nerve-graft junction in one of two ways.

1. It is sutured at the original operation. Then, just in advance of the calculated arrival of regenerating axons, the junctional zone is excised, the nerve ends are "freshened," and then resutured. In this way the regenerating axon tips are confronted with a relatively fresh suture line, which, it is believed, favors their passage to the distal stump.

2. The distal graft and nerve ends are not sutured at the original operation but are tagged and left in juxtaposition. With the arrival of regenerating axons at the distal end of the graft, a neuroma forms at that site. At this time the graft and nerve ends are freshened and sutured.

Modifying graft repair in these ways is open to a number of objections.

1. Timing the arrival of regenerating axon tips at the distal level presents difficulties. Calculations based on the graft length and regeneration rates can be best be only approximate. If the nerve contains sensory fibers, tracking a Tinel's sign down the graft is a useful guide. Electrophysiological techniques for detecting the presence of regenerating axons and of following their growth distally have been proposed by Kline and his associates,[18,20] and it would be interesting to know how reliable these have proved to be in practice. The formation of a neuroma at the distal end of the graft is also evidence of active regeneration and the arrival of axons at that site.

2. If the distal anastomosis is performed too soon, then there is still time for the postulated damaging fibrosis to reform before axons arrive. If, on the other hand, axons have already crossed the suture site, then what might have been satisfactory regeneration would have been lost by the second operation. This second possibility is, of course, avoided by not anastomosing the distal graft-nerve ends at the original operation.

3. There is the risk, when refreshening the graft and nerve ends, of creating a gap that then requires tension to close it. Furthermore, this delayed repair could be followed later by a constrictive fibrosis little different from that originally inferred to be present.

4. It is also pertinent to inquire if harmful fibrosis is an inevitable complication of distal suture line healing, particularly when union is tension free. There is both experimental and clinical evidence that this does not necessarily occur.

Taking all factors into consideration the preferable course of action is to complete the entire grafting procedure at the one operation. If testing confirms the passage of axons across the distal suture line, then no further action is required. It is only when axon growth is arrested at this site that the distal suture line should be resected and resutured.

Further investigations directed at devising dependable methods of tracking the descent of regenerating axons should be encouraged.

HETEROGRAFTING

Although research into heterografting may be biologically satisfying, it has no clinical relevance to nerve repair and we should cease talking about it.

HOMOGRAFTING

One of the greatest achievements in nerve repair would be to find a nerve replacement that is readily available in any given quantity, length, and thickness, ideally structured to bridge the gap between the two ends of a severed nerve and guaranteed to succeed.

Could homografting be relied on to succeed consistently this would represent a tremendous advance in nerve repair. Regrettably such is not the case, and the method has been largely discredited both on experimental and clinical grounds. The recent clinical evaluation of the method in West Germany has been mentioned earlier.

Attempts to overcome the antigenic properties of the graft have been disappointing, and intensive immunosuppressive therapy is hardly justified for supporting a measure that is not lifesaving and is of dubious value. The reinnervation that occasionally follows homografting is very incomplete and could be a reflection of the propensity of regenerating axons to overcome remarkable obstacles to reach the distal stump.

However, despite the pessimism currently attaching to this method of repair, it is too early to abandon efforts in this field. Work should be continued because the benefits that would flow from a successful outcome would be considerable.

AUTOGRAFTING

It is generally agreed, one of the few points of agreement, that autografting is the method of choice for bridging gaps in nerves with options covering inlay, full-thickness, free vas-cularized, pedicle, and cable grafting. Comment will be confined largely to cable autografting which is the "workhorse" of the group.

While all are agreed on the merits of autografting, there are some striking differences in management policy that are of particular concern to the clinician.

Abandoning end-to-end suture in favor of autografting

There are some, and Dr. Millesi is the most experienced and strongest advocate of this group, who insist that even the slightest tension of the suture line is harmful and that all but clean transections and gaps of less than 1 cm should be repaired by grafting. He has, in this volume, outlined his reasons for adopting this policy, which are based on his experimental study of suture line fibrosis, a serious obstacle to regeneration. His contention is that even the slightest tension promotes harmful suture line fibrosis, and it is to eliminate this complication that small defects are grafted in order to avoid all tension at the nerve-graft junctions, which also facilitates group funicular repair.

All would now agree that suture under great tension aided by limb positioning and mobilization is to be avoided. Not only is scarring increased at the suture line, but the postoperative stretching of the nerve that occurs as the limb is extended can rupture nerve fibers within the funiculi even if the suture line holds. However, the point to be decided is whether even slight tension at the suture line is incompatible with a good recovery.

As we have seen, a nerve trunk is an elastic structure, which explains why the nerve ends retract and become separated by a centimeter or so following a clean transection. Removing a segment of 1 cm from a nerve leaves a gap of 2 to 3 cm. Limb movement after the injury may increase this distance. However, because of the elasticity of the nerve, the retracted nerve ends are easily drawn together and held by sutures. The question is whether the tension required to do this prejudices recovery.

Clinical experience confirms that gaps of 3

to 5 cm can be closed under slight tension, perhaps supplemented by mild degrees of limb flexion, and that such repairs are followed by good recovery.

Clearly the allegedly harmful effects of suture under tension are difficult to evaluate because, with so many factors contributing to the end result, it is impossible to decide to what extent the residual disability is directly attributable to the tension. Comparative recovery evaluations following end-to-end suture and grafting under identical conditions are not yet available, although there is no doubt that the results of autografting have greatly improved in recent years and to a degree that justifies an objective comparison between the two methods. In this respect, however, it is not sufficient that grafting should give good results. It must consistently give better results.

Having said all this, two questions remain unanswered.

1. At what point does acceptable tension become unacceptable? Tension at the suture line has not yet been the subject of precise measurement so that there is no basis of equating it with the quality of the recovery. We are, therefore, forced to rely on subjective assessments using the best of human experience and judgment.

2. What is the largest gap that can be safely closed by end-to-end union without prejudicing a successful outcome. My own conclusion is that it will be somewhere between 3 and 5 cm, at the most 7 cm, but in any given situation one should rely more on the ease with which the nerve ends can be brought together.

Finally, one should carefully weigh the "pros and cons" of converting a repair with one suture line into one involving two suture lines. In the latter the chances of regenerating axons going astray are greatly increased despite the advantages conferred by group funicular suture at the nerve-graft junctions.

When nerve grafting should no longer be considered worthwhile

We now shift our concern from the small gap to the very large defect. Large defects are usually associated with considerable soft tissue destruction, which involves delays in treating the nerve defect. Before giving any thought to the latter, the residual function should be carefully and thoroughly assessed. Sometimes a surprisingly good degree of function is retained because of anomalous innervations and other factors (for example, Martin-Gruber anastomosis) and the availability of tendon transfers, all of which make any attempt at a complicated nerve repair of questionable value.

Having decided that procedures to reinnervate the denervated distal segment are indicated, there are three options open to the surgeon:

1. To repair the defect with a cable autograft using group funicular suture
2. To repair the defect by means of a free vascularized nerve graft[32]
3. To reinnervate the distal segment from another source using some form of nerve cross-anastomosis[29]

The merits of each of these options will be briefly examined, using as an example the extreme conditions imposed by extensive destruction of the median nerve and associated soft tissue in the forearm.

Free cable autografting

Under the conditions of free cable autografting two problems in particular complicate this method of repair:

1. Obtaining sufficient nerve strands to bridge the gap
2. The unfavorable nature of the nerve bed and the associated hazards to graft revascularization and graft survival (In this respect we need more information on critical funicular size in relation to graft survival and on the precise manner in which very long grafts are revascularized.)

Dr. Millesi, however, has reported favorable recovery after a 2 cm graft replacement, which appears to be the outside limit for grafting. However, whether grafting such large defects can be expected to give consistently satisfactory results remains an open question.

Free vascularized nerve grafting

Free vascularized nerve grafting was introduced to ensure the survival of the graft in a poor bed.[32] Briefly the method involves transposing the superficial radial nerve, and the related radial artery serving it with nutrient vessels, from the sound side to replace the lost segments of the corresponding artery and median nerve in the forearm on the affected side. The nerve-graft junctions are completed by group funicular suture, and continuity between the stumps of the radial artery is restored by microvascular anastomoses. In this way the circulation to the transposed nerve autograft is preserved.

Nerve cross-anastomosis

Attention was directed earlier to features of the funicular anatomy of the median and ulnar nerves at the wrist, which suggested the possibility of reinnervating the distal median stump from the dorsal cutaneous branch of the ulnar nerve by a method of group funicular union at the wrist. This method has the following advantages.

1. Both the distal stump of the median nerve and the dorsal cutaneous nerve of the hand branch of the ulnar nerve can be cleanly severed, which gives the best possible conditions at the suture line.

2. The regenerating sensory processes have only one suture line to negotiate.

3. The regenerating sensory processes have short distances to grow to reach cutaneous terminations.

4. The funiculi in the dorsal cutaneous donor stump are composed solely of cutaneous nerve fibers.

5. The fiber localization obtaining in the median nerve at this level permits the reasonable approximation of sensory funiculi to those in the median nerve whose constituent fibers serve the thumb and index finger.

6. Funicular group suture under magnification reduces the wasteful regeneration of sensory processes into the interfunicular tissues of the median stump.

7. The resulting sensory defect on the ulnar side of the dorsum of the hand is minimal in extent and depth and affects an area of skin where the cutaneous innervation is not of special importance. Furthermore, the dorsal cutaneous nerve of the hand does not innervate skin that adjoins the area denervated by the median injury.

8. All in all, the method offers the best prospects of getting large numbers of regenerating sensory processes to the thumb and index finger with the least possible delay.

While the most effective way of repairing large defects in nerves has by no means been settled, free vascularized grafting and nerve cross-anastomosis have increased the options open to the surgeon. It remains to extend the search to other regions for arrangements that would facilitate nerve repair by these methods.

ANIMAL EXPERIMENTATION

Finally, a concluding and somewhat controversial comment on another facet of nerve repair, namely, the place of animal experimentation in the solution of clinical problems.

There is now a dangerous belief, particularly among younger investigators, that animal experimentation, and animal experimentation alone, can provide the answers to all clinical problems. Lest I be misunderstood in what I have to say, I acknowledge the ousstanding contributions that animal experimentation has made and continues to make to progress in this field. They are too obvious to be questioned. I have never hesitated to use this approach when I felt it was indicated. At the same time it should be remembered that the clinical approach still has much to offer, while the results derived from animal experimentation can at times be misleading when they are transposed to the human situation.

The model so conveniently offered by the experimental animal for the study of nerve repair often fails to meet the complicated conditions obtaining in clinical practice. Often the subject of study is a nerve composed of a single funiculus, gap distances are short, the wounds are clean, and the nerve is cleanly transected so that conditions in no way resemble the mutilating injuries of civilian accidents and battle casualties.

Animal experimentation has certainly told us much about axon regeneration and related biological processes, but in man the emphasis is now moving from axon regeneration per se to the study of the more complex processes on which the restoration of useful function depends, including, importantly, reeducation to overcome the residual motor and sensory disability of imperfect and incomplete regeneration. Here studies and estimates of the quality of recovery after nerve repair in the experimental animal bear little relation to the human situation. The function of the forepaw or hindlimb of the rat, rabbit, dog, and cat is in no way comparable to the manual dexterity of man, while the stereognostic sense, as we understand it, is a peculiarly human attribute.

Lest, therefore, the clinician should at times despair, he would do well to remember that valuable information is still to be obtained by the intelligent and persistent clinical investigator with the capacity to recognize in unusual clinical situations those unique experiments by which nature reveals its secrets. In this respect I cannot do better than quote that distinguished English surgeon, James Paget, who wrote, "Receiving thankfully all the help that physiology or chemistry or any other sciences more advanced than our own can give us, and pursuing all our studies with the precision and circumspection that we may best learn from them, let us still hold that, within our range of study, that alone is true which is proved clinically, and that which is clinically proved needs no other evidence."

REFERENCES

1. Abercrombie, M., and Johnson, M. L.: The outwandering of cells in tissue cultures of nerves undergoing Wallerian degeneration, J. Exp. Biol. **19**:266, 1942.
2. Almquist, E. E., Smith, O., and Fry, L.: Nerve conduction velocity, microscopic and electron microscopic studies comparing repaired adult and baby monkey median nerves, J. Bone Joint Surg. **55A**:883, 1973.
3. Bentley, F. H., and Hill, M.: Experimental surgery. Nerve grafting, Br. J. Surg. **24**:368, 1936.
4. Berger, A., Meissl, G., and Samii, J.: Experimentelle Erfahrungen mit Kollagenfolien über nahtlose Nervenanastomosen, Acta Neurochir. **23**:141, 1970.
5. Braun, R.: Experimental peripheral nerve repair-tubulation, Surg. Forum **15**:452, 1964.
6. Braun, R. M.: Comparative studies of neurorrhaphy and sutureless peripheral nerve repair. Surg. Gynecol. Obstet. **122**:15, 1966.
7. Collier, J.: Facial paralysis and its operative treatment, Lancet **2**:91, 1940.
8. Cravioto, H.: Wallerian degeneration. Ultrastructural and histochemical studies, Bull. Los Angeles Neurol. Soc. **34**:233, 1969.
9. Ducker, T. B.: Metabolic factors in surgery of peripheral nerves, Surg. Clin. North Am. **52**:1109, 1972.
10. Ducker, T. B., Kempe, L. G., and Hayes, G. J.: The metabolic background for peripheral nerve surgery, J. Neurosurg. **30**:270, 1969.
11. Eng, G. D.: Brachial plexus palsy in new born infants, Pediatrics **48**:18, 1971.
12. Forman, D. S., and Berenberg, R. A.: Regeneration in the rat sciatic nerve studied by labeling the motor fibers with axonally transported radio-active proteins, Soc. Neurosci. Abstr. **3**:425, 1977.
13. Jacoby, W.: Beuteilung und Behandlung traumatischer Nervenschädigungen, Klin. Wschr. **50**:747, 1972.
14. Jacoby, W.: Diagnostik und Behandlung traumatischer Nervenschädigungen, Z. Allgemeinmedizin, Landarzt **48**:993, 1972.
15. Jacoby, W., Fahlbusch, R., and Mackert, B.: Transplantation Lyophilisierter homoioplastischer Nerven zur Überbrückung peripherer Nervendefekte beim Menschen, Fortschr. Med. **88**:183, 1970.
16. Jacoby, W., et al.: Überbruckung peripherer Nervedefekte mit lyophilisierten und desantigenisierten homologen Transplantaten, Münch. Med. Wschr. **112**:586, 1970.
17. Jacoby, W., et al.: Fortschritte in der Behandlung peripherer Nervenverletzungen. 1. Diagnostik, nervanaht, Fortschr. Med. **89**:181, 1971.
18. Kline, D. G., and DeJonge, B. R.: Evoked potentials to evaluate peripheral nerve injuries, Surg. Gynecol. Obstet. **127**:1239, 1963.
19. Kline, D. G., and Hayes, G. J.: Use of resorbable wrapper for peripheral-nerve repair, J. Neurosurg. **21**:737, 1964.
20. Kline, D. G., Hackett, E. R., and May, P. R.: Evaluation of nerve injuries by evoked potentials and electromyography, J. Neurosurg. **31**:128, 1969.
21. Kuhlendahl, H., et al.: The treatment of peripheral nerve injuries with homologous nerve grafts, Acta Neurochir. **26**:339, 1972.
22. McQuarrie, I. G., and Graftstein, B.: Axon outgrowth enhanced by a previous nerve injury, Arch. Neurol. **29**:53, 1973.

23. McQuarrie, I. G., Graftstein, B., and Gershon, M. D.: Axonal regeneration in the rat sciatic nerve: effect of a conditioning lesion and of dbcAMP, Brain Res. **132:**443, 1977.

24. McQuarrie, I. G., et al.: Regeneration of adrenergic axons in rat sciatic nerve: effect of a conditioning lesion, Brain Res. **141:**21, 1978.

25. Marinacci, A. A.: Clinical electromyography. A review, Bull. Los Angeles Neurol. Soc. **35:**181, 1970.

26. Metz, R., and Seeger, W.: Collagen wrapping of nerve homotransplants in dogs, Eur. Surg. Res. **1:**157, 1969.

27. Proebster, R.: Ueber Muskelaktionsstrome am gesunden und kranken Menschen, Stuttgart. Enke. (Suppl. to vol. 50 of Z. Orthop. Chir.), 1928.

28. Sunderland, S.: Capacity of reinnervated muscles to function efficiently after prolonged denervation, Arch. Neurol. Psychiatry **64:**755, 1950.

29. Sunderland, S.: The restoration of median nerve function after destructive lesions which preclude end-to-end repair, Brain **97:**1, 1974.

30. Sunderland, S.: Nerves and nerve injuries, ed. 2, Edinburgh, 1978, Churchill Livingstone. (This reference should be consulted for the details on which statements made in the text are based.)

31. Sunderland, S., and Ray, L. J.: Denervation changes in mammalian striated muscle, J. Neurol. Neurosurg. Psychiatry **13:**159, 1950.

32. Taylor, G. I., and Ham, F. J.: The free vascularized nerve graft. A further experimental and clinical application of microvascular techniques, Plast. Reconstr. Surg. **57:**413, 1976.

33. Weddell, G., Feinstein, B., and Pattle, R. E.: The electrical activity of voluntary muscle in man under normal and pathological conditions, Brain **67:**178, 1944.

34. Wickstrom, J.: Comment on the paper by Adler, J. B., and Patterson, R. L.: Erb's palsy. Long-term results of treatment in eight-eight cases, J. Bone Joint Surg. **49A:**1064, 1967.

35. Zalis, O. S., et al.: Motor patterning following transitory sensory-motor deprivations, Arch. Neurol. **13:**487, 1965.

INDEX